METHODS IN MOLECULAR BIOLOGY

Series Editor
John M. Walker
School of Life and Medical Sciences
University of Hertfordshire
Hatfield, Hertfordshire, AL10 9AB, UK

For further volumes:
http://www.springer.com/series/7651

RNA Structure Determination

Methods and Protocols

Edited by

Douglas H. Turner

Department of Chemistry and Center for RNA Biology, University of Rochester
College of Arts and Sciences, Rochester, NY, USA

David H. Mathews

Department of Biochemistry and Biophysics and Center for RNA Biology,
University of Rochester Medical Center, Rochester, NY, USA

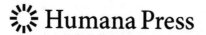 Humana Press

Editors
Douglas H. Turner
Department of Chemistry and Center
  for RNA Biology
University of Rochester College
  of Arts and Sciences
Rochester, NY, USA

David H. Mathews
Department of Biochemistry and Biophysics
  and Center for RNA Biology
University of Rochester Medical Center
Rochester, NY, USA

ISSN 1064-3745   ISSN 1940-6029   (electronic)
Methods in Molecular Biology
ISBN 978-1-4939-8198-4   ISBN 978-1-4939-6433-8   (eBook)
DOI 10.1007/978-1-4939-6433-8

Printed on acid-free paper

This Humana Press imprint is published by Springer Nature
The registered company is Springer Science+Business Media LLC New York

Preface

Research in the last 30 years has revealed that an unexpectedly large fraction of genomic DNA is transcribed into RNA [1]. Moreover, many new functions of RNA are being discovered [2]. This has provided a need for ways to rapidly translate sequence into structural information.

The twenty-first century witnessed many advances in modeling and determining RNA structures. Secondary structure prediction on the basis of sequences alone is increasingly accurate. New methods have been developed for experimentally probing secondary structure to identify paired and unpaired nucleotides for restraining predictions. Multiple methods are being developed to model three-dimensional structure. At the same time, more and more three-dimensional structures are being determined. The new structures are providing benchmarks for improving predictions of three-dimensional structure from sequence.

Twenty-First Century Advances

Secondary structure prediction improved in accuracy as a result of several innovations. New parameter sets were derived to quantify structure quality [3–5]. New algorithms were invented to consider folding of structural ensembles, rather than only most likely structures [4, 6–10]. Additionally, new approaches are available to determine the conserved secondary structure for multiple homologous sequences, thus increasing accuracy relative to single sequence structure prediction [11–17].

Probing structure by enzymatic and chemical methods is a cornerstone of determining RNA secondary structure [18–20]. New methods for probing structure were developed. In particular, a new class of chemical probing agents, based on selective 2′-hydroxyl acylation and primer extension readout (SHAPE), was developed to identify RNA nucleotides in flexible regions of the structure. The most reactive nucleotides tend to be in loops [21–23]. Unlike base-specific agents, SHAPE attacks flexible 2′-hydroxyl groups and thus interrogates all nucleotides. SHAPE was also coupled with quantification of the reactivity per nucleotide, and these data provide restraints that dramatically improve the accuracy of secondary structure prediction [24–27]. At the same time, traditional probing agents were applied in new ways. Enzymatic cleavage was coupled with next-generation sequencing to probe structure across the transcriptome [28, 29]. The extent of dimethyl sulfate (DMS) reactivity was quantified and also used as restraints for structure prediction [30]. SHAPE reagents were shown to be effective at in vivo mapping [31, 32], as previously shown for DMS [33]. Finally, DMS and SHAPE were coupled with next-generation sequencing to probe RNA structure in vivo across the transcriptome [34–36].

Modeling of three-dimensional RNA structure has also advanced. As for protein structure prediction [37], RNA structure prediction uses blind modeling to assess advances in the field by employing new benchmarks, called RNA Puzzles [38, 39]. A number of groups participate in the blind predictions, using approaches ranging from physics-based to knowledge-based [40–49]. The second RNA Puzzles comparison concluded that overall topologies are correctly modeled, but that noncanonical pair interactions are not yet well predicted [39].

At the start of the century, x-ray crystal structures of ribosomes were solved. Since that time, ongoing advances in x-ray crystallography [50–52], nuclear magnetic resonance (NMR) [53–55], and cryo-electron microscopy (cryo-EM) [56–58] have all led to the determination of more complex and higher resolution structures. Small angle x-ray scattering (SAXS) is being applied to RNA to determine molecular envelopes in solution [59, 60]. The advances extend to new approaches to consider ensembles and structural flexibility [61, 62]. Importantly, this work was enabled by development of new modeling methods, including improved methods for validating structures [63].

Organization of the Book

This book provides protocols for RNA structure modeling and determination. The first chapters provide protocols for RNA secondary structure prediction. Chapters 1 and 2 discuss single sequence modeling with the software packages, Crumple [64] and RNAstructure [65], respectively. Chapter 3 discusses using RNAstructure to model conserved secondary structures with multiple homologs. The prediction of bimolecular secondary structures with RNAstructure is presented in Chapter 4 and with Vfold [42] in Chapter 5. Chapter 6 presents STarMir [66], an application of secondary structure prediction to miRNA target prediction.

Chapters 7, 8, and 9 provide protocols for structure mapping, with traditional chemical agents [18], with enzymatic mapping across the transcriptome [29], and with SHAPE reagents [67], respectively. Chapter 10 provides protocols for using mapping data to constrain or restrain RNA secondary structure prediction with RNAstructure. Chapter 11 gives the protocol for using unassigned NMR resonances to improve secondary structure prediction and to provide initial assignments of some resonances to start solving a three-dimensional structure [68].

The book concludes with protocols focusing on three-dimensional structure. Chapters 12, 13, 14, and 15 provide modeling protocols for FARFAR [43], RNAComposer [40], ModeRNA [41], and MC-Fold [46], respectively. Chapter 16 provides an introduction to structure determination by NMR. Chapter 17 provides a protocol for x-ray crystallography determination of RNA structure.

Rochester, NY, USA   *David H. Mathews*
Rochester, NY, USA   *Douglas H. Turner*

References

1. Birney E, Stamatoyannopoulos JA, Dutta A, Guigo R, Gingeras TR, Margulies EH, Weng Z, Snyder M, Dermitzakis ET, Thurman RE, Kuehn MS, Taylor CM, Neph S, Koch CM, Asthana S, Malhotra A, Adzhubei I, Greenbaum JA, Andrews RM, Flicek P, Boyle PJ, Cao H, Carter NP, Clelland GK, Davis S, Day N, Dhami P, Dillon SC, Dorschner MO, Fiegler H, Giresi PG, Goldy J, Hawrylycz M, Haydock A, Humbert R, James KD, Johnson BE, Johnson EM, Frum TT, Rosenzweig ER, Karnani N, Lee K, Lefebvre GC, Navas PA, Neri F, Parker SC, Sabo PJ, Sandstrom R, Shafer A, Vetrie D, Weaver M, Wilcox S, Yu M, Collins FS, Dekker J, Lieb JD, Tullius TD, Crawford GE, Sunyaev S, Noble WS, Dunham I, Denoeud F, Reymond A, Kapranov P, Rozowsky J, Zheng D, Castelo R, Frankish A, Harrow J, Ghosh S, Sandelin A, Hofacker IL, Baertsch R, Keefe D, Dike S, Cheng J, Hirsch HA, Sekinger EA, Lagarde J, Abril JF, Shahab A, Flamm C, Fried C, Hackermuller J, Hertel

J, Lindemeyer M, Missal K, Tanzer A, Washietl S, Korbel J, Emanuelsson O, Pedersen JS, Holroyd N, Taylor R, Swarbreck D, Matthews N, Dickson MC, Thomas DJ, Weirauch MT, Gilbert J, Drenkow J, Bell I, Zhao X, Srinivasan KG, Sung WK, Ooi HS, Chiu KP, Foissac S, Alioto T, Brent M, Pachter L, Tress ML, Valencia A, Choo SW, Choo CY, Ucla C, Manzano C, Wyss C, Cheung E, Clark TG, Brown JB, Ganesh M, Patel S, Tammana H, Chrast J, Henrichsen CN, Kai C, Kawai J, Nagalakshmi U, Wu J, Lian Z, Lian J, Newburger P, Zhang X, Bickel P, Mattick JS, Carninci P, Hayashizaki Y, Weissman S, Hubbard T, Myers RM, Rogers J, Stadler PF, Lowe TM, Wei CL, Ruan Y, Struhl K, Gerstein M, Antonarakis SE, Fu Y, Green ED, Karaoz U, Siepel A, Taylor J, Liefer LA, Wetterstrand KA, Good PJ, Feingold EA, Guyer MS, Cooper GM, Asimenos G, Dewey CN, Hou M, Nikolaev S, Montoya-Burgos JI, Loytynoja A, Whelan S, Pardi F, Massingham T, Huang H, Zhang NR, Holmes I, Mullikin JC, Ureta-Vidal A, Paten B, Seringhaus M, Church D, Rosenbloom K, Kent WJ, Stone EA, Batzoglou S, Goldman N, Hardison RC, Haussler D, Miller W, Sidow A, Trinklein ND, Zhang ZD, Barrera L, Stuart R, King DC, Ameur A, Enroth S, Bieda MC, Kim J, Bhinge AA, Jiang N, Liu J, Yao F, Vega VB, Lee CW, Ng P, Shahab A, Yang A, Moqtaderi Z, Zhu Z, Xu X, Squazzo S, Oberley MJ, Inman D, Singer MA, Richmond TA, Munn KJ, Rada-Iglesias A, Wallerman O, Komorowski J, Fowler JC, Couttet P, Bruce AW, Dovey OM, Ellis PD, Langford CF, Nix DA, Euskirchen G, Hartman S, Urban AE, Kraus P, Van Calcar S, Heintzman N, Kim TH, Wang K, Qu C, Hon G, Luna R, Glass CK, Rosenfeld MG, Aldred SF, Cooper SJ, Halees A, Lin JM, Shulha HP, Zhang X, Xu M, Haidar JN, Yu Y, Ruan Y, Iyer VR, Green RD, Wadelius C, Farnham PJ, Ren B, Harte RA, Hinrichs AS, Trumbower H, Clawson H, Hillman-Jackson J, Zweig AS, Smith K, Thakkapallayil A, Barber G, Kuhn RM, Karolchik D, Armengol L, Bird CP, de Bakker PI, Kern AD, Lopez-Bigas N, Martin JD, Stranger BE, Woodroffe A, Davydov E, Dimas A, Eyras E, Hallgrimsdottir IB, Huppert J, Zody MC, Abecasis GR, Estivill X, Bouffard GG, Guan X, Hansen NF, Idol JR, Maduro VV, Maskeri B, McDowell JC, Park M, Thomas PJ, Young AC, Blakesley RW, Muzny DM, Sodergren E, Wheeler DA, Worley KC, Jiang H, Weinstock GM, Gibbs RA, Graves T, Fulton R, Mardis ER, Wilson RK, Clamp M, Cuff J, Gnerre S, Jaffe DB, Chang JL, Lindblad-Toh K, Lander ES, Koriabine M, Nefedov M, Osoegawa K, Yoshinaga Y, Zhu B, de Jong PJ (2007) Identification and analysis of functional elements in 1% of the human genome by the ENCODE pilot project. Nature 447(7146):799–816

2. Atkins JF, Gesteland RF, Cech TR (2010) RNA worlds: from life's origins to diversity in gene regulation. Cold Spring Harbor Laboratory Press, Cold Spring Harbor, NY

3. Mathews DH, Disney MD, Childs JL, Schroeder SJ, Zuker M, Turner DH (2004) Incorporating chemical modification constraints into a dynamic programming algorithm for prediction of RNA secondary structure. Proc Natl Acad Sci U S A 101:7287–7292

4. Do CB, Woods DA, Batzoglou S (2006) CONTRAfold: RNA secondary structure prediction without physics-based models. Bioinformatics 22(14):e90–e98

5. Rivas E, Lang R, Eddy SR (2012) A range of complex probabilistic models for RNA secondary structure prediction that includes the nearest-neighbor model and more. RNA 18(2):193–212. doi:10.1261/rna.030049.111

6. Ding Y, Lawrence CE (2003) A statistical sampling algorithm for RNA secondary structure prediction. Nucleic Acids Res 31(24):7280–7301

7. Hamada M, Kiryu H, Sato K, Mituyama T, Asai K (2009) Prediction of RNA secondary structure using generalized centroid estimators. Bioinformatics 25(4):465–473. doi:10.1093/bioinformatics/btn601

8. Lu ZJ, Gloor JW, Mathews DH (2009) Improved RNA secondary structure prediction by maximizing expected pair accuracy. RNA 15:1805–1813

9. Bellaousov S, Mathews DH (2010) ProbKnot: fast prediction of RNA secondary structure including pseudoknots. RNA 16:1870–1880. doi:10.1261/rna.2125310

10. Knudsen B, Hein J (2003) Pfold: RNA secondary structure prediction using stochastic context-free grammars. Nucleic Acids Res 31(13):3423–3428

11. Mathews DH, Turner DH (2002) Dynalign: an algorithm for finding the secondary structure common to two RNA sequences. J Mol Biol 317:191–203

12. Hofacker IL, Fekete M, Stadler PF (2002) Secondary structure prediction for aligned RNA sequences. J Mol Biol 319:1059–1066

13. Will S, Reiche K, Hofacker IL, Stadler PF, Backofen R (2007) Inferring noncoding RNA families and classes by means of genome-scale structure-based clustering. PLoS Comput Biol 3(4):e65

14. Seetin MG, Mathews DH (2012) RNA structure prediction: an overview of methods. Methods Mol Biol 905:99–122. doi:10.1007/978-1-61779-949-5_8

15. Harmanci AO, Sharma G, Mathews DH (2008) PARTS: probabilistic alignment for RNA joinT secondary structure prediction. Nucleic Acids Res 36:2406–2417. doi:PMC2367733

16. Harmanci AO, Sharma G, Mathews DH (2011) TurboFold: iterative probabilistic estimation of secondary structures for multiple RNA sequences. BMC Bioinformatics 12(1):108. doi:10.1186/1471-2105-12-108

17. Reeder J, Giegerich R (2005) Consensus shapes: an alternative to the Sankoff algorithm for RNA consensus structure prediction. Bioinformatics 21(17):3516–3523

18. Ehresmann C, Baudin F, Mougel M, Romby P, Ebel J, Ehresmann B (1987) Probing the structure of RNAs in solution. Nucleic Acids Res 15:9109–9128

19. Knapp G (1989) Enzymatic approaches to probing RNA secondary and tertiary structure. Methods Enzymol 180:192–212

20. Sloma MF, Mathews DH (2015) Improving RNA secondary structure prediction with structure mapping data. Methods Enzymol 553:91–114. doi:10.1016/bs.mie.2014.10.053

21. Merino EJ, Wilkinson KA, Coughlan JL, Weeks KM (2005) RNA structure analysis at single nucleotide resolution by selective 2′-hydroxyl acylation and primer extension (SHAPE). J Am Chem Soc 127(12):4223–4231

22. Sukosd Z, Swenson MS, Kjems J, Heitsch CE (2013) Evaluating the accuracy of SHAPE-directed RNA secondary structure predictions. Nucleic Acids Res 41(5):2807–2816. doi:10.1093/nar/gks1283

23. Low JT, Weeks KM (2010) SHAPE-directed RNA secondary structure prediction. Methods 52(2):150–158. doi:10.1016/j.ymeth.2010.06.007

24. Deigan KE, Li TW, Mathews DH, Weeks KM (2009) Accurate SHAPE-directed RNA structure determination. Proc Natl Acad Sci U S A 106(1):97–102. doi:10.1073/pnas.0806929106

25. Hajdin CE, Bellaousov S, Huggins W, Leonard CW, Mathews DH, Weeks KM (2013) Accurate SHAPE-directed RNA secondary structure modeling, including pseudoknots. Proc Natl Acad Sci U S A 110(14):5498–5503. doi:10.1073/pnas.1219988110

26. Wu Y, Shi B, Ding X, Liu T, Hu X, Yip KY, Yang ZR, Mathews DH, Lu ZJ (2015) Improved prediction of RNA secondary structure by integrating the free energy model with restraints derived from experimental probing data. Nucleic Acids Res 43(15):7247–7259. doi:10.1093/nar/gkv706

27. Eddy SR (2014) Computational analysis of conserved RNA secondary structure in transcriptomes and genomes. Annu Rev Biophys 43:433–456. doi:10.1146/annurev-biophys-051013-022950

28. Kertesz M, Wan Y, Mazor E, Rinn JL, Nutter RC, Chang HY, Segal E (2010) Genome-wide measurement of RNA secondary structure in yeast. Nature 467(7311):103–107. doi:10.1038/nature09322

29. Underwood JG, Uzilov AV, Katzman S, Onodera CS, Mainzer JE, Mathews DH, Lowe TM, Salama SR, Haussler D (2010) FragSeq: transcriptome-wide RNA structure probing using high-throughput sequencing. Nat Methods 7(12):995–1001. doi:10.1038/nmeth.1529

30. Cordero P, Kladwang W, VanLang CC, Das R (2012) Quantitative dimethyl sulfate mapping for automated RNA secondary structure inference. Biochemistry 51(36):7037–7039. doi:10.1021/bi3008802

31. Spitale RC, Crisalli P, Flynn RA, Torre EA, Kool ET, Chang HY (2013) RNA SHAPE analysis in living cells. Nat Chem Biol 9(1):18–20. doi:10.1038/nchembio.1131

32. Tyrrell J, McGinnis JL, Weeks KM, Pielak GJ (2013) The cellular environment stabilizes adenine riboswitch RNA structure. Biochemistry 52(48):8777–8785. doi:10.1021/bi401207q

33. Zaug AJ, Cech TR (1995) Analysis of the structure of Tetrahymena nuclear RNAs in vivo: telomerase RNA, the self-splicing rRNA intron, and U2 snRNA. RNA 1:363–374

34. Ding Y, Tang Y, Kwok CK, Zhang Y, Bevilacqua PC, Assmann SM (2014) In vivo genome-wide profiling of RNA secondary structure reveals novel regulatory features. Nature 505(7485):696–700. doi:10.1038/nature12756

35. Rouskin S, Zubradt M, Washietl S, Kellis M, Weissman JS (2014) Genome-wide probing of RNA structure reveals active unfolding of mRNA structures in vivo. Nature 505(7485):701–705. doi:10.1038/nature12894

36. Flynn RA, Zhang QC, Spitale RC, Lee B, Mumbach MR, Chang HY (2016) Transcriptome-wide interrogation of RNA secondary structure in living cells with icSHAPE. Nat Protoc 11(2):273–290. doi:10.1038/nprot.2016.011

37. Moult J, Fidelis K, Kryshtafovych A, Rost B, Tramontano A (2009) Critical assessment of methods of protein structure prediction—round VIII. Proteins 77(Suppl 9):1–4. doi:10.1002/prot.22589

38. Cruz JA, Blanchet MF, Boniecki M, Bujnicki JM, Chen SJ, Cao S, Das R, Ding F, Dokholyan NV, Flores SC, Huang L, Lavender CA, Lisi V, Major F, Mikolajczak K, Patel DJ, Philips A, Puton T, Santalucia J, Sijenyi F, Hermann T, Rother K, Rother M, Serganov A, Skorupski M, Soltysinski T, Sripakdeevong P, Tuszynska I, Weeks KM, Waldsich C, Wildauer M, Leontis NB, Westhof E (2012) RNA-Puzzles: a CASP-like evaluation of RNA three-dimensional structure prediction. RNA 18(4):610–625. doi:10.1261/rna.031054.111

39. Miao Z, Adamiak RW, Blanchet MF, Boniecki M, Bujnicki JM, Chen SJ, Cheng C, Chojnowski G, Chou FC, Cordero P, Cruz JA, Ferre-D'Amare AR, Das R, Ding F, Dokholyan NV, Dunin-Horkawicz S, Kladwang W, Krokhotin A, Lach G, Magnus M, Major F, Mann TH, Masquida B, Matelska D, Meyer M, Peselis A, Popenda M, Purzycka KJ, Serganov A, Stasiewicz J, Szachniuk M, Tandon A, Tian S, Wang J, Xiao Y, Xu X, Zhang J, Zhao P, Zok T, Westhof E (2015) RNA-puzzles round II: assessment of RNA structure prediction programs applied to three large RNA structures. RNA 21(6):1066–1084. doi:10.1261/rna.049502.114

40. Popenda M, Szachniuk M, Antczak M, Purzycka KJ, Lukasiak P, Bartol N, Blazewicz J, Adamiak RW (2012) Automated 3D structure composition for large RNAs. Nucleic Acids Res 40(14):e112. doi:10.1093/nar/gks339

41. Rother M, Rother K, Puton T, Bujnicki JM (2011) ModeRNA: a tool for comparative modeling of RNA 3D structure. Nucleic Acids Res 39(10):4007–4022. doi:10.1093/nar/gkq1320

42. Xu X, Zhao P, Chen SJ (2014) Vfold: a web server for RNA structure and folding thermodynamics prediction. PLoS One 9(9):e107504. doi:10.1371/journal.pone.0107504

43. Das R, Karanicolas J, Baker D (2010) Atomic accuracy in predicting and designing noncanonical RNA structure. Nat Methods 7(4):291–294. doi:10.1038/nmeth.1433

44. Sripakdeevong P, Kladwang W, Das R (2011) An enumerative stepwise ansatz enables atomic-accuracy RNA loop modeling. Proc Natl Acad Sci U S A 108(51):20573–20578. doi:10.1073/pnas.1106516108

45. Ding F, Sharma S, Chalasani P, Demidov VV, Broude NE, Dokholyan NV (2008) Ab initio RNA folding by discrete molecular dynamics: from structure prediction to folding mechanisms. RNA 14(6):1164–1173. doi:10.1261/rna.894608

46. Parisien M, Major F (2008) The MC-Fold and MC-Sym pipeline infers RNA structure from sequence data. Nature 452(7183):51–55. doi:10.1038/nature06684

47. Zhao Y, Huang Y, Gong Z, Wang Y, Man J, Xiao Y (2012) Automated and fast building of three-dimensional RNA structures. Sci Rep 2:734. doi:10.1038/srep00734

48. Flores SC, Altman RB (2010) Turning limited experimental information into 3D models of RNA. RNA 16(9):1769–1778. doi:10.1261/rna.2112110

49. Sijenyi F, Saro P, Ouyang Z, Damm-Ganamet K, Wood M, Jiang J, Santalucia J, Jr (2012) The RNA folding problems: different levels of RNA structure prediction. In: Leontis NB, Westhof E (eds) RNA 3D structure analysis and prediction. Springer-Verlag, Berlin

50. Zhang J, Ferre-D'Amare AR (2014) New molecular engineering approaches for crystallographic studies of large RNAs. Curr Opin Struct Biol 26:9–15. doi:10.1016/j.sbi.2014.02.001

51. Golden BL, Kundrot CE (2003) RNA crystallization. J Struct Biol 142(1):98–107

52. Holbrook SR, Holbrook EL, Walukiewicz HE (2001) Crystallization of RNA. Cell Mol Life Sci 58(2):234–243

53. Foster MP, McElroy CA, Amero CD (2007) Solution NMR of large molecules and assemblies. Biochemistry 46(2):331–340. doi:10.1021/bi0621314

54. Latham MP, Brown DJ, McCallum SA, Pardi A (2005) NMR methods for studying the structure and dynamics of RNA. Chembiochem 6(9):1492–1505. doi:10.1002/cbic.200500123

55. Furtig B, Richter C, Wohnert J, Schwalbe H (2003) NMR spectroscopy of RNA. Chembiochem 4(10):936–962. doi:10.1002/cbic.200300700

56. Zhou ZH (2008) Towards atomic resolution structural determination by single-particle cryo-electron microscopy. Curr Opin Struct Biol 18(2):218–228. doi:10.1016/j.sbi.2008.03.004

57. Bai XC, McMullan G, Scheres SH (2015) How cryo-EM is revolutionizing structural biology. Trends Biochem Sci 40(1):49–57. doi:10.1016/j.tibs.2014.10.005

58. Frank J (2002) Single-particle imaging of macromolecules by cryo-electron microscopy. Annu Rev Biophys Biomol Struct 31:303–319. doi:10.1146/annurev.biophys.31.082901.134202

59. Rambo RP, Tainer JA (2010) Bridging the solution divide: comprehensive structural analyses of dynamic RNA, DNA, and protein assemblies by small-angle X-ray scattering. Curr Opin Struct Biol 20(1):128–137. doi:10.1016/j.sbi.2009.12.015

60. Fang X, Stagno JR, Bhandari YR, Zuo X, Wang YX (2015) Small-angle X-ray scattering: a bridge between RNA secondary structures and three-dimensional topological structures. Curr Opin Struct Biol 30:147–160. doi:10.1016/j.sbi.2015.02.010

61. Salmon L, Yang S, Al-Hashimi HM (2014) Advances in the determination of nucleic acid conformational ensembles. Annu Rev Phys Chem 65:293–316. doi:10.1146/annurev-physchem-040412-110059

62. Al-Hashimi HM (2005) Dynamics-based amplification of RNA function and its characterization by using NMR spectroscopy. Chembiochem 6(9):1506–1519. doi:10.1002/cbic.200500002

63. Adams PD, Baker D, Brunger AT, Das R, DiMaio F, Read RJ, Richardson DC, Richardson JS, Terwilliger TC (2013) Advances, interactions, and future developments in the CNS, Phenix, and Rosetta structural biology software systems. Annu Rev Biophys 42:265–287. doi:10.1146/annurev-biophys-083012-130253

64. Bleckley S, Stone JW, Schroeder SJ (2012) Crumple: a method for complete enumeration of all possible pseudoknot-free RNA secondary structures. PLoS One 7(12):e52414. doi:10.1371/journal.pone.0052414

65. Reuter JS, Mathews DH (2010) RNAstructure: software for RNA secondary structure prediction and analysis. BMC Bioinformatics 11:129

66. Rennie W, Liu C, Carmack CS, Wolenc A, Kanoria S, Lu J, Long D, Ding Y (2014) STarMir: a web server for prediction of microRNA binding sites. Nucleic Acids Res 42(Web Server issue):W114–W118. doi:10.1093/nar/gku376

67. Lucks JB, Mortimer SA, Trapnell C, Luo S, Aviran S, Schroth GP, Pachter L, Doudna JA, Arkin AP (2011) Multiplexed RNA structure characterization with selective 2′-hydroxyl acylation analyzed by primer extension sequencing (SHAPE-Seq). Proc Natl Acad Sci U S A 108(27):11063–11068. doi:10.1073/pnas.1106501108

68. Chen JL, Bellaousov S, Tubbs JD, Kennedy SD, Lopez MJ, Mathews DH, Turner DH (2015) Nuclear magnetic resonance-assisted prediction of secondary structure for RNA: incorporation of direction-dependent chemical shift constraints. Biochemistry 54(45):6769–6782. doi:10.1021/acs.biochem.5b00833

Contents

Contributors

RYSZARD W. ADAMIAK • *Department of Structural Chemistry and Biology of Nucleic Acids, Institute of Bioorganic Chemistry, Polish Academy of Sciences, Poznan, Poland*

STANISLAV BELLAOUSOV • *Center for RNA Biology, University of Rochester, Rochester, NY, USA; Department of Biochemistry & Biophysics, University of Rochester Medical Center, Rochester, NY, USA*

MARCIN BIESIADA • *European Center for Bioinformatics and Genomics, Institute of Computing Science, Poznan University of Technology, Poznan, Poland; Department of Structural Chemistry and Biology of Nucleic Acids, Institute of Bioorganic Chemistry, Polish Academy of Sciences, Poznan, Poland*

JACEK BLAZEWICZ • *Institute of Computing Science, Poznan University of Technology, Poznan, Poland*

JANUSZ M. BUJNICKI • *Laboratory of Bioinformatics and Protein Engineering, International Institute of Molecular and Cell Biology, Warsaw, Poland; Laboratory of Bioinformatics, Institute of Molecular Biology and Biotechnology, Adam Mickiewicz University, Poznan, Poland*

C. STEVEN CARMACK • *Wadsworth Center, New York State Department of Health, Center for Medical Science, Albany, NY, USA*

JONATHAN L. CHEN • *Department of Chemistry, University of Rochester, Rochester, NY, USA; Center for RNA Biology, University of Rochester, Rochester, NY, USA*

SHI-JIE CHEN • *Department of Physics, Informatics Institute, University of Missouri, Columbia, MI, USA; Department of Biochemistry, Informatics Institute, University of Missouri, Columbia, MI, USA*

GRZEGORZ CHOJNOWSKI • *Laboratory of Bioinformatics and Protein Engineering, International Institute of Molecular and Cell Biology, Warsaw, Poland*

PAUL DALLAIRE • *Department of Computer Science and Operations Research, Institute for Research in Immunology and Cancer, Université de Montréal, Montréal, QC, Canada*

RHIJU DAS • *Biochemistry Department, Stanford University, Stanford, CA, USA*

LAURA DICHIACCHIO • *Department of Biochemistry & Biophysics, University of Rochester Medical Center, Rochester, NY, USA; Center for RNA Biology, University of Rochester Medical Center, Rochester, NY, USA*

YE DING • *Wadsworth Center, New York State Department of Health, Center for Medical Science, Albany, NY, USA*

PIERRE FECHTER • *Biotechnologie et Signalisation Cellulaire, CNRS-INSERM, ESBS, Université de Strasbourg, Illkirch, France*

OLIVIER FUCHSBAUER • *Architecture et Réactivité de l'ARN, CNRS, IBMC, Université de Strasbourg, Strasbourg, France*

IVAN GUERRA • *Department of Chemistry & Biochemistry, Department of Microbiology & Plant Biology, University of Oklahoma, Norman, OK, USA*

JERMAINE L. JENKINS • *Department of Biochemistry & Biophysics, University of Rochester School of Medicine and Dentistry, Rochester, NY, USA; Center for RNA Biology, University of Rochester School of Medicine and Dentistry, Rochester, NY, USA; The Structural Biology and Biophysics Facility, University of Rochester School of Medicine and Dentistry, Rochester, NY, USA*

SHAVETA KANORIA • *Wadsworth Center, New York State Department of Health, Center for Medical Science, Albany, NY, USA*

JOANNA M. KASPRZAK • *Laboratory of Bioinformatics and Protein Engineering, International Institute of Molecular and Cell Biology, Warsaw, Poland; Laboratory of Bioinformatics, Institute of Molecular Biology and Biotechnology, Adam Mickiewicz University, Poznan, Poland*

SCOTT D. KENNEDY • *Department of Biochemistry & Biophysics, School of Medicine and Dentistry, University of Rochester Medical Center, Rochester, NY, USA*

DEEPAK KUMAR • *Laboratory of Bioinformatics, Institute of Molecular Biology and Biotechnology, Adam Mickiewicz University, Poznan, Poland*

CHAOCHUN LIU • *Wadsworth Center, New York State Department of Health, Center for Medical Science, Albany, NY, USA*

JUN LU • *Department of Genetics and Yale Stem Cell Center, Yale University, New Haven, CT, USA*

JULIUS B. LUCKS • *Robert F. Smith School of Chemical and Biomolecular Engineering, Cornell University, Ithaca, NY, USA*

MARCIN MAGNUS • *Laboratory of Bioinformatics and Protein Engineering, International Institute of Molecular and Cell Biology, Warsaw, Poland*

FRANÇOIS MAJOR • *Department of Computer Science and Operations Research, Institute for Research in Immunology and Cancer, Université de Montréal, Montréal, QC, Canada*

STEFANO MARZI • *Architecture et Réactivité de l'ARN, CNRS, IBMC, Université de Strasbourg, Strasbourg, France*

DAVID H. MATHEWS • *Department of Biochemistry and Biophysics, Center for RNA Biology, University of Rochester Medical Center, Rochester, NY, USA; Department of Biostatistics & Computational Biology, University of Rochester Medical Center, Rochester, NY, USA*

DELPHINE PARMENTIER • *Architecture et Réactivité de l'ARN, CNRS, IBMC, Université de Strasbourg, Strasbourg, France*

PAWEL PIATKOWSKI • *Laboratory of Bioinformatics and Protein Engineering, International Institute of Molecular and Cell Biology, Warsaw, Poland*

KATARZYNA J. PURZYCKA • *Department of Structural Chemistry and Biology of Nucleic Acids, Institute of Bioorganic Chemistry, Polish Academy of Sciences, Poznan, Poland*

WILLIAM RENNIE • *Wadsworth Center, New York State Department of Health, Center for Medical Science, Albany, NY, USA*

PASCALE ROMBY • *Architecture et Réactivité de l'ARN, CNRS, IBMC, Université de Strasbourg, Strasbourg, France*

SUSAN J. SCHROEDER • *Department of Chemistry & Biochemistry, Department of Microbiology & Plant Biology, University of Oklahoma, Norman, OK, USA*

MARTA SZACHNIUK • *Institute of Computing Science, Poznan University of Technology, Poznan, Poland*

DOUGLAS H. TURNER • *Department of Chemistry and Center for RNA Biology, University of Rochester College of Arts and Sciences, Rochester, NY, USA*

JASON G. UNDERWOOD • *Research and Development, Pacific Biosciences, Menlo Park, CA, USA*

ANDREW V. UZILOV • *Department of Genetics and Genomic Sciences, Icahn School of Medicine at Mount Sinai, New York, NY, USA*

KYLE E. WATTERS • *Robert F. Smith School of Chemical and Biomolecular Engineering, Cornell University, Ithaca, NY, USA*

JOSEPH E. WEDEKIND • *Department of Biochemistry & Biophysics, University of Rochester School of Medicine and Dentistry, Rochester, NY, USA; Center for RNA Biology, University of Rochester School of Medicine and Dentistry, Rochester, NY, USA;*

The Structural Biology and Biophysics Facility, University of Rochester School of Medicine and Dentistry, Rochester, NY, USA

ZONGFU WU • *College of Veterinary Medicine, Nanjing Agricultural University, Nanjing, China*

XIAOJUN ZECH XU • *Department of Physics, Informatics Institute, University of Missouri, Columbia, MI, USA; Department of Biochemistry, Informatics Institute, University of Missouri, Columbia, MI, USA; Center for RNA Biology, University of Rochester Medical Center, Rochester, NY, USA*

ZHENJIANG ZECH XU • *Department of Biochemistry & Biophysics, University of Rochester Medical Center, Rochester, NY, USA; Center for RNA Biology, University of Rochester Medical Center, Rochester, NY, USA*

JOSEPH D. YESSELMAN • *Biochemistry Department, Stanford University, Stanford, CA, USA*

Chapter 1

Crumple: An Efficient Tool to Explore Thoroughly the RNA Folding Landscape

Ivan Guerra and Susan J. Schroeder

Abstract

The folding landscape for an RNA sequence contains many diverse structures and motifs, which are often sampled rather than completely explored. Today's supercomputers make the complete enumeration of all possible folds for an RNA and a detailed description of the RNA folding landscape a more feasible task. This chapter provides protocols for using the Crumple folding algorithm, an efficient tool to generate all possible non-pseudoknotted folds for an RNA sequence. Crumple in conjunction with Sliding Windows and Assembly can incorporate experimental constraints on the global features of an RNA, such as the minimum number and lengths of helices, which may be determined by crystallography or cryo-electron microscopy. This complete enumeration method is independent of free-energy minimization and allows the user to incorporate experimental data such as chemical probing, SELEX data on RNA–protein binding motifs, and phylogenetic covariation.

Key words Viral RNA, Global RNA helical constraints, Parallel computing, RNA structure prediction, RNA ensembles, Complete enumeration of RNA secondary structures

---

1 Introduction

Folding an RNA sequence is like folding a piece of paper. Imagine crumpling identical pieces of paper in every possible way and then picking which structures fit in the right waste basket. This task generates a lot of garbage, but if all possible ways of crumpling a piece of paper have been completely and accurately explored, then the correct folds will surely be somewhere in the garbage pile. The Crumple approach for RNA folding is to generate all possible structures rapidly and efficiently and then filter with appropriate experimental constraints. Although complete enumeration methods often produce large quantities of output that may not be of practical use for many biologists, this approach is useful for disproving logic true/false statements about possible RNA folds and evaluating alternative folding approaches[1, 2]. Complete enumeration can help evaluate the effects of different kinds of experimental data on reducing the possible conformational space.

Douglas H. Turner and David H. Mathews (eds.), *RNA Structure Determination: Methods and Protocols*, Methods in Molecular Biology, vol. 1490, DOI 10.1007/978-1-4939-6433-8_1, © Springer Science+Business Media New York 2016

The Crumple program offers an efficient tool to explore all possible folds for an RNA sequence and incorporate experimental constraints to reduce conformational space.

The satellite tobacco mosaic virus (STMV) RNA folding problem inspired recent developments in complete enumeration methods and applications of supercomputing power, but these methods have general applications to RNA folding. The first complete enumeration method was developed by Pipas and McMahon [3] to study all the possible folds of tRNA. The Wuchty algorithm computes all possible folds for an RNA sequence within a given free energy range of the minimum free energy (MFE) structure [4]. Recent parallelization and incorporation of filters for multibranch loops and the minimum number of helices have expanded the free energy range of possible structures to be explored [5]. The Crumple algorithm is an efficient tool for enumerating all possible structures independently of free energy minimization [2].

Complete enumeration methods currently are limited more by the availability of experimental constraints than the computing time or the length of the sequence. For example, in the case of STMV RNA, 30 helices of nine pairs are observed in a high-resolution crystal structure of the virus particle [6, 7]. The complete enumeration approach of Helix Find & Combine, which allows multibranch loops and pseudoknots, disproved the hypothesis that all 30 helices consisted of only Watson–Crick and GU pairs. The computations revealed 86 possible helices of nine Watson–Crick or GU pairs, but no possible simultaneous combination of 30 of these helices. Thus, the helices observed in the crystal structure must contain some mismatched pairs [1]. In the STMV case, the experimental constraint on the minimum number and lengths of helices reduces significantly the possible folding space even for a viral RNA genome of 1058 nucleotides. With sufficient experimental constraints, any RNA sequence can be evaluated with complete enumeration methods.

The Crumple method can accommodate a wide variety of experimental data in RNA structure predictions. Global features of the RNA fold for an encapsidated viral RNA genome may be known from crystallography or cryo-electron microscopy experiments. For example, amazing 1.8 Å resolution crystallography data revealed 30 helices of at least nine base pairs in STMV particles [6, 7]. For MS2 bacteriophage RNA, cryo-electron microscopy and crystallography revealed 60 helices of at least five pairs in the 3569-nucleotide RNA genome [8, 9]. Crumple, Sliding Windows, and Assembly generated secondary structures for encapsidated MS2 bacteriophage that include data from cryo-electron microscopy and SELEX data on protein–RNA interactions [10]. RNA viruses such as canine parvovirus, flock house virus, mouse minute virus, pariacoto virus, Q-beta bacteriophage, hepatitis B pregenomic RNA, and cowpea chlorotic mottle virus (CCMV) also show electron density for ordered RNA helices within the viral capsid, which suggests that structured encapsidated nucleic acid occurs throughout a wide range of viruses [11]. Thus, a helix filter and the Crumple, Sliding Windows, and Assembly approach will be useful for modeling other encapsidated viral genomes.

The Crumple approach allows a user to moderate or remove thermodynamic parameters when the assumptions of free energy minimization may not hold true. For example, in the case of encapsidated viral RNA genomes, the RNA folding may be determined by kinetics rather than thermodynamics, and protein binding may create kinetic traps for RNA folds [12]. In the case of STMV RNA, a hypothesis of cotranscriptional folding and viral assembly proposes that a series of hairpins form and bind virus coat proteins [1, 13]. Based on this hypothesis, Crumple, in combination with Sliding Windows and Assembly, generated a model that is the basis for the first all-atom three-dimensional structure of an RNA virus [14]. These modeling studies showed that STMV RNA secondary structures based on the cotranscriptional folding and virus assembly hypothesis fit crystallography data better than secondary structures based on free energy minimization [14]. The Crumple approach allows examination of alternative hypotheses that may not include free-energy minimization as the driving force for the functional RNA structure.

Thermodynamic parameters remain an important part of experimental data in RNA structure predictions, although the database of thermodynamic parameters is continually being updated [15]. In the case of *Trypanosome brucei* guide RNA, the RNA sequence has few cytosines, and thus many possible structures form with AU and GU pairs. The thermodynamic parameters for GU pairs are notoriously idiosyncratic [16–19]. The Crumple method is able to generate many structures consistent with the chemical and enzymatic probing experiments on *T. brucei* guide RNA [2]. Thus, the Crumple method offers additional insights into the RNA folding landscape. Crumple is best used in conjunction with several RNA structure prediction methods when exploring possible RNA folds. Each folding prediction method has advantages and disadvantages [20], and when multiple tools converge on a consensus structure, then the highest-confidence predictions are generated. The following protocols outline the use and utility of the Crumple method in generating hypothesis of RNA structure and function.

2 Materials

Crumple can be run locally using an executable compiled from the source code (Subheading 3.1). To compile Crumple, a standard C compiler, such as the GNU gcc, is required. Many Linux distributions come with the gcc preinstalled. The Crumple build system recommends the user download GNU make, an open-source program for controlling the generation of executables and other non-source files of the program from the program's source files (http://www.gnu.org/software/make/). A machine running a Linux distribution, such as Ubuntu or Fedora, is recommended in order to meet the above requirements. Alternatively, a virtual machine can be setup to run a Linux operating system from a Mac or PC.

3   Methods

3.1   Crumple Local Installation

This protocol outlines the steps to setup Crumple through the terminal on a Linux system running Ubuntu 14.04. Similar procedures can be followed using other Linux distributions. Using your preferred web browser, navigate to https://figshare.com/articles/Crumple_RNA/3471767 or http://adenosine.chem.ou.edu/software.html. Scroll down to the Crumple section and click the download link to access the package.

3.1.1   Downloading and Extracting the Crumple Package

Using the terminal or the right-click context menu with the 'Extract Here' option, extract the contents of crumple.tgz to the preferred directory. Alternatively, navigate to the package directory: using the console with the command cd /directory/name and then extract the file with the command tar –xvzf crumple.tgz. Figure 1 summarizes the options for extracting the Crumple package using GUI and CLI methods.

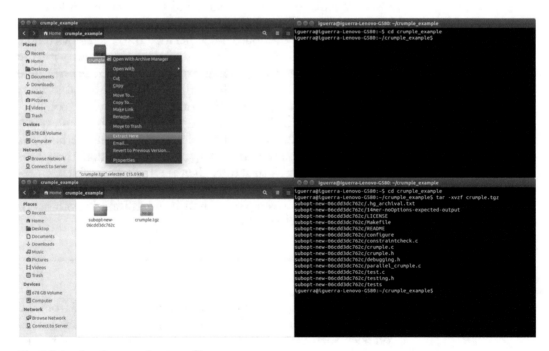

Fig. 1 Extracting the crumple source file

3.1.2   Installing GNU Make and Compiling Crumple

To compile the Crumple source, use the GNU make tool. After reading the documentation on the GNU make website (http://www.gnu.org/software/make/), download make using one of the mirrors provided on the site. Following the same procedure for the console outlined in Subheading 3.1.1, extract the compressed files. Once the files are extracted, move the working directory into the new directory and execute the commands as listed in Fig. 2.

After make has successfully installed, compile Crumple using the command make from a terminal within the subopt directory extracted in Subheading 3.1.1. The result will be a new executable file titled crumple found within the subopt directory. Figures 3 and 4 demonstrate this process. Note that a C compiler must be present on the system for make to compile the program successfully. Many Linux distributions come with the gcc preinstalled. Check the documentation for the system if compilation errors occur.

3.2   Using Crumple Features and Commands

This section describes a few sample runs of Crumple using various constraints and commands. The following sample runs will use the sequence

5′GCUCUAAAAGAGAGGCUCUAAAAGAGAG

For the sake of conciseness, we denote this sequence as 28mer throughout the following sections. 14mer, the first half of this sequence, was specifically designed to include an example of each possible context for dimethyl sulfate (DMS) modification of adenines. The 28mer sequence allows the possibility of multibranch loop formation. Thus this example sequence aptly demonstrates several features of Crumple.

3.2.1   Crumple Output Syntax

Crumple's output takes the form of strings of characters where a return to a newline indicates the completion of a structure. Table 1 provides definitions for the meaning of each individual output character as well as some significant character combinations.

3.2.2   Crumple Input and Output

Crumple supports input and output via the terminal and text files or any combination of the two. The first step in running Crumple

Building and Installing GNU Make
./configure
sh ./build.sh
./make check
./make install

Fig. 2 Building and installing GNU make, part I

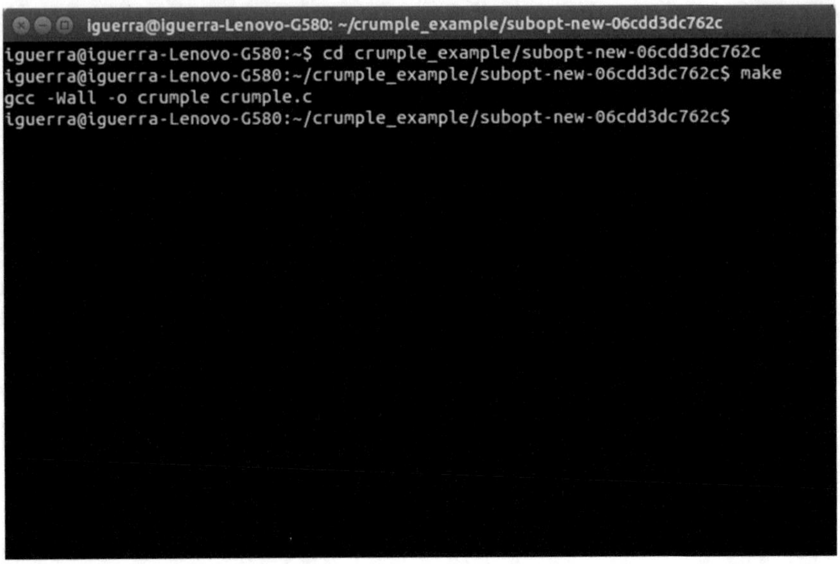

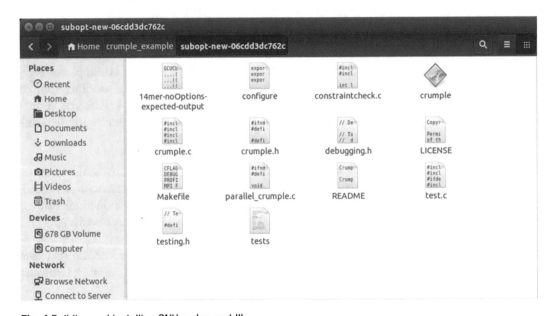

Fig. 3 Building and installing GNU make, part II

Fig. 4 Building and installing GNU make, part III

is opening a terminal window within the directory of the crumple executable. To display all possible structures for the given sample sequence, enter the command

echo "28mer" | ./crumple.

After a few seconds, all possible secondary structures will be printed to the console as well as a count of how many total structures were printed. Alternatively, in order to printout only the

Table 1
Crumple output syntax

Crumple symbol table	
.	Single dots are undetermined or unpaired nucleotides
(and)	Parentheses indicate base pairing
...(...)...	A parenthesis surrounded by unpaired nucleotides is a lonely pair
((((...))))	Helices are denoted by an opening parenthesis followed by its corresponding closing parenthesis. This example contains a helix of four pairs and a hairpin loop of three unpaired nucleotides

number of total structures, the parameter --count can be included, such as in the following command:

echo "28mer" | ./crumple --count

that generates the output FINAL COUNT: 124926. Similarly, parameters can be used in conjunction to reduce the output in meaningful ways. For instance, the command

echo"28mer" | ./crumple --helix-count 1 --helix-length 3

will display all structures with at least one or more helices of three nucleotides: . A list of all possible parameters, their syntax, and their purpose can be viewed by entering the following command as illustrated in Fig. 5

./crumple –h

Crumple can also take an input sequence from a file and output all possible structures, filtered through any constraints specified, to a user specified text file. To be a valid input file, the file must be plain text and contain a single line with only the sample sequence. As an example, the command

./crumple –i 28mer.txt

will provide the same output as

echo "28mer" | ./crumple

assuming all the previously outlined input file constraints have been met.

Outputting the results of a Crumple run to a text file: is possible and may be the preferred method for output solutions. To output results to a file, use the command

–o filename.txt.

The output will follow the same formatting procedure as is seen in the console. After executing the command, the resulting file will be located within the directory of the crumple executable. Figures 6 and 7 demonstrate how to use file I/O in Crumple.

```
iguerra@iguerra-Lenovo-G580:~/crumple_example/subopt-new-06cdd3dc762c$ ./crumple
-h

    usage:
    crumple [-noLP] [-noGU] [-max-dist #] [-noML]
            [-count [-b #]] [-i] [-o] [-help | -h]

    -b #         : If -count is used, b determines the 'breadcrumb' rate.
                   If -b 1000, solutions will print once ever 1000 seconds.
    -c           : Uses constraints from input: M for solvent-
                   accessible bases; X or x for modified, unpairing
                   bases; ( and ) for covarying, must-pair bases; . for
                   unconstrained bases.
    -help | -h   : Prints this message and exits.
    -i FILE      : Defines an input file, containing a sequence.

    -max-dist #  : Restricts to only solutions where all pairings
                   are between bases # or fewer bases apart.
    -noLP        : Restricts to only solutions with no lonely pairs.
    -noGU        : Disallows G-U pairing.
    -noML        : Restricts to only solutions without multiloops.
    -o FILE      : Defines an output file, to overwrite with solutions.

    --count        : Does not print solutions --- only the number of total
                     solutions found.
    --helix-count #      : Print only solutions with # helices.
    --helix-length #     : Print only solutions with helices # bases long.
    --helix-bulge #      : Print only solutions with <= # bulges per helix.
    --helix-mismatches # : Print only solutions with <= # mismatches per helix.

    --polling-interval # : MPI only; how many states to process before
                           sending work to needy nodes.


iguerra@iguerra-Lenovo-G580:~/crumple_example/subopt-new-06cdd3dc762c$ █
```

Fig. 5 The command ./crumple –h shows all possible parameters, syntax, and purpose

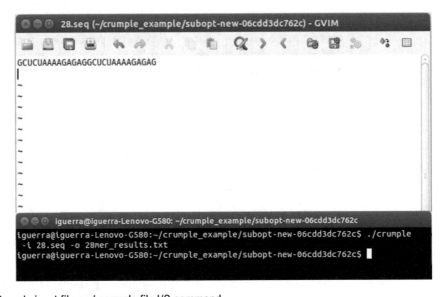

Fig. 6 Sample input file and crumple file I/O command

To better understand the way that Crumple explores the space of possible secondary structures, try the online, interactive demo at http://adenosine.chem.ou.edu/explore.html. For short sequences such as the 14-mer sequence 5′GCUCUAAAAGAGAG, the entire tree of possible folds can be visualized.

```
⊗ ⊖ ⊡   28mer_results.txt (~/crumple_ex...e/subopt-new-06cdd3dc762c) - GVIM1

🖿 🖿 🖿 🖿   ↩ ↪   ✂ 🗎 📋   🔍 ⟩ ⟨   🖿 🖿 ✂   ✦ ▦

.................(.(.......).)
.................(.(........))
.................(..........)
.................((...))....
.................(.....)....
.................((...)..)..
.................((....).)..
.................((.....))..
.................(.......)..
.................((...)....)
.................((....)...)
.................((....)..)
.................((......).)
.................((......))
.................(.......)
.................(...).....
.................(...)....
.................(......)...
.................(......)..
.................(......).
.................(.......)

FINAL COUNT:12492█
                                              124927,18    Bot
```

Fig. 7 Sample text file results

3.3 Running Parallelized Crumple

Crumple can be run both in serial and in parallel. The previous examples execute Crumple in serial on a single machine with no further distribution of the computation. Crumple supports parallelization based on a ring graph system using Message Passing Interface (MPI): and is capable of linear speedup times depending on the amount of work and the number of processors.

3.3.1 Materials and Compilation

In order to run parallelized Crumple, a multiprocessor computer or a computer cluster is necessary. Parallel Crumple was tested on the Sooner supercomputer, an Intel Xeon E5405 2.0 GHz Linux MPI cluster. Contact a university's information technology department in order to learn more about local resources that fulfill this requirement.

To compile for parallel execution, first ensure that libMPI is available. Next, check that GNU make is installed on the compiling machine. Finally, in order to create the executable, enter the command

make mpi

3.3.2 Parallel Output Efficiency

In implementation, the Crumple algorithm has been transformed into a completely iterative process, and then parallelized, for the sake of speed. Crumple's implementation follows a ring graph system. In the ring graph format, the work of the call stack is shared among a ring of nodes, which request work from one neighboring node and pass requests for work on to the other neighboring node. Work can be distributed between any node in the ring. A message passing algorithm from Dijsktra's work on token rings is used to recognize the end of the computation [21, 22]. The ultimate result is that computer resources are used more efficiently resulting in a linear speedup in execution.

Speedup is the ratio of times for the serial computation and the parallel computation. Using a 48-nucleotide guide RNA sequence from *Trypanosome brucei*, the speedup is almost perfectly linear until 32 processes [2]. For the 48-nucleotide *T. brucei* guide RNA sequence, the actual computation time was 47.5 h in serial and 30.9 min with 512 cores on the Sooner supercomputer (Intel Xeon E5405 2.06 GHz Linux MPI cluster). In the best case, Crumple completed computations for an unconstrained 60-nucleotide sequence with 1024 processes in 48 h on the Sooner computer. The point at which the graph of speedup versus cores shows nonlinearity will vary with the sequence and sequence length.

For a problem with exponential complexity and ideally linear speedup, doubling the number of processes approximately allows the consideration of a sequence one nucleotide longer in the same amount of time. Adding additional constraints greatly increases the efficiency of the computation. For example, Crumple computations for a 72-nucleotide noncoding RNA MicA sequence took longer than 48 h without any filters using 256 processes on the Sooner computer but required only 53 min and 27 s to generate 410, 270, 854 structures consistent with 27 single strand constraints, 1 covarying pair, and no isolated pairs [2]. The ability to incorporate selectively experimental constraints without reliance on thermodynamic parameters is one of the strengths of the Crumple method.

4 Notes

4.1 Use with Sliding Windows and Assembly

Sliding Windows and Assembly can be run in conjunction with Crumple to approximate a hypothesis of cotranscriptional folding and generate a series of hairpins with only local pairing. Sliding Windows performs Crumple computations on windows, or subsections, of a sequence and identifies the best-scoring structure in each window. Assembly is a dynamic algorithm that finds the best-scoring combination of a specific number of hairpins selected from the output of Sliding Windows. Configuration files include the parameters for incorporation of experimental constraints. Sliding Windows and Assembly and examples of the configuration files used to generate models for STMV and MS2 viral RNA genomes are available at http://adenosine.chem.ou.edu. This option is run in conjunction with the Vienna RNA package [23], which is available at http://www.tbi.univie.ac.at/RNA/. The Sliding Windows step calls the rna_eval function in the Vienna Package.

Begin by downloading Sliding Windows and Assembly and the Vienna RNA package. Install the Vienna RNA package in a $PATH folder. Extract the Sliding Windows and Assembly program using the following commands:

tar xvfz sliding_windows.tgz

cd sliding_windows-RN

make

./sliding_windows.sh sequence.conf

The program is run with the command

.sliding_windows sequence.conf

The output from Sliding Windows and Assembly includes the best-scoring structure in each window and a single structure composed of the best-scoring, nonoverlapping combination: of helices. The best-scoring structure per window is stored in a folder labeled "best" with filenames labeled by position and length. For example 83x24.lab is the name for a structure 24 nucleotides long and starting at nucleotide 83 in the sequence. The best structure per window may also be visualized in a "pilegram" with the x-axis representing the sequence; bars representing the length and position of the hairpin structure; and the color of the bars representing the score of the hairpin structure (Fig. 8). The "labeled" folder contains the processed output for each window from which the best-scoring hairpin structures are selected. The "structs" folder contains the raw Crumple output for each window.

The configuration files are designed by the user and incorporate any type of available experimental data that the user can express as a constraint. The SEQ parameter contains the RNA sequence of A, U, C, and G. The WINDOW parameter is the number of nucleotides in each subsection of the sequence. For example, a window

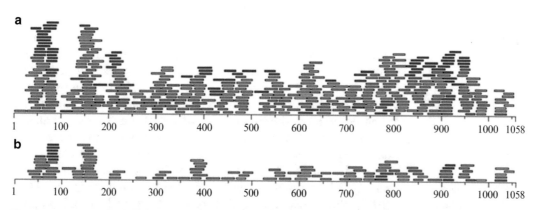

Fig. 8 Pilegrams for STMV RNA sequence. (**a**) The constraints allow up to two noncanonical pairs per helix. (**b**) The constraints allow up to one noncanonical pair per helix

size of 30 would Crumple the first 30 nucleotides of a sequence, ie nucleotides 1–30 in the first window, and then nucleotides 2–31 in the next window.

Chemical modification constraints can be incorporated as a series of periods "." for unconstrained nucleotides, "X" for nucleotides forced to remain unpaired, and "M" for modifications that are conditional on the position in a helix. The "M" option allows nucleotides that have chemical modification constraints to pair at the end of a helix or adjacent to an internal loop, bulge loop: , or GU pair [24]. The string of periods, X's, and M's must have the number of characters as the sequence.

Crystallography and cryo-electron microscopy can provide experimental data on the minimum number, lengths, and features of helices. The LENGTH and HELICES parameters define the minimum length and exact number of helices that will be output in the best scoring structure. The geometry of an icosahedral virus particle or predicted Hamiltonian paths on an icosahedral lattice [10, 25] may provide information on the minimum number of nucleotides between helices that can be included as the parameter, BETWEEN_HELICES. This parameter may be constant or may vary for each space between helices. The maximum number of internal base pair mismatches and terminal mismatches are defined by the parameters MISMATCHES and TERMINAL_ MISMATCHES, respectively. The parameter ASYMMETRY defines the maximum asymmetry in internal loops. Additional constraints may be included in SCORE_MODIFIER parameters. For example, data from SELEX experiments for RNA–protein binding that identify a preference for a hairpin loop size or a specific nucleotide at a particular position in a loop can be included in a user-defined SCORE_MODIFIER function. The flexibility of the scoring functions in Sliding Windows an Assembly is limited only by the user and the available experimental data.

4.2 Use with Thermodynamic Parameters

The output from Crumple may be evaluated based on thermodynamics, and free energy may be included in the scoring function for Sliding Windows and Assembly. The rna_eval function in the Vienna package returns the free energy of forming a structure given a specific sequence and structure [23]. Similar functions are available in RNAstructure [26] and other RNA folding programs. In some cases, computing all the structures first with Crumple and then computing the free energy of formation for each structure may be more efficient than considering thermodynamic parameters at each step of determining a base pair. In the case of STMV RNA, the order in which biophysical experimental parameters or free energy is incorporated can alter the best-scoring structure. Thus, the flexibility of Crumple, Sliding Windows, and Assembly allows users to modulate the influence of free energy minimization on the generation of possible structures for the development of hypotheses about function.

Acknowledgements

The authors would like to thank Jonathan W. Stone, Samuel Bleckley, and Jui-wen Liu for the development of the Crumple algorithm and RNA folding software in the Schroeder lab. We thank Kimberly Ughamadu for helpful comments on this manuscript and Fig. 8 pilegrams. We thank Henry Neeman and the staff at the Oklahoma Supercomputing Center for Education and Research (OSCER) for advice, assistance, and access to the Sooner and Boomer supercomputers. This work was supported by NSF CAREER award 0844913.

References

1. Schroeder SJ, Stone JW, Bleckley S, Gibbons T, Mathews DM (2011) Ensemble of secondary structures for encapsidated satellite tobacco mosaic virus RNA consistent with chemical probing and crystallography constraints. Biophys J 101:167–175

2. Bleckley S, Stone JW, Schroeder SJ (2012) Crumple: a method for complete enumeration of all possible pseudoknot-free RNA secondary structures. PLoS One 7:e52414

3. Pipas J, McMahon J (1975) Methods for predicting RNA secondary structure. Proc Natl Acad Sci U S A 72:2017–2021

4. Wuchty S, Fontana W, Hofacker IL, Schuster P (1999) Complete suboptimal folding of RNA and the stability of secondary structures. Biopolymers 49:145–165

5. Stone JW, Bleckley S, Lavelle S, Schroeder SJ (2015) A parallel implementation of the Wuchty algorithm with additional experimental filters to more thoroughly explore RNA conformational space. PLoS One 10:e0117217

6. Larson NB, Day J, Greenwood A, McPherson A (1998) Refined structure of satellite tobacco mosaic virus at 1.8 A resolution. J Mol Biol 277:37–59

7. Larson SB, Koszelak S, Day J, Greenwood A, Dodds JA, McPherson A (1993) Double helical RNA in satellite tobacco mosaic virus. Nature 361:179–182

8. Golmohammadi R, Valegard K, Fridborg K, Liljas L (1993) The refined structure of bacteriophage MS2 at 2.8 A resolution. J Mol Biol 234:620–639

9. Valegard K, Liljas L, Fridborg K, Unge T (1990) The three-dimensional structure of the bacterial virus MS2. Nature 345:36–41

10. Bleckley S, Schroeder SJ (2012) Incorporating global features of RNA motifs in predictions for an ensemble of secondary structures for encapsidated MS2 bacteriophage RNA. RNA 18:1309–1318

11. Shepherd CM, Borelli IA, Lander G, Natarajan P, Siddavanahalli V, Bajaj C, Johnson JE, Brooks CL, Reddy VS (2006) VIPERdb: a relational database for structural virology. Nucleic Acids Res 34:D386–D389

12. Schroeder SJ (2014) Alternative viewpoints and alternative structures for satellite tobacco mosaic virus RNA. Biochemistry 53:6728–6737

13. Larson SB, McPherson A (2001) Satellite tobacco mosaic virus RNA: structure and implications for assembly. Curr Opin Struct Biol 11:59–65

14. Zeng Y, Larson SB, Heitsch CE, McPherson A, Harvey SC (2012) A model for the structure of satellite tobacco mosaic virus. J Struct Biol 180:110–116

15. Turner DH, Mathews DH (2009) NNDB: the nearest neighbor parameter database for predicting stability of nucleic acid secondary structure. Nucleic Acids Res 38:D280–D282

16. Nguyen M-T, Schroeder SJ (2010) Consecutive terminal GU pairs stabilize RNA helices. Biochemistry 49:10574–10581

17. Chen JL, Dishler AL, Kennedy SD, Yildirim I, Liu B, Turner DH, Serra MJ (2012) Testing the nearest neighbor model for canonical RNA base pairs: revision of GU parameters. Biochemistry 51:3508–3522

18. Schroeder SJ, Turner DH (2001) Thermodynamic stabilities of internal loops with GU closing pairs in RNA. Biochemistry 40:11509–11517

19. Gu X, Mooers BH, Thomas LM, Malone J, Harris S et al (2015) Structures and energetics of four adjacent G.U pairs that stabilize an RNA helix. J Phys Chem B 119:13252–13261

20. Schroeder SJ (2009) Advances in RNA structure prediction from sequence: new tools for generating hypotheses about viral RNA structure-function relationships. J Virol 83:6326–6334

21. Dijkstra EW, Scholten CS (1980) Termination detection for diffusing computations. Inform Process Lett 11:1–4

22. Dinan J, Olivier S, Sabin G, Prins J, Sadayappan P, Tseng C-W (2007) Dynamic load balancing of unbalanced computations using message passing; March 2007. Long Beach, CA. IEEE

23. Lorenz R, Bernhart SH, Honer Zu Siederdissen C, Tafer H, Flamm C, Stadler PF, Hofacker IL (2011) ViennaRNA package 2.0. Algorithms Mol Biol 6:26

24. Mathews DH, Disney MD, Childs JL, Schroeder SJ, Zuker M, Turner DH (2004) Incorporating chemical modification constraints into a dynamic programming algorithm for prediction of RNA secondary structure. Proc Natl Acad Sci U S A 101:7287–7292

25. Dykeman EC, Grayson NE, Toropova K, Ranson NA, Stockley PG et al (2011) Simple rules for efficient assembly predict the layout of a packaged viral RNA. J Mol Biol 408:399–407

26. Reuter JS, Mathews DH (2010) RNAstructure: software for RNA secondary structure prediction and analysis. BMC Bioinformatics 11:129

Chapter 2

Secondary Structure Prediction of Single Sequences Using RNAstructure

Zhenjiang Zech Xu and David H. Mathews

Abstract

RNA secondary structure is often predicted using folding thermodynamics. RNAstructure is a software package that includes structure prediction by free energy minimization, prediction of base pairing probabilities, prediction of structures composed of highly probably base pairs, and prediction of structures with pseudoknots. A user-friendly graphical user interface is provided, and this interface works on Windows, Apple OS X, and Linux. This chapter provides protocols for using RNAstructure for structure prediction.

Key words RNA structure prediction, RNA folding thermodynamics, RNA statistical mechanics

1 Introduction

Computational prediction of RNA secondary structure is a cost-effective approach to design structures [1–3], discover non-coding RNAs [4–6], study folding [7], and design siRNA sequences [8–10]. This chapter provides protocols for using RNAstructure to predict a secondary structure [11]. Prediction methods, including free energy minimization, suboptimal structure prediction, partition function calculation, and pseudoknot prediction, are described in detail with examples. Their merits are also explained for users to choose the appropriate tools for their own problems. The performance of the prediction methods are benchmarked by comparing the predicted structures to reference secondary structures derived from comparative sequence analysis [12]. Their accuracies are measured with two statistics—sensitivity and positive predictive value (PPV). Sensitivity is the percentage of true base pairs that are predicted and PPV is the percentage of predicted base pairs that are in the reference structure.

Douglas H. Turner and David H. Mathews (eds.), *RNA Structure Determination: Methods and Protocols*, Methods in Molecular Biology, vol. 1490, DOI 10.1007/978-1-4939-6433-8_2, © Springer Science+Business Media New York 2016

1.1 Free Energy Minimization

Free energy minimization is a popular computational method to predict secondary structure. It is based on the assumption that an RNA finds the most thermodynamically favorable conformation [13]. Typically, a nearest neighbor free energy model with empirical parameters, based on optical melting experiments of small model RNAs, is used for this approach [14–16]. The thermodynamic model can also be improved by accounting for the sequences that occur frequently in loops in the database of RNA sequences with known structures [17–19]. The model assumes that the stability of an RNA secondary structure mainly depends on the sequence of a motif and the sequence of the neighboring base pairs, and the total free energy change is the sum of these nearest neighbor terms.

Using the nearest neighbor model, a dynamic programming algorithm is commonly used to find the RNA secondary structures with lowest free energy because it guarantees the lowest free energy structure will be found. It implicitly considers all possible structures to identify the lowest free energy structure, but does not need to explicitly enumerate all the structures. The process is divided into two steps, fill and trace back [20, 21]. In the fill step, the optimal folding free energies for increasingly longer overlapping segments of the sequence are stored into a matrix. At the end of the fill step, the optimal folding free energy is known, but the structure that has that folding free energy is not yet determined. Then, in the second (trace back) step, the base pairs in the lowest free energy structure are determined and the optimal secondary structure is thus generated. This dynamic programming algorithm scales $O(N^2)$ in storage and $O(N^3)$ in time, where N is the sequence length. This means that a doubling of sequence length would require four times the computer memory and eight times the computer time.

In addition to the minimum free energy structure, low free energy structures can also be generated. They provide important alternative hypotheses for the secondary structure because the minimum free energy structure is not perfect due to experimental errors in the free energy parameters [21], the fact that not all sequences find their lowest free energy conformation, and most algorithms cannot predict pseudoknots (see section 1.3). Several methods exist for generating the low free energy structures, which are generally called suboptimal structures. For example, an exhaustive set of structures can be predicted within an energy increment above the minimum free energy [22] or a smaller heuristic sample of diverse structures can be generated [23, 24]. It is often convenient, if structures will be inspected manually, to use the heuristic approach to generate representative structures because the exhaustive set is often quite large for even small energy increments (such as the thermal noise increment of kT, where k is the Boltzmann constant and T is the absolute temperature).

1.2 Partition Functions

To understand the structures that are reasonable for a sequence to adopt according to the nearest neighbor model, dynamic programming algorithms have been developed to characterize the ensemble of structures by calculating their partition functions [25, 26]. Partition functions sum the equilibrium constants of all the possible secondary structures in thermodynamic equilibrium. The probability of a structure occurring in the ensemble is then the equilibrium constant for that structure, divided by the partition function. The partition function, Q, for a RNA secondary structure ensemble is:

$$Q = \sum_i \exp\left(-\Delta G\left(S_i\right) / RT\right),$$

where R is the gas constant, T is the absolute temperature, $\Delta G(S_k)$ is the Gibbs free energy change for the secondary structure S_k, and the sum is over all secondary structures. The probability for a base pair is then the sum of the probabilities of all the structures containing this base pair:

$$P_{i,j} = \sum_n \exp\left(-\Delta G\left(S_n\right) / RT\right) / Q,$$

where i and j are nucleotide indices with i canonically base paired with j, and S_n indicates a secondary structure containing the i-j base pair [26]. Highly probable base pairs are more likely to be in the actual secondary structure. For example, it was shown that the fraction of predicted pairs in lowest free energy structures that are correctly predicted increased from 65.8 to 91.0% when only the base pairs with high probabilities (≥ 0.99 pairing probability) are considered [26]. Base pairs in predicted structures can be color-annotated to show the fidelity of the predicted pairs.

A number of algorithms were developed to use partition function calculations. A representative set of structures can be sampled from the ensemble according to their computed Boltzmann probabilities [27]. This sample is statistically reproducible with even a moderate size (~100 structures). Alternative conformations that are adopted by RNA under different conditions can be readily revealed by classifying the structures into various clusters. Furthermore, a single centroid structure for the ensemble can be identified from the sample, which has higher PPV than the minimum free energy structure [28, 29]. Individual RNA motifs, besides the whole structure, are also able to be probabilistically predicted with the sampling algorithm [27]. Another algorithm, called Maximum Expected Accuracy (MEA), was also applied to predict RNA secondary structures [19], using base paring probabilities calculated from the partition function [30].

1.3 Pseudoknot Prediction

The algorithms described above are not able to predicted pseudoknots. A pseudoknot is defined by at least two base pairs, with indices i-j and i'-j', where $i < i' < j < j'$. Pseudoknots are well structurally conserved and functionally important topologies [31, 32] in RNA structures such as telomerase RNA [33, 34] and ribozymes [35]. Their prediction, however, remains notoriously difficult. It is proven that predicting the lowest free energy structure with pseudoknots is NP-complete [36], which in practice means that the prediction of lowest free energy structures is not solvable in realistic computation time for most sequences long enough to be important for biology. By sacrificing computational time efficiency compared to algorithms that neglect pseudoknots, dynamic programming algorithms are able to predict lowest free energy RNA secondary structures for restricted classes of pseudoknots [37–39]. Other algorithms are also proposed to predict pseudoknotted structures quickly, but with heuristics such as assembling structures from probable base pairs [40], helices or pseudoknot-free substructures [41–44]. These algorithms allow pseudoknots of more diverse topologies, but they do not guarantee the minimum free energy structure will be found. A third class of algorithms combines graph algorithms with dynamic programming algorithms for optimal pseudoknotted structure prediction to improve the computation efficiency [45, 46]. Although algorithms for pseudoknot prediction are now computationally tractable, it was shown that the accuracy of pseudoknot prediction is poor [40], suggesting the need for improvement.

The RNAstructure package is an integrated collection of computational tools for RNA or DNA analysis, including secondary structure prediction, folding free energy calculations, structure visualization, and siRNA design [11]. It uses the latest nearest neighbor parameters obtained at 37 °C and a set of folding enthalpy changes for extrapolating the free energy changes to other temperatures. The following protocols explain how to predict RNA secondary structure with tools in the package ranging from free energy minimization to partition function calculation, either considering or not considering pseudoknots.

2 Protocols

2.1 Installing the Graphical User Interface

RNAstructure is freely available at the website http://rna.urmc.rochester.edu. The graphical interface (GUI) installs and runs on Microsoft Windows, Mac (OS X 10.7 Lion or higher), or Unix / Linux platforms. First, download the version for the operating system being used (Windows, OS X, or Linux). The GUI relies on JAVA, and it is crucial that JAVA 1.7 or higher is installed. You can check what Java version is installed by going to the website http://www.java.com/en/download/installed.jsp.

The help page for installation and usage is also available at http://rna.urmc.rochester.edu/RNAstructureHelp.html.   On   Windows, install RNAstructure by double-clicking RNAstructureWindows Installer.exe. When complete, RNAstructure can be run by choosing RNAstructure on the start menu. On Mac, the program can then be started by double-clicking the RNAstructure app. Note that the security settings need to be changed on the Mac so that a downloaded program can be run. To do this, click on "System Properties". Go into "Security & Privacy". Click on the lock to allow changes to be made. Select "Anywhere" under "Allow applications downloaded from:" On Linux, a gzipped tar is downloaded. This can be extracted using "tar -xzvf RNAstructureForLinux.tgz". Then the GUI can be launched by running "RNAstructure/exe/RNAstructureScript".

2.2 Sequence Input and Editing

RNAstructure provides a convenient interface for users to input or edit nucleic acid sequences. Users can click menu "File" → "New Sequence" to manually type in sequences or paste what is copied into the system clipboard. A sequence title and comment can also be specified. Or users can click menu "File" → "Open Sequence" to open an existing file for editing (the RNAstructure SEQ format or FASTA format can be read). After a sequence is input and edited, users can click "Format Sequence" as shown in Fig. 1. The sequence will be read out by clicking "Read Sequence" to check for possible typographical errors. Finally, the sequence is saved to disk by clicking "File" → "Save Sequence" to overwrite the opened file or "File" → "Save Sequence As …" to save to a new file. In the same

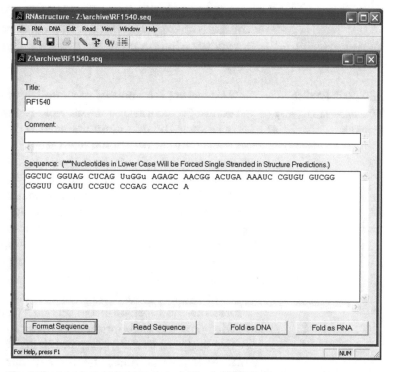

Fig. 1 The interface of the sequence editor in RNAstructure

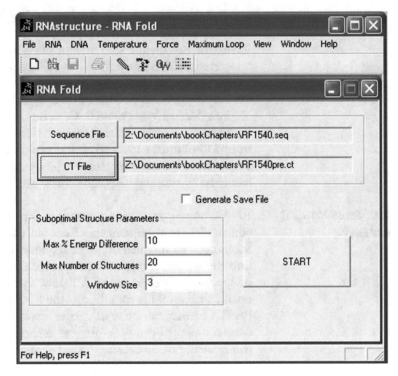

Fig. 2 The Fold module window, used to specify input, output, and parameters

dialog window, users can click "Fold as RNA" to predict the minimum free energy structure for the sequence. Before the prediction, a window will pop up to ask users whether to save the changes of the sequence.

2.3 Fold: Predict Minimum Free Energy Structure

RNAstructure is composed of a number of modules for performing structure prediction or analysis. Fold is a module in RNAstructure that predicts the minimum free energy structure for a single RNA sequence. By clicking "Fold RNA Single Strand" under the "RNA" menu, the Fold input form pops up (Fig. 2). Users click the "Sequence File" button to provide the RNA sequence file in SEQ or FASTA format. A default output file name is then generated, but the file name and save directory can be changed by clicking the "CT File" button. Users can save the predicted energy information to the same file name in the same directory with a .sav suffix by checking the box "Generate Save File". The .sav file is needed to produce the energy dot plot as described below.

Besides the predicted minimum free energy structure, which represents the most probable secondary structure at equilibrium, Fold also predicts suboptimal secondary structures, providing alternative solutions to the folding problem. The prediction of suboptimal structures is tuned by three parameters, which are given reasonable default values based on the length of the input sequence.

"Max % Energy Difference" sets the maximum increment in percentage above the computed lowest free energy. Only the predicted structures with free energies falling into this interval are output. Increasing this parameter can result in a greater number of suboptimal structures. "Max Number of Structures" defines the maximum number of structures that can be generated. "Window Size" controls how different the suboptimal structures must be from each other. It can be set to the minimum value of zero to allow outputting structures with small variations or to higher values for greater variations. Alternatively, all suboptimal structures within a small increment of the lowest free energy structure could be generated by clicking "RNA" → "Generate All Suboptimal Structures" to choose a different module of the program.

After clicking "Fold RNA Single Strand", several additional menu items appear. "Temperature" allows users to specify the temperature at which the folding occurs. Temperature changes should be used with caution. The enthalpy parameters for predicting free energy changes at temperatures other than 37 °C are prone to significant errors outside the range of about 20–50 °C [47]. Note that the change in temperature applies only to a single calculation. Subsequent predictions will return to the default of 37 °C. The maximum size of the internal/bulge loops can be changed at "Maximum Loop". The default is 30, and this is usually sufficient for structure predictions. Folding constraints from chemical/enzymatic mapping and/or SHAPE experiments can also be incorporated into prediction under the "Force" menu (described in detail in Chapter 10 of this volume). These additional features are available in many of the following RNA prediction tools in RNAstructure.

The prediction is initiated by clicking the "Start" button. A progress bar then appears to show the progress of the calculation. After prediction is done, the structure can be drawn, as shown in Fig. 3 using the drawing module. All the predicted structures are presented in ascending order of their free energies. By default the first structure, i.e., the predicted lowest free energy structure, is drawn. Users can choose to draw alternative structures by clicking "Draw" → "Go to Structure..." or by pressing ctrl + up/down arrows. The view can be zoomed in or out it with ctrl + right/left arrows or by clicking "Zoom" under "Draw" menu. In addition, the structure diagram can be color annotated according to its nucleotide SHAPE reactivity (*see* Chapter 10 of this volume) or base pair probabilities (*see* Subheading 2.5) by clicking "Add SHAPE Annotation" or "Add Probability Color Annotation" under the menu "Annotations". Furthermore, the structure can be output to a helix file by clicking "Draw" → "Write Helix File". The helix file can be read by XRNA for creating publication-quality figures (http://rna.ucsc.edu/rnacenter/xrna/xrna.html).

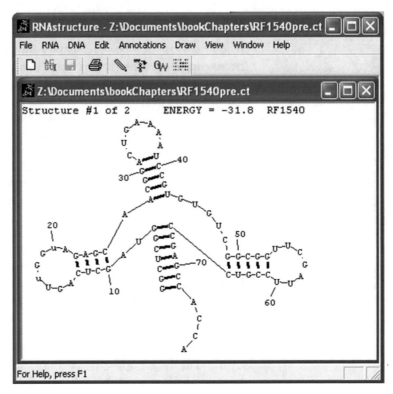

Fig. 3 Screenshot of the minimum free energy secondary structure predicted by Fold. Above the drawing, the number of structures, the predicted free energy in kcal/mol and the sequence name are shown. This tRNA[Ser] from *Bacillus subtilis* is perfectly predicted, agreeing with the reference structure from comparative sequence analysis

Because the energy save file with .sav suffix contains predicted energy information for a given sequence, it can be used to output secondary structures by clicking "File" → "Refold from Save File", which is much faster than predicting from scratch.

2.4 Energy Dot Plot: Show Well-Defined ness of Predicted RNA Motifs

The saved energy file with the .sav suffix can be used to produce an energy dot plot by choosing "File" → "DotPlot". The dots in the plot represent all possible base pairs predicted between the nucleotides i on the x axis and j on the y axis (Fig. 4). The color indicates the energy of the lowest free energy structure that is predicted to contain that pair [23]. The legend shows the folding free energy ranges associated with each color. The plot provides information about all alternative secondary structures. The emptiness of the dot plot indicates how well defined the RNA structure is. The color patterns, such as the line composed of red dots in Fig. 4, reveal possible helices that can form in low free energy structures. Although the algorithm cannot predict pseudoknots,

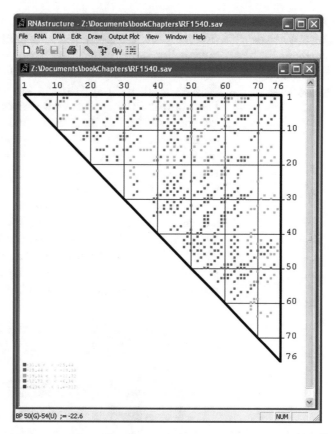

Fig. 4 RNA energy dot plot for the same tRNA sequence in Fig. 3. Each *dot* indicates a base pair between the nucleotides indexed on *horizontal* and *vertical* axes. Each *dot* is color annotated according to the folding free energy of the optimal structure containing this base pair. The color legend is shown in *bottom left corner*, which can be zoomed in with ctrl + right arrow. The nucleotide indices and identity and lowest free energy involving the base pair are shown in the *bottom* status bar by clicking a dot in the dot plot

the well-defined regions and color patterns in the dot plot that are absent in minimum free energy structures may imply potential pseudoknotted helices. The appearance of the dot plot can be modified using the "Draw" menu options. It is often useful, for example, to restrict the range of energies shown on the plot by choosing "Plot Range" under "Draw". By default, all pairs are shown, up to an energy of 0 kcal/mol, but this can be changed to something closer to the lowest free energy structure. A difference in energy above the lowest free energy of about 2 kT (1.2 kcal/mol at 37 °C) shows most pairs of interest [47]. Finally, the dot-plot can be output to a plain text file by clicking "Output Plot". The resulting file will contain each base pair in the plot and an energy value of the lowest free energy structure containing that base pair.

2.5   Partition Function Calculation: Color Annotate Structure with Base Pair Probabilities

A dynamic programming algorithm for partition function calculation for a single RNA sequence is implemented in RNAstructure. It is accessible under "RNA" → "Partition Function RNA". After clicking it, a window appears for controlling input, output, and options. As with Fold, the user selects a sequence file using the "Sequence File" button. The output of this calculation is a partition function save file (.pfs suffix). By default, the result of partition function calculation is stored to the same file name with the input file but with a .pfs suffix, but this can be changed by clicking the "Save File" button. "Temperature" and "Force" menus become visible and act similarly as in Fold module.

The calculation is started by pressing the "Start" button. After the calculation is complete, a base pairing probability dot plot is shown as in Fig. 5. A .pfs file could be reopened subsequently by "File" → "DotPlot Partition Function" to draw the dot plot. The probability dot plot is similar to an energy dot plot, except that color indicates the probability of base pairs instead of free energy.

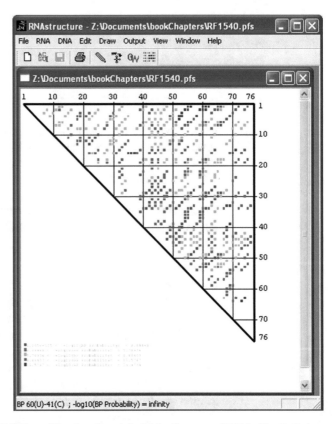

Fig. 5 RNA partition function dot plot for the same tRNA in Fig. 3. *Dots* are color annotated according to their base pair probabilities. The color legend is shown in *bottom left corner*, which can be zoomed in with ctrl + right arrow. The nucleotides indices and identity and pairing probability of the base pair are shown in the *bottom* status bar by clicking a dot in the dot plot

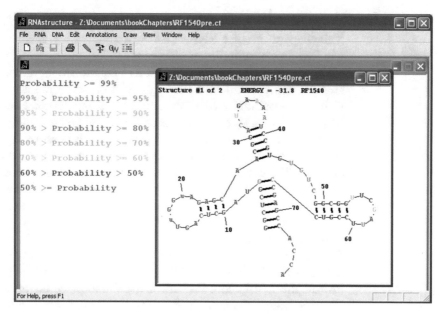

Fig. 6 Color annotated structure. The structure is for the same tRNA in Fig. 3 predicted by the Fold module

In the "Draw" menu, similar tools are also available to customize the dot plot. The only difference is that the plot range now is on scale of $-\log_{10}$(base pair probability) instead of free energy. In most cases, the base pairing probability dot plot is more useful than the energy dot plot because it provides an overall picture of the RNA structural ensemble [48]. It is especially important for RNAs that have multiple conformations. The probability plot is also useful to derive helices for pseudoknot prediction [49].

For any given secondary structure diagram opened in RNAstructure, the .pfs file can also be used to annotate the base pairs according to their predicted probabilities by choosing menu "Annotations" → "Add Probability Color Annotations" (Fig. 6) [50]. The color annotation provides confidence estimates in the base pairs of the structure. Structural motifs composed of highly probable base pairs are likely to be in the actual structure. The average fraction of correctly predicted pairs in lowest free energy structures increased from 65.8 to 91.0 % when only the base pairs with high probabilities (≥ 0.99) were considered [26].

2.6 MaxExpect: Predict a Structure Composed of Probable Pairs

RNAstructure offers a module, MaxExpect, which uses the partition function calculation [30] to predict secondary structures that maximize the expected base pair accuracy. This structure maximizes a score that balances the probabilities of base pairing and being unpaired. A scaling factor, gamma, can favor or disfavor base pair formation. The default value for gamma is 1, and making gamma larger than 1 results in more base pairs. Gamma controls a trade-off between sensitivity and PPV of the prediction, where higher gamma results in higher sensitivity at the cost of PPV.

MaxExpect is accessible under the "RNA" menu option as "MaxExpect: Predict RNA MEA Structure". This opens an input window for choosing input files, output files, and option. It takes a pfs file from a prior partition function calculation as input and generates the optimal structure (having maximum expected accuracy) as well as suboptimal structures until either the "Max Number of Structures" is reached or the score differs by greater than "Max % Score Difference" from the structure with the best score. Again, the "Window Size" parameter ensures the suboptimal structures are sufficiently different from each other, where larger integer values result in structures more different from each other and the minimum is zero. The calculation is started by clicking the "Start" button.

It has been shown that MaxExpect has higher average PPV than minimum free energy prediction [30]. Taking the tRNA sequence RF1540 in Fig. 3 as an example, the same perfect structure is predicted as that by Fold. The "ENERGY" reported for MaxExpect is instead the MEA score instead of the folding free energy change. The free energy change, however, can be calculated by inputting the predicted structure to the program Efn2 (Subheading 2.9).

2.7 Stochastic Sampling: Sample a Set of Structures

Another module in RNAstructure uses the results of a partition function calculation to sample a representative set of secondary structures, with the probability of choosing a secondary structure equal to its Boltzmann probability of occurrence in the complete folding ensemble [27]. This module is chosen with "RNA" → "Stochastic Sampling". A .pfs file from a prior partition function calculation is provided as input file by clicking "Partition Function Save File". Again, an output file name will be generated automatically and users are able to change it by clicking the "CT File" button. "Ensemble Size" is a parameter to specify how many structures to sample. "Random Seed" is an integer used to set the starting point for generating a series of random numbers for the sampling. The same random seed number will always output the same sampled structures on the same computer system. It can be changed to sample an alternative set of structures.

2.8 ProbKnot: Predict Structures That May Contain Pseudoknots

The structure prediction methods described previously in the chapter are incapable of predicting one important topology for RNA secondary structure, the pseudoknot. ProbKnot is a simple yet powerful algorithm to predict pseudoknotted RNA structures [40]. It assembles maximum expected accuracy structures from base-pairing probabilities computed from a non-pseudoknotted partition function. A base pair i-j is included in the predicted structure only if the probability of i-j is higher than any i-k or j-k base pairs, where k is any other nucleotide in the sequence. The key observation is that the pseudoknot motif is usually thermodynamically stable and often is predicted in the set of suboptimal structures.

ProbKnot is accessible under the "RNA" menu as "ProbKnot: Predict RNA Structures Including Pseudoknots". This opens a window for selecting the input sequence, the file to which the predicted structure is output, and the parameters. Additional iterations, specified by the "iterations" parameter, are supported to find additional base pairs by repeating the calculation only on the remaining unpaired nucleotides. After structure assembly, a post-processing step is used to remove short helices. The minimum number of base pairs in a helix can be specified as parameter "Minimum helix length". By default, helices composed of two or one base will be removed. The calculation is started by clicking the "Start" button.

ProbKnot is fast, and it scales the same as the free energy minimization method. It is one of the best algorithms capable of pseudoknot prediction because it does not sacrifice overall prediction accuracy. Figure 7 shows an example of prediction by ProbKnot on the *Tetrahymena thermophila* group I intron. Its sensitivity and PPV are 86% and 76%, higher than the 82% and 75% of the

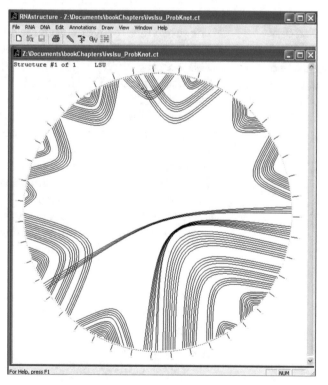

Fig. 7 The visualization of *Tetrahymena thermophila* group I intron secondary structure predicted by ProbKnot. Pseudoknotted structures are drawn by RNAstructure in this circular diagram instead of the radial representation, as in Fig. 3. The sequence backbone is arranged in a *circle* and paired bases are connected with chords. The *nested chords* denote helices and the crossing *chords* denote pseudoknots. One of the two pseudoknots (the lower one) is correctly predicted by ProbKnot

Fold-predicted structure. This improvement upon Fold mainly results from a correctly predicted pseudoknot. Note that structures with pseudoknots are drawn by RNAstructure with the backbone around a circle.

2.9 Efn2: Calculate The Free Energy Change of a Given Structure

Efn2 is a module in RNAstructure to predict the folding free energy change of an inputted structure. It utilizes a full nearest neighbor model, including coaxial stacking, an end-to-end stacking of adjacent helices in multibranch and exterior loops. The module is available under menu "RNA" → "Efn2 RNA". It outputs a free energy change for each structure in the input file provided by the user clicking "CT File". An output file name is automatically generated, but users are free to change it. With the option "Write Thermodynamic Details File" checked, more thermodynamic details of substructure in each structure is reported, including the stabilities of each loop and stacking base pair. The calculation is initiated by clicking the "Start" button. The output file can be opened as a plain text file. On Windows, WordPad is a convenient programming for viewing the results. On OS X, TextEdit can be used.

2.10 Text User Interface (TUI) (Command Line Interface)

The procedures provided above are for the graphical user interface (GUI). All the functionalities, however, are also available in the TUI for the three major operating systems. The options and parameters for the TUI are explained online in help pages, http://rna.urmc.rochester.edu/Text/index.html.

The TUI is user-friendly, and uses a standard Makefile to compile each program. After downloading the source code in Unix format. The package can be unzipped, and users can change to the package directory ("RNAstructure") and issue the command "make [program name]" to create an executable or "make instructions" to list all available programs in the terminal. The compiled executables will be located in the "exe" directory ready for use. To run the programs, an environment variable needs to be defined to specify the location of the nearest neighbor parameters. This is done with the following:

In BASH:

export DATAPATH = [directory where RNAstructure resides]/ RNAstructure/data_tables

In CSH:

setenv DATAPATH [directory where RNAstructure resides]/ RNAstructure/data_tables

In DOS/Windows:

set DATAPATH = [driver letter on which RNAstructure resides]:\ [directory where RNAstructure resides]\RNAstructure\ data_tables

Users of Linux and OS X can also put this statement in their login shell script and source it to make the environment variable permanently defined.

```
─────────── SEQ Sample File ───────────

; (first line of file) Comments must start with a semicolon.
;
; There can be any number lines of comments
A title line must imediately follow
AA      GCGG UUTGTT UTCUTaaTCTXXXXUCAGG1
```

```
─────────── CT Sample File ───────────

13  ENERGY = -2.9  fake seq
  1 C    0         2    13    1
  2 C    1         3    12    2
  3 A    2         4    11    3
  4 G    3         5    10    4
  5 A    4         6     0    5
  6 C    5         7     0    6
  7 U    6         8     0    7
  8 C    7         9     0    8
  9 A    8        10     0    9
 10 C    9        11     4   10
 11 U   10        12     3   11
 12 G   11        13     2   12
 13 G   12         0     1   13
```

Fig. 8 Examples of the SEQ and CT file formats

Documentation for the source code of the underlying C++ classes is also available at http://rna.urmc.rochester.edu/RNA_class/html/index.html . Advanced users can customize the programs or build their own tools with the source code.

2.11 SEQ and CT File Formats

RNAstructure takes sequence files of SEQ format or FASTA format as input and outputs secondary structures in CT format.

A SEQ file is a file containing a nucleotide sequence, typically with a .seq extension. It must conform to the following specifications (Fig. 8):

1. Comment lines must be at the beginning of the file. There needs to be at least one comment line.

2. Each comment line must start with a semicolon.

3. A single title line not starting with a semicolon must immediately follow comments lines.

4. Any number of lines of sequence must immediately follow the title line. The sequence should contain nucleotides in capital letters from 5′ to 3′. The letter "T" is treated as "U" for RNA

sequences. The letter "X" is used to indicate unknown nucleotides that will not be allowed to pair. Lowercase letter(s) are used to force nucleotide(s) to be single-stranded in the prediction. Any number of white space characters is allowed in the sequences.

5. The sequence must end with "1".

A CT (connectivity table) file contains secondary structure information for a sequence with a .ct extension. It must comply with these specifications (Fig. 8):

1. The first line must start with the sequence length, followed by the title of the structure.

2. Each of the following lines provides the information on each nucleotide in the sequence. It must contain six fields separated by an arbitrary number of spaces: (1) nucleotide position i; (2) a single letter for nucleotide (A, U, T, G, C, or X) in either lower or upper case; (3) the preceding nucleotide to this nucleotide (position i-1 or 0 for the 5′ end); (4) the following nucleotide in the sequence (position i+1 or 0 at the 3′ end); (5) position of the nucleotide to which this nucleotide is base paired, where no pairing is indicated by 0; (6) natural numbering, which is ignored by RNAstructure and usually set to repeat i.

3. One CT file can contain multiple structures for the same sequence, with all structures, in the format above, concatenated.

2.12 DOT2CT and CT2DOT: Structure File Conversions

Some RNA structure prediction algorithms, such as the Vienna RNA package (http://www.tbi.univie.ac.at/RNA/), report secondary structures in the dot-bracket format. The dot-bracket format is a string notation for a nested RNA secondary structure, with an unpaired nucleotide denoted with a dot and a base pair with an opening and closing brackets. This format is succinct, but needs to be extended to denote pseudoknots. The full file contains a header line starting with a '>' sign, a RNA sequence on a single line and its dot-bracket structure on another single line. DOT2CT and CT2DOT are two programs in RNAstructure to make the file convertible to or from the CT file format for pseudoknot-free structures. They are only available as text interfaces, although a dot-bracket file can be generated in the GUI using "Draw" → "Write to Dot-Bracket Notation" to get a dot-bracket file of a structure being displayed in the draw module.

2.13 CircleCompare: To Visually Compare Two Structures

RNAstructure offers a facility called CircleCompare to visually compare two secondary structures of the same sequence. It takes two structures as input and outputs a postscript image of them in a circle with one on top of the other, especially making pseudoknotted base pairs conveniently visible. The base pairs are colored differently according to whether they exist in the first structure, in the second structure or in both of the structures. As

```
Predicted Structure file name: /home/zane/Desktop/ivslsu.ct
Accepted Structure file name:  /home/zane/archive/ivslsu.ct

Predicted Structure: LSU
Accepted Structure:  Warring et.al. (Nature 321, 13

Green: Pair in both structures
Black: Pair in Accepted Structure only
Red:   Pair in Predicted Structure only
```

Sensitivity: 111 / 129 = 86.05%
PPV: 112 / 148 = 75.68%

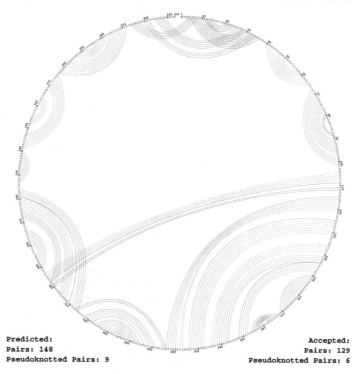

Predicted: Accepted:
Pairs: 148   Pairs: 129
Pseudoknotted Pairs: 9   Pseudoknotted Pairs: 6

Fig. 9 The comparison of *Tetrahymena thermophila* group I intron secondary structure predicted by ProbKnot with the reference structure from comparative analysis

an example, the reference structure and the ProbKnot-predicted structures are overlaid with CircleCompare (Fig. 9). CircleCompare is only available with a text interface.

3 Notes

Currently, on average, 73 % of known base pairs are correctly predicted for RNA sequences shorter than 700 nucleotides [16]. Several factors limit the accuracy of free energy minimization method:

1. The nearest neighbor model in incomplete. Little is known about non-nearest neighbor effects [51, 52] and stabilities of modified nucleotides such as inosine and pseudouridine [13].

2. The thermodynamic parameters are imperfect. This is because of experimental errors, non-nearest neighbor effects that are neglected, and salt concentrations that are different from physiological conditions [13, 47].

3. There may be a kinetic influence on the folding. Riboswitches have two or more functional structures for a given sequence [53]. In addition, sequential folding during the transcription was reported to affect the final structure [54], although this may be less of a concern for in vivo folding [55].

4. Higher order interactions are ignored. Tertiary interactions [2] and cellular components in vivo [56] may impact RNA folding, which is neglected in computational prediction.

5. Pseudoknots are often not predicted, and the prediction accuracy is generally low if they are included.

Methods such as the partition function calculation and energy dot plot can complement the free energy minimization method. It is also recommended that multiple methods are used depending on the situation. For example, Fold, energy dot plot, partition function, and stochastic sampling could be run on a riboswitch RNA [57] to develop hypotheses about its different conformations. If homologous sequences are available, prediction algorithms of multiple sequences, such as Multilign [58] and TurboFold [59], are more accurate. Experimental data from chemical modifications, enzymatic mapping, and SHAPE are shown to improve prediction quality dramatically. The tools for these analyses are also included in RNAstructure, and their usages are described in subsequent chapters (Chapter 3 for using multiple homologous sequences and Chapter 10 for using experimental data).

Acknowledgement

This protocol was developed with the support of National Institutes of Health Grant R01GM076485 to D.H.M.

References

1. Aguirre-Hernandez R, Hoos H, Condon A (2007) Computational RNA secondary structure design: empirical complexity and improved methods. BMC Bioinformatics 8:34

2. Diamond JM, Turner DH, Mathews DH (2001) Thermodynamics of three-way multibranch loops in RNA. Biochemistry 40:6971–6981

3. Dirks RM, Lin M, Winfree E, Pierce NA (2004) Paradigms for computational nucleic acid design. Nucleic Acids Res 32:1392–1403

4. Washietl S, Hofacker IL, Stadler PF (2005) Fast and reliable prediction of noncoding RNAs. Proc Natl Acad Sci U S A 102:2454–2459

5. Gorodkin J, Hofacker IL, Torarinsson E, Yao Z, Havgaard JH, Ruzzo WL (2010) De novo prediction of structured RNAs from genomic sequences. Trends Biotechnol 28:9–19

6. Uzilov AV, Keegan JM, Mathews DH (2006) Detection of non-coding RNAs on the basis of

predicted secondary structure formation free energy change. BMC Bioinformatics 7:173

7. Li PTX, Bustamante C, Tinoco I (2007) Real-time control of the energy landscape by force directs the folding of RNA molecules. Proc Natl Acad Sci U S A 104:7039–7044

8. Long D, Lee R, Williams P, Chan CY, Ambros V, Ding Y (2007) Potent effect of target structure on microRNA function. Nat Struct Mol Biol 14:287–294

9. Lu ZJ, Mathews DH (2008) Efficient siRNA selection using hybridization thermodynamics. Nucleic Acids Res 36:640–647

10. Tafer H, Ameres SL, Obernosterer G, Gebeshuber CA, Schroeder R, Martinez J, Hofacker IL (2008) The impact of target site accessibility on the design of effective siRNAs. Nat Biotechnol 26:578–583

11. Reuter JS, Mathews DH (2010) RNAstructure: software for RNA secondary structure prediction and analysis. BMC Bioinformatics 11:129

12. James BD, Olsen GJ, Pace NR (1989) Phylogenetic comparative analysis of RNA secondary structure. Methods Enzymol 180:227–239

13. Mathews DH, Turner D (2006) Prediction of RNA secondary structure by free energy minimization. Curr Opin Struct Biol 16:270–278

14. Mathews DH, Sabina J, Zuker M, Turner DH (1999) Expanded sequence dependence of thermodynamic parameters improves prediction of RNA secondary structure. J Mol Biol 288:911–940

15. Xia T, SantaLucia J, Burkard ME, Kierzek R, Schroeder SJ, Jiao X, Cox C, Turner DH (1998) Thermodynamic parameters for an expanded nearest-neighbor model for formation of RNA duplexes with Watson-Crick base pairs. Biochemistry 37:14719–14735

16. Mathews DH, Disney MD, Childs JL, Schroeder SJ, Zuker M, Turner DH (2004) Incorporating chemical modification constraints into a dynamic programming algorithm for prediction of RNA secondary structure. Proc Natl Acad Sci U S A 101:7287–7292

17. Andronescu M, Condon A, Hoos HH, Mathews DH, Murphy KP (2010) Computational approaches for RNA energy parameter estimation. RNA 16:2304–2318

18. Gardner DP, Ren P, Ozer S, Gutell RR (2011) Statistical potentials for hairpin and internal loops improve the accuracy of the predicted RNA structure. J Mol Biol 413:473–483

19. Do CB, Woods DA, Batzoglou S (2006) CONTRAfold: RNA secondary structure prediction without physics-based models. Bioinformatics 22:e90–e98

20. Eddy SR (2004) How do RNA folding algorithms work? Nat Biotechnol 22:1457–1458

21. Mathews DH (2006) Revolutions in RNA secondary structure prediction. J Mol Biol 359:526–532

22. Wuchty S, Fontana W, Hofacker IL, Schuster P (1999) Complete suboptimal folding of RNA and the stability of secondary structures. Biopolymers 49:145–165

23. Zuker M (1989) On finding all suboptimal foldings of an RNA molecule. Science 244:48–52

24. Steger G, Hofmann H, Förtsch J, Gross HJ, Randles JW, Sänger HL, Riesner D (1984) Conformational transitions in viroids and virusoids: comparison of results from energy minimization algorithm and from experimental data. J Biomol Struct Dyn 2:543–571

25. McCaskill JS (1990) The equilibrium partition function and base pair binding probabilities for RNA secondary structure. Biopolymers 29:1105–1119

26. Mathews DH (2004) Using an RNA secondary structure partition function to determine confidence in base pairs predicted by free energy minimization. RNA 10:1178–1190

27. Ding Y, Lawrence CE (2003) A statistical sampling algorithm for RNA secondary structure prediction. Nucleic Acids Res 31:7280–7301

28. Ding Y, Chan CY, Lawrence CE (2005) RNA secondary structure prediction by centroids in a Boltzmann weighted ensemble. RNA 11:1157–1166

29. Ding Y, Chan CY, Lawrence CE (2004) Sfold web server for statistical folding and rational design of nucleic acids. Nucleic Acids Res 32:W135–W141

30. Lu ZJ, Gloor JW, Mathews DH (2009) Improved RNA secondary structure prediction by maximizing expected pair accuracy. RNA 15:1805–1813

31. Staple DW, Butcher SE (2005) Pseudoknots: RNA structures with diverse functions. PLoS Biol 3:e213

32. Liu B, Mathews DH, Turner DH (2010) RNA pseudoknots: folding and finding. F1000 Biol Rep 2:8

33. Chen J-L, Greider CW (2005) Functional analysis of the pseudoknot structure in human telomerase RNA. Proc Natl Acad Sci U S A 102:8080–8085

34. Mihalusova M, Wu JY, Zhuang X (2011) Functional importance of telomerase pseudoknot revealed by single-molecule analysis. Proc Natl Acad Sci U S A 108:20339–20344

35. Wadkins TS, Perrotta AT, Ferré-D'Amaré AR, Doudna JA, Been MD (1999) A nested double pseudoknot is required for self-cleavage activity of both the genomic and antigenomic hepatitis delta virus ribozymes. RNA 5:720–727

36. Lyngsø RB, Pedersen CN (2000) RNA pseudoknot prediction in energy-based models. J Comput Biol 7:409–427

37. Rivas E, Eddy SR (1999) A dynamic programming algorithm for RNA structure prediction including pseudoknots. J Mol Biol 285:2053–2068

38. Reeder J, Giegerich R (2004) Design, implementation and evaluation of a practical pseudoknot folding algorithm based on thermodynamics. BMC Bioinformatics 5:104

39. Dirks RM, Pierce NA (2003) A partition function algorithm for nucleic acid secondary structure including pseudoknots. J Comput Chem 24:1664–1677

40. Bellaousov S, Mathews DH (2010) ProbKnot: fast prediction of RNA secondary structure including pseudoknots. RNA 16:1870–1880

41. Chen X, He S-M, Bu D, Zhang F, Wang Z, Chen R, Gao W (2008) FlexStem: improving predictions of RNA secondary structures with pseudoknots by reducing the search space. Bioinformatics 24:1994–2001

42. Sato K, Kato Y, Hamada M, Akutsu T, Asai K (2011) IPknot: fast and accurate prediction of RNA secondary structures with pseudoknots using integer programming. Bioinformatics 27:i85–i93

43. Ruan J, Stormo GD, Zhang W (2004) An iterated loop matching approach to the prediction of RNA secondary structures with pseudoknots. Bioinformatics 20:58–66

44. Ren J, Rastegari B, Condon A, Hoos HH (2005) HotKnots: Heuristic prediction of RNA secondary structures including pseudoknots. RNA 11:1494–1504

45. Bon M, Orland H (2011) TT2NE: a novel algorithm to predict RNA secondary structures with pseudoknots. Nucleic Acids Res 39:e93

46. Zhao J, Malmberg RL, Cai L (2007) Rapid ab initio prediction of RNA pseudoknots via graph tree decomposition. J Math Biol 56:145–159

47. Lu ZJ, Turner DH, Mathews DH (2006) A set of nearest neighbor parameters for predicting the enthalpy change of RNA secondary structure formation. Nucleic Acids Res 34:4912–4924

48. Halvorsen M, Martin JS, Broadaway S, Laederach A (2010) Disease-associated mutations that alter the RNA structural ensemble. PLoS Genet 6:e1001074

49. Sperschneider J, Datta A (2010) DotKnot: pseudoknot prediction using the probability dot plot under a refined energy model. Nucleic Acids Res 38:e103

50. Zuker M, Jacobson AB (1998) Using reliability information to annotate RNA secondary structures. RNA 4:669–679

51. Theimer CA, Wang Y, Hoffman DW, Krisch HM, Giedroc DP (1998) Non-nearest neighbor effects on the thermodynamics of unfolding of a model mRNA pseudoknot. J Mol Biol 279:545–564

52. Blose JM, Manni ML, Klapec KA, Stranger-Jones Y, Zyra AC, Sim V, Griffith CA, Long JD, Serra MJ (2007) Non-nearest-neighbor dependence of the stability for RNA bulge loops based on the complete set of group I single-nucleotide bulge loops. Biochemistry 46:15123–15135

53. Tucker BJ, Breaker RR (2005) Riboswitches as versatile gene control elements. Curr Opin Struct Biol 15:342–348

54. Heilman-Miller SL, Woodson SA (2003) Effect of transcription on folding of the Tetrahymena ribozyme. RNA 9:722–733

55. Mahen EM, Harger JW, Calderon EM, Fedor MJ (2005) Kinetics and thermodynamics make different contributions to RNA folding in vitro and in yeast. Mol Cell 19:27–37

56. Stone MD, Mihalusova M, O'Connor CM, Prathapam R, Collins K, Zhuang X (2007) Stepwise protein-mediated RNA folding directs assembly of telomerase ribonucleoprotein. Nature 446:458–461

57. Mandal M, Breaker RR (2004) Gene regulation by riboswitches. Nat Rev Mol Cell Biol 5:451–463

58. Xu Z, Mathews DH (2011) Multilign: an algorithm to predict secondary structures conserved in multiple RNA sequences. Bioinformatics 27:626–632

59. Harmanci AO, Sharma G, Mathews DH (2011) TurboFold: iterative probabilistic estimation of secondary structures for multiple RNA sequences. BMC Bioinformatics 12:108

Chapter 3

Prediction of Secondary Structures Conserved in Multiple RNA Sequences

Zhenjiang Zech Xu and David H. Mathews

Abstract

RNA structure is conserved by evolution to a greater extent than sequence. Predicting the conserved structure for multiple homologous sequences can be much more accurate than predicting the structure for a single sequence. RNAstructure is a software package that includes the programs Dynalign, Multilign, TurboFold, and PARTS for predicting conserved RNA secondary structure. This chapter provides protocols for using these programs.

Key words RNA structure prediction, RNA homology, Comparative sequence analysis

1 Introduction

RNA secondary structure forms much faster and is more stable than tertiary structure, thus providing important scaffolds and constraints for tertiary structure. Although homologous RNA molecules vary in sequence across species, their conserved function requires them to fold into a common structure. The nucleotides base paired with each other usually covary in evolution in order to preserve the structure. For example, a GC base pair in one sequence is replaced by a homologous AU pair in another sequence. Comparative sequence analysis employs this information, called compensating base pair changes, in multiple homologous sequences to infer the consensus secondary structure [1, 2]. Currently it is the most reliable method to predict RNA secondary structure, with 97 % accuracy as demonstrated by crystal structures of ribosomal RNAs [3]. But it requires large sets of homologous sequences, special expertise, and intensive labor [2].

As explained in Chapter 2, secondary structure prediction for a single RNA sequence is limited in accuracy because of the imperfect nearest neighbor model, higher-order molecular interactions, and kinetic effects. It is well known that the prediction of consensus

Douglas H. Turner and David H. Mathews (eds.), *RNA Structure Determination: Methods and Protocols*, Methods in Molecular Biology, vol. 1490, DOI 10.1007/978-1-4939-6433-8_3, © Springer Science+Business Media New York 2016

structures conserved in multiple homologous RNA sequences is much more accurate, although it tends to take more computer time and memory than single sequence structure prediction. Many algorithms combine free energy minimization with detection of base pair covariation to automate the process of comparative sequence analysis. Some require a fixed alignment as input [4–6], which is usually determined by sequence pattern matching. While methods that require an input alignment predict reliable secondary structures fast, their accuracy is restricted by the quality of the initial sequence alignment, which may be confounded by compensating base pair changes.

Another type of algorithm folds and aligns sequences simultaneously. Generally they are more robust since they are not constrained by an initial alignment. Sankoff first reported such an algorithm to predict consensus structures of lowest free energy for multiple homologous RNA sequences [7]. This algorithm is implemented in several programs, such as Dynalign [8] and Foldalign [9], to predict secondary structures for a pair of sequences. They can be accurate for structure prediction for RNA sequences with low pairwise sequence identity because they optimize the common structure prediction and alignment simultaneously.

Dynalign is a component of the RNAstructure package. It uses the latest nearest neighbor rules for estimating the folding free energy change. Its prediction accuracy is greatly improved upon single sequence free energy minimization methods [8]. It is also extended to predict suboptimal structures common to two sequences. Experimental constraints from chemical modification and enzymatic cleavage can also be imposed as constraints in Dynalign structure prediction [10]. Two pre-filtering steps are implemented to improve the computation efficiency of Dynalign by restricting the space of solutions that Dynalign needs to consider. One is to only allow base pairs that appear in the near-optimal secondary structures in single sequence free energy minimization prediction [11]. The other constrains the alignment space with a probabilistic alignment using a Hidden Markov Model [12].

Including more homologous sequences in prediction should improve structure prediction accuracy because more compensating base pair changes are available. Generalizing Sankoff's algorithm to over two sequences, however, is too computationally prohibitive for most sequences of interest; its computation requirement of time and memory increases exponentially to the number of sequences ($O(N^{3S})$ in time and $O(N^{2S})$) in memory for S sequences of length N. In fact, an X-Dynalign was reported to fold and align three sequences [13]. It improves predictions but is extremely computationally demanding even for sequences as short as 5S rRNA, which are about 150 nucleotides long.

A popular solution to the problem of including more than two sequences is to construct structures and alignments progressively based on the pairwise predictions. Another attempt to extend Dynalign takes this approach with a profile alignment algorithm to find common base pairs in all the input sequences. Its prediction, however, depends highly on the quality of the guide tree that is used to guide the progressive alignment [14]. Also based on Dynalign, the Multilign algorithm implemented in RNAstructure predicts secondary structures conserved in three or more sequences [15]. It uses multiple Dynalign calculations to progressively construct conserved structures with one sequence used in all Dynalign calculations. It improves upon Dynalign prediction by only allowing base pairs existing in suboptimal secondary structures across all of the progressive Dynalign calculations. It is especially powerful for some sequences where Dynalign performs poorly. Multilign scales linearly to the number of sequences in time and scales the same with Dynalign in memory.

Instead of trying to predict structure and alignment simultaneously, some algorithms calculate base pair probabilities for each individual sequence (*see* partition function calculations in Chapter 2 of this volume) and then match sequences via sequence and base pair alignment to predict their common secondary structure. There are several programs implemented to align two base pair probability matrices to search for the maximum weight common structures and their associated alignment [16–18]. These methods are applied to more than two sequences by progressively constructing a multiple sequence alignment.

An RNAstructure module, PARTS (*P*robabilistic *A*lignment for *R*NA join*T* *S*econdary structure prediction), is also an algorithm that uses base pair probabilities and alignment probabilities to predict alignment and secondary structures for two sequences [19]. It uses a probabilistic model with pseudo free energies calculated from base pairing and alignment probabilities that are pre-computed independently. It uses a generalized alignment concept, called a matched helical region, to treat a base pair of one sequence as inserted or aligned to unpaired nucleotides or paired nucleotides in the other sequence. This generalization confers PARTS the advantage to correctly handle diversity in the helical branches among homologous sequences. It was shown PARTS performs significantly better in both alignment and structure prediction than other benchmarked methods over RNA families with structural diversity, such as RNase P RNA.

Another RNAstructure module, TurboFold, is also a method capable of RNA secondary structure prediction for two or more sequences [20]. TurboFold takes a set of homologous RNA sequences as input and computes the base pairing probabilities for each sequence. The pairing probabilities for each sequence are calculated with the partition function for the sequence itself and updated information derived from the partition function calculations for the other sequences, called extrinsic information. The extrinsic information from each of the other sequences is applied as a pseudo free energy change by mapping its base pairing probabilities to the current sequence through alignment probabilities predicted with a Hidden Markov Model between sequences. The updated base pairing probabilities are then used to recompute extrinsic information, resulting in an iterative procedure. The calculated base pairing probabilities can be used to assemble secondary structures by either thresholding the probabilities or maximizing expected accuracy. Evaluation showed it performs favorably to other methods in accuracy with less computational and memory requirements.

Another class of prediction methods is based on probabilistic sampling using the partition function calculation. This category includes RNA Sampler [21], RNAG [22], and MASTR [23]. RNAshapes [24] provides another unique algorithm to predict abstract shapes of RNA structures and search for the best common shape for all the sequences.

All the methods introduced so far are unable to predict pseudoknotted secondary structures. Pseudoknot prediction is already difficult and computationally intensive for a single sequence, let alone the prediction of a conserved pseudoknot in multiple sequences. Several programs, however, are able to take a multiple-sequence alignment and predict secondary structures that may contain pseudoknots [25–27]. As the non-pseudoknot predicting methods that take alignments as input, they are also highly dependent on the quality of the input alignment. The inaccuracies caused by sequence alignment prediction may make them even worse in accuracy than single sequence pseudoknot prediction methods [28]. To our knowledge, there are two algorithms that are able to predict pseudoknotted structures for multiple unaligned sequences. SimulFold [29] uses a Monte Carlo method to sample from the joint distribution of RNA secondary structures, multiple-sequence alignments and evolutionary trees in a Bayesian framework. The other method, TurboKnot [28], which is implemented in RNAstructure, combines the ProbKnot [30] algorithm with TurboFold [20]. It assembles secondary structure in the same manner as ProbKnot by forming base pairs of nucleotide pairs with mutually maximal pairing probability, where the base pair probabilities are calculated by TurboFold. It retains the high prediction accuracy of TurboFold and predicts more correct pseudoknotted base pairs with fewer false positives than ProbKnot, especially for transfer-messenger RNA (tmRNA) sequences. Nonetheless, even with the comparative information from multiple sequences, the pseudoknot prediction methods are all still relatively poor in accuracy, missing many true pseudoknotted base pairs and predicting many false positives.

This chapter provides a practical guide for using the RNAstructure package to facilitate prediction of RNA secondary structure conserved in multiple homologous sequences. The merits of the tools are also explained for users to choose the appropriate one for their real problems. The performance of the prediction methods are benchmarked by comparing the predicted structures to reference secondary structures derived from comparative sequence analysis [2]. Their accuracies are measured with two statistics—sensitivity and positive predictive value (PPV) [31]. Sensitivity is the percentage of true base pairs that are predicted and PPV is the percentage of predicted base pairs that are in the reference structure. Benchmarks demonstrate that the prediction accuracies of the methods in RNAstructure are among the best. The download and installation of the RNAstructure package is described in detail in Chapter 2. The help page, with additional installation information, is available at http://rna.urmc.rochester.edu/RNAstructureHelp.html.

2 Protocols

2.1 Dynalign: Predict Consensus Structures of a Pair of Sequences and Its Associated Alignment

Dynalign is a module in RNAstructure to predict consensus secondary structures for two RNA sequences. It implements Sankoff's simultaneous fold and align algorithm using the nearest neighbor model for folding thermodynamics. It minimizes the total free energy:

$$\Delta G_{total} = \Delta G_1 + \Delta G_2 + \Delta G_{gap} \times n \tag{1}$$

where ΔG°_1 and ΔG°_2 are the free energy changes of the consensus structures for the two sequences, respectively, ΔG°_{gap} is the gap penalty in the form of pseudo free energy, and n is the total number of gaps in the pairwise alignment. Dynalign improves prediction accuracy compared to single sequence prediction methods [8]. Compared with other multiple structure prediction methods that separate structure and alignment predictions, it performs better on sequences with low identity. Besides the serial program, Dynalign has a parallel version, which can take the advantage of multiple CPU cores to accelerate the calculation.

The module is available in the graphical user interface under "RNA" → "RNA Dynalign". The input window pops up as shown in Fig. 1. Users click "Sequence File 1" and "Sequence File 2" to specify the two input sequence files in SEQ format (refer to the previous chapter for SEQ and CT formats). Default output file names to store predicted structures are then generated, but the file names and save directories can be changed by clicking the "CT File 1" and "CT File 2" buttons. An alignment file name is also automatically entered and can be changed by clicking "Alignment File".

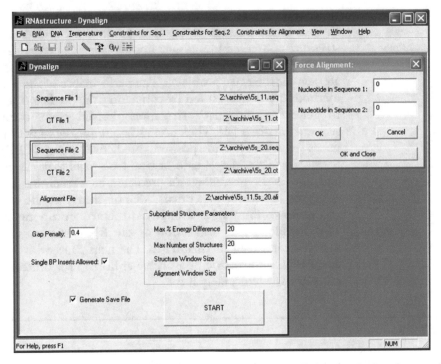

Fig. 1 The user interface window for the Dynalign module, used to specify input, output, and parameters

After specifying the input and output files, users can set the following parameters to achieve best prediction result:

1. Gap penalty. Gaps are locations in a sequence alignment where a nucleotide in one sequence has no matching nucleotide in the other. Users can customize the penalty per gapped nucleotide in "Gap Penalty" box. The default value is 0.4 in the unit of kcal/mol/gap, and this provides the best average performance.

2. Single base pair insertion. Dynalign allows the insertion of a single base pair between two conserved base pairs. Generally, allowing single base pair insertions improves prediction accuracy. Users can uncheck "Single BP inserts allowed" box to prohibit it.

3. Dynalign save file. A Dynalign save file stores the predicted energy information for every possible alignment and structure of the two sequences. It is needed to make Dynalign energy dot plots. Users can uncheck "Generate Save File" to not create the Dynalign Save file.

4. Parameters to control the prediction of suboptimal structures. Dynalign was extended to predict a set of low free energy structures to provide alternative hypotheses in addition to the lowest free energy structures. There are several parameters to tune the prediction: (1) "Max % Energy Difference" sets the maximum increment in percentage above the computed lowest

free energy. Only the predicted structures with free energies falling into this interval are output. (2) "Max Number of Structures" defines the maximum number of structures that can be generated. (3) "Structure Window Size" and "Alignment Window Size" control how different the suboptimal structures must be from each other. The minimum values are 0, and the suboptimal structures and alignments are required to be more different from each other as larger values are used.

After the Dynalign input window pops up, several new menus appear, including "Temperature", "Constraints for Sequence 1", "Constraints for Sequence 2", and "Constraints for Alignment". "Temperature" allows users to specify the temperature at which the RNA folding occurs. Temperature changes should be used with caution. The enthalpy parameters for predicting free energy changes at temperatures other than 37 °C are prone to significant errors outside the range of about 20–50 °C. Note that the change in temperature applies only to a single calculation. Subsequent predictions will return to the default of 37 °C. Constraints from experimental data or other knowledge can be specified under menu "Constraints for Sequence 1" and "Constraints for Sequence 2" (described in detail in Chapter 10). User can also force nucleotides of the input sequences to be aligned by clicking "Constraints for Alignment" → "Force Alignment". Then the indices of the two nucleotides to be aligned are entered. Users can press "OK" to force the alignment of additional nucleotides or press "OK and close" to finish inputting. The inputted alignment constraints can be saved to disk for future usage by clicking "Constraints for Alignment" → "Save Alignment". Users can review the alignment constraints to make sure there are no errors by clicking "Constraints for Alignment" → "Show Current Alignment Constraints".

After setting the parameters and constraints, users click "Start" to run the prediction and a progress bar will show the progress of the calculation. When the calculation is done, users are asked whether to draw the predicted structures using the drawing module. On the drawing (Fig. 2), the shown energy values are the ΔG°_{total} in Eq. (1) rather than the predicted energy change of the structures, which can be calculated with the Efn2 module under the "RNA" menu (*see* Efn2 in Chapter 2). All pairs of predicted common structures are stored in the CT files in ascending order of their ΔG°_{total}. By default the first structure, the predicted lowest free energy common structure, is drawn. User can choose to draw alternative structures by clicking "Draw" → "Goto Structure Number" or by pressing ctrl + up/down arrows. The drawings can be zoomed in or out with ctrl + right/left arrows or by clicking "Zoom" under "Draw" menu. The structure can be output to a helix file by clicking "Draw" → "Write Helix File". The helix file can be used by XRNA for creating publication-quality figures (http://rna.ucsc.edu/rnacenter/xrna/xrna.html).

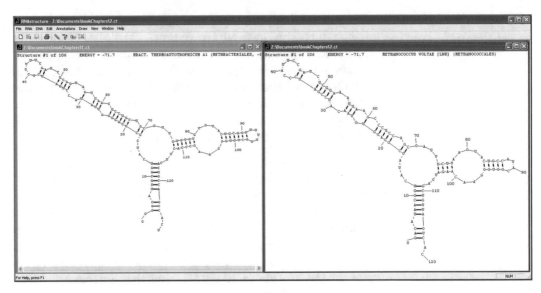

Fig. 2 The Dynalign-predicted structures for two 5S rRNA from *Methanobacterium thermoautotrophicum A1* and *Methanococcus voltae [lnk]*, respectively. The prediction accuracies are 0.94 sensitivity and 0.80 PPV for the first sequence, and 0.91 sensitivity and 0.81 PPV for the second sequence, while the accuracies of Fold, the single sequence free energy minimization method in RNAstructure is 0.91 sensitivity and 0.73 PPV for the first sequence, and 0.82 sensitivity and 0.69 PPV for the second sequence

The common secondary structures can also be predicted from the Dynalign Save file by clicking "File" → "Refold from Dynalign Save File". Because the save file contains energy information, only the step of trace back in the dynamic programming algorithm is needed to generate structures. Thus it is much faster than the prediction from scratch. Refolding is useful if a different set of suboptimal structures is needed than for the original structure prediction.

The Dynalign save file can also be used to draw Dynalign energy dot plots with the dotplot module by clicking "File" → "DotPlot Dynalign". Dynalign energy dot plots are analogous to the dot plots produced by secondary structure prediction of single sequences described in Chapter 2. They are originally 4-dimensional plots because they contain information of a base pair (i-j) in one sequence aligned to the possible base pair (k-l) in the other sequence. They are then projected into two dimensions to display all base pairs for each sequence in a separate dot plot as shown in Fig. 3. The dots in a plot represent all possible base pairs predicted between the nucleotides i on the x axis and j on the y axis in one sequence. The color indicates the $\Delta G°_{total}$ of the lowest free energy common structures that are predicted to contain that pair. The legend shows the folding free energy ranges associated with each color. The plot provides information about all alternative secondary structures. The emptiness of the dot plot indicates how well defined the RNA structure is. The color patterns, such as the line composed of red dots in Fig. 3, reveal possible helices that can form in low free energy structures. Although the algorithm cannot

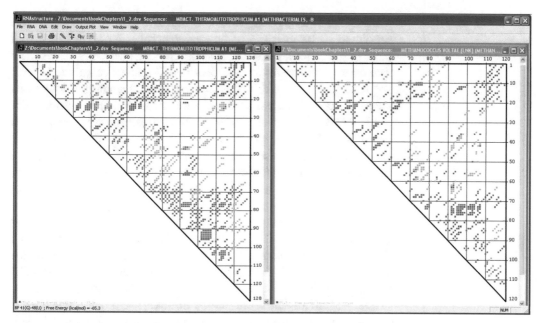

Fig. 3 Dynalign-predicted energy dot plot for two 5S rRNA from *Methanobacterium thermoautotrophicum* A1 and *Methanococcus voltae* [lnk], respectively. Each dot indicates a base pair between the nucleotides indexed on horizontal and vertical axes. Each dot is color annotated according to the total free energy of the optimal structure containing this base pair in the sequence that is either inserted or aligned to any possible base pair in the other sequences. The color legend is shown in *bottom left corner*, which can be zoomed in with ctrl + right arrow. The nucleotide indices and identity and lowest total free energy involving the base pair can be shown in the bottom status bar by clicking a dot in the dot plot

predict pseudoknots, the well-defined regions and color patterns in the dot plot that are absent in minimum free energy structures may imply potential pseudoknotted motifs. The Dynalign dot plots are usually much cleaner and better defined than single sequence dot plots because many possible base pairs from each single sequence cannot be aligned to a pair in the other sequence. The appearance of the dot plot can be modified using the "Draw" menu options. It is often useful, for example, to restrict the range of energies shown on the plot by choosing "Plot Range" under "Draw". By default, all possible pairs are shown before the plot range is changed.

2.2 Multilign: Predict Consensus Structures of Multiple Sequences and Associated Alignments

Multilign predicts structures and alignments based on multiple progressive Dynalign calculations [15]. For a given set of input sequences, Multilign chooses the first as an index sequence and compares it with each of the other sequences with Dynalign. The current Dynalign calculation is templated according to information from the previous Dynalign calculation. Specifically, a base pair in the index sequences is allowed in the current Dynalign calculation only if it is predicted to be in the low free energy common structures in the prior Dynalign calculations. The idea behind this progressive Multilign algorithm is that the genuine base pairs are predicted to be in low free energy structures by Dynalign for all pairs of sequences, while the false competing base pairs exist in low free energy structures in one or a few Dynalign calculations with sequence pairs. Thus this style of progressive Dynalign calculations keeps genuine base pairs in the prediction while preventing false ones. Thus, if there are more than two homologous sequences available, Multilign predicts structures more accurately than Dynalign, especially for some occasional cases where Dynalign performs poorly. Because Multilign uses Dynalign internally, it is able to take the advantage of the parallelized Dynalign to accelerate predictions on computers with multiple compute cores.

The Multilign module is started in the graphical interface by clicking "RNA"→"RNA Multilign". Users must provide sequence files and their corresponding output CT files by clicking "Sequence File" and "CT File" as shown in Fig. 4. The pairs of sequence/CT file names will then be listed in the box on the right after clicking "ADD -->". If any file is entered by mistake, it can be removed from the list by specifying its index number and clicking "Delete Sequence". Generally, Multilign prediction accuracy is independent of the choice of index sequence and the order of the Dynalign calculations. Other parameters, however, could have a large impact on Multilign prediction accuracy and can be tuned in the interface

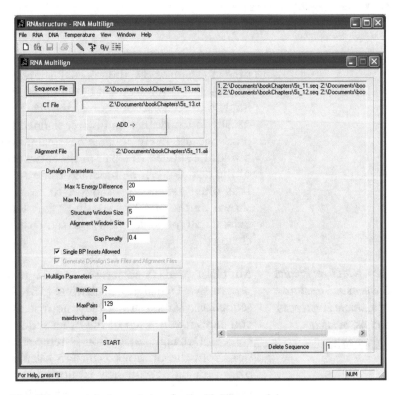

Fig. 4 The user interface window for the Multilign module

window. "Iterations" is the number of cycles the index sequence compared with the other sequences. Usually the first few Dynalign calculations are not well improved because not many false base pairs are removed yet. Thus a second iteration is helpful and the default iteration number is set to 2. "MaxPairs" and "maxdsvchange" are parameters used to exclude as many as possible false base pairs from prediction while allowing true base pairs. "MaxPairs" defines the number of base pairs to be allowed. "maxdsvchange" defines a percentage. The base pairs in the index sequence will be allowed if they are predicted into common structures with the ΔG°_{total} less than "maxdsvchange" percent above the minimum ΔG°_{total}. At each Dynalign step, base pairs for the index sequence are allowed with free energy above the minimum free energy defined by "maxdsvchange", up to a maximum number of pairs equal to "MaxPairs". These two parameters are key to prediction accuracy. Setting them to small values risks excluding true base pairs while setting them to large values might not exclude false pairs effectively. Their default values provide best average performance.

Multilign outputs predicted secondary structure during the last iteration of Dynalign calculations. Thus Dynalign parameters also impact the final prediction result. Users are able to adjust those parameters in the box named "Dynalign Parameters". Users are also free to change the temperature of the prediction by clicking the "Temperature" menu. All these are the same as Dynalign and explained in the previous section.

The prediction is initiated by clicking "START". A progress bar will show the progress. The predicted structures can be drawn with draw module in RNAstructure. The subsequent manipulations are exactly the same as those described in the previous section.

2.3 TurboFold: Predict Structures of Multiple Sequences

TurboFold is an iterative method that takes multiple sequences as input and outputs estimates of base pair probabilities [20]. For a given sequence in the input, the base pair probabilities are initially predicted by a partition function calculation. The pair probabilities are then refined using pair probabilities estimated by all other sequences in a way that conserved pairs become more likely. To map the base pair probabilities from other sequences, pairwise probabilistic alignment between two sequences is used. This refinement step can be iterated to update base pair probabilities multiple times. The concept of this iterative update used in TurboFold is analogous to iterative error-correction coding methods in digital communications [32], specifically Turbo decoding, in the sense that homologous sequences "encode" a common secondary structure with some noise [33]. With base pair probabilities calculated, TurboFold can predict secondary structures for each sequence in three ways. One is to assemble structures with base pairs that have pairing probabilities larger than a threshold. The second is to use the Maximum Expected Accuracy (MEA) algorithm to search for structures that maximize the expected base pair accuracy [34, 35].

The third is to use the ProbKnot approach [28], which is capable of predicting pseudoknotted base pairs. In the ProbKnot approach, pairs are made between nucleotides that are mutually the most probable pairing partner.

The advantage of TurboFold, as compared to most other approaches that predict conserved structure, is that it does not enforce strict commonality of structures and is therefore useful for homologous sequences with diverse structures. Unlike Multilign, however, it does not output sequence alignments.

TurboFold has a similar user interface to Multilign (Fig. 5). Users specify the input and output file names in the same way as for Multilign; by choosing one sequence at a time and clicking the "ADD -->" button to add the sequence to the list on the right. One difference is that at least three sequences must be inputted for TurboFold to run. The "Maximum Expected Accuracy" mode, the "ProbKnot/TurboKnot" mode, or the "Probability Threshold" mode must be chosen. The default, "Maximum Expected Accuracy" is the best choice for most users, although "ProbKnot/TurboKnot" is an important alternative if a pseudoknot is expected. There are different sets of parameters for the three modes. For Maximum Expected Accuracy mode, "Max % Energy Difference", "Max Number of Structures", and "Structure Window Size" have the same meaning as their corresponding parameters in the Dynalign module described in

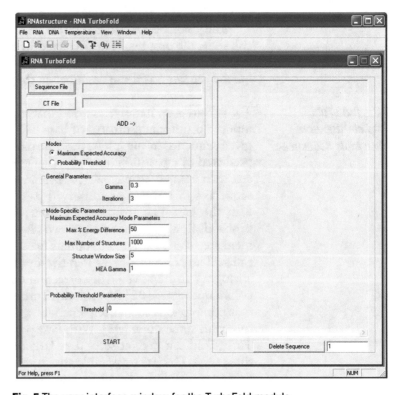

Fig. 5 The user interface window for the TurboFold module

the previous section. "MEA Gamma" is a scaling factor that balances the number of unpaired and paired nucleotides in the predicted structure, and thus provides a trade-off between sensitivity and PPV of the prediction. Larger gamma will result in more base pairs, higher sensitivity and lower PPV. The default value of 1 is best for most users. For the ProbKnot/TurboKnot mode, the number of iterations and the minimum helix length can be chosen. Increasing the number of iterations above 1 can result in more pairs, although the average accuracy of the pairs will be reduced. Additional iterations reconsider whether additional nucleotides are mutually the maximum probability pairing partner after the nucleotides in prior iterations are ignored. The minimum helix length ensures that short helices, which are empirically found to often be incorrect predictions, are not allowed. The default length of 3 is best on average. For Probability Threshold mode, there is only one parameter, "Threshold". It sets a cutoff value and only base pairs with estimated pairing probabilities larger than the cutoff are included in the structure prediction. Increasing the threshold improves PPV at the cost of sensitivity, and the minimum value is 0.5. There are also two parameters common to both modes, "Gamma" and "Iterations". "Gamma" defines the relative contributions of information from each sequence on its own structure prediction and those from other sequences. "Gamma" has a default of 0.3, and setting it larger will result in more consistent structures across all sequences. The default value provides a good balance between finding the common structure, but also allowing for base pairs that are specific to a single sequence. "Iterations" defines how many times the base pair probabilities will be refined. The default value of 3 works well for most calculations. The temperature at which structures are predicted is set by clicking "Temperature" menu.

The TurboFold calculation is run by clicking "START" and then a progress bar appears. The structure visualization and annotation are the same as those explained in Dynalign.

2.4 PARTS

PARTS is a module that predicts secondary structure and alignment for two sequences [19]. It generalizes Sankoff's structure and alignment model to allow base pair insertions anywhere in matched helical regions. It also allows the alignment of paired nucleotides in one sequence to either paired or unpaired nucleotides in the other. Combining this advanced alignment model with base pair probabilities calculated from the single sequence partition function, PARTS devised a pseudo free energy scoring function to predict the most probable structural alignment for the two sequences. It is shown that PARTS performs significantly better than Dynalign in alignments. As it handles structural alignment in a sophisticated way and relaxes the commonality imposed on consensus structure prediction, it improves structure prediction accuracy especially for sequence families with diverse structures, such as RNase P.

Besides predicting the lowest pseudo free energy structures, PARTS can compute the pseudo Boltzmann partition function and then the probabilities for all possible structures. Thus PARTS is able to probabilistically sample the ensemble for structures according to their probabilities. PARTS can also estimate the probability of a base pair by summarizing the probabilities of all the structures that contain that pair. With base pair probabilities, PARTS can set a probability threshold and use only base pairs that have larger probabilities to assemble secondary structures.

PARTS is only available with a command-line interface. The input configuration file for PARTS is explained on the online help page: http://rna.urmc.rochester.edu/Text/PARTS.html.

3 Notes

All the modules described above have command-line interfaces for Windows, GNU/Linux, and Mac OS X platforms. The command-line versions have the same sets of parameters as the graphical interface versions, and thus, the output is identical.

While RNAstructure depends on the nearest neighbor model for folding free energy changes and on dynamic programming algorithms, there are many alternative methods. Some use a probabilistic framework called a stochastic context-free grammar (SCFG) instead of nearest neighbor parameters to model RNA structures [36–38]. Other methods take a more generalized conditional log-linear model and can then use a more feature-rich scoring scheme [35, 39]. Another type of method combines the nearest neighbor model with a genetic algorithm rather than a dynamic programming algorithm [40]. It is not guaranteed to find the most stable secondary structure.

Although significant effort has been made to improve RNA secondary structure prediction accuracy for conserved structure, the accuracy is still not as good as manual comparative sequence analysis. This gap in performance is largest for RNA families that have great structural diversity, such as RNase P and SRP RNA. It remains a challenge to balance commonality and variation during the consensus structure prediction. The available methods, however, are generally more accurate than predictions made with a single sequence, and these methods are an excellent starting point for further manual refinement.

Acknowledgement

This protocol was developed with the support of National Institutes of Health Grant R01GM076485 to D.H.M.

References

1. James BD, Olsen GJ, Pace NR (1989) Phylogenetic comparative analysis of RNA secondary structure. Methods Enzymol 180:227–239

2. Cannone JJ, Subramanian S, Schnare MN, Collett JR, D'Souza LM, Du Y, Feng B, Lin N, Madabusi LV, Müller KM et al (2002) The Comparative RNA Web (CRW) Site: an online database of comparative sequence and structure information for ribosomal, intron, and other RNAs. BMC Bioinformatics 3:2

3. Gutell RR, Lee JC, Cannone JJ (2002) The accuracy of ribosomal RNA comparative structure models. Curr Opin Struct Biol 12:301–310

4. Bernhart SH, Hofacker IL, Will S, Gruber AR, Stadler PF (2008) RNAalifold: improved consensus structure prediction for RNA alignments. BMC Bioinformatics 9:474

5. Hofacker IL (2007) RNA consensus structure prediction with RNAalifold. Methods Mol Biol 395:527–544

6. Knight R, Birmingham A, Yarus M (2004) BayesFold: rational 2° folds that combine thermodynamic, covariation, and chemical data for aligned RNA sequences. RNA 10:1323–1336

7. Sankoff D (1985) Simultaneous solution of the RNA folding, alignment and protosequence problems. SIAM J Appl Math 45:810–825

8. Mathews DH, Turner DH (2002) Dynalign: an algorithm for finding the secondary structure common to two RNA sequences. J Mol Biol 317:191–203

9. Havgaard JH, Lyngso RB, Gorodkin J (2005) The FOLDALIGN web server for pairwise structural RNA alignment and mutual motif search. Nucleic Acids Res 33:W650–W653

10. Mathews DH (2005) Predicting a set of minimal free energy RNA secondary structures common to two sequences. Bioinformatics 21:2246–2253

11. Uzilov AV, Keegan JM, Mathews DH (2006) Detection of non-coding RNAs on the basis of predicted secondary structure formation free energy change. BMC Bioinformatics 7:173

12. Harmanci AO, Sharma G, Mathews DH (2007) Efficient pairwise RNA structure prediction using probabilistic alignment constraints in Dynalign. BMC Bioinformatics 8:130

13. Masoumi B, Turcotte M (2005) Simultaneous alignment and structure prediction of three RNA sequences. Int J Bioinform Res Appl 1:230–245

14. Bellamy-Royds AB, Turcotte M (2007) Can Clustal-style progressive pairwise alignment of multiple sequences be used in RNA secondary structure prediction? BMC Bioinformatics 8:190

15. Xu Z, Mathews DH (2011) Multilign: an algorithm to predict secondary structures conserved in multiple RNA sequences. Bioinformatics 27:626–632

16. Hofacker IL, Bernhart SHF, Stadler PF (2004) Alignment of RNA base pairing probability matrices. Bioinformatics 20:2222–2227

17. Will S, Reiche K, Hofacker IL, Stadler PF, Backofen R (2007) Inferring noncoding RNA families and classes by means of genome-scale structure-based clustering. PLoS Comput Biol 3:e65

18. Torarinsson E, Havgaard JH, Gorodkin J (2007) Multiple structural alignment and clustering of RNA sequences. Bioinformatics 23:926–932

19. Harmanci AO, Sharma G, Mathews DH (2008) PARTS: probabilistic alignment for RNA joinT secondary structure prediction. Nucleic Acids Res 36:2406

20. Harmanci AO, Sharma G, Mathews DH (2011) TurboFold: iterative probabilistic estimation of secondary structures for multiple RNA sequences. BMC Bioinformatics 12:108

21. Xu X, Ji Y, Stormo GD (2007) RNA Sampler: a new sampling based algorithm for common RNA secondary structure prediction and structural alignment. Bioinformatics 23:1883–1891

22. Wei D, Alpert LV, Lawrence CE (2011) RNAG: a new Gibbs sampler for predicting RNA secondary structure for unaligned sequences. Bioinformatics 27:2486–2493

23. Lindgreen S, Gardner PP, Krogh A (2007) MASTR: multiple alignment and structure prediction of non-coding RNAs using simulated annealing. Bioinformatics 23:3304–3311

24. Steffen P, Voss B, Rehmsmeier M, Reeder J, Giegerich R (2006) RNAshapes: an integrated RNA analysis package based on abstract shapes. Bioinformatics 22:500–503

25. Ruan J, Stormo GD, Zhang W (2004) An iterated loop matching approach to the prediction of RNA secondary structures with pseudoknots. Bioinformatics 20:58–66

26. Sato K, Kato Y, Hamada M, Akutsu T, Asai K (2011) IPknot: fast and accurate prediction of RNA secondary structures with pseudoknots using integer programming. Bioinformatics 27:i85–i93

27. Witwer C, Hofacker IL, Stadler PF (2004) Prediction of consensus RNA secondary

structures including pseudoknots. IEEE/ACM Trans Comput Biol Bioinform 1:66–77

28. Seetin MG, Mathews DH (2012) TurboKnot: rapid prediction of conserved RNA secondary structures including pseudoknots. Bioinformatics 28:792–798

29. Meyer IM, Miklós I (2007) SimulFold: simultaneously inferring RNA structures including pseudoknots, alignments, and trees using a Bayesian MCMC framework. PLoS Comput Biol 3:e149

30. Bellaousov S, Mathews DH (2010) ProbKnot: fast prediction of RNA secondary structure including pseudoknots. RNA 16:1870–1880

31. Mathews DH, Sabina J, Zuker M, Turner DH (1999) Expanded sequence dependence of thermodynamic parameters improves prediction of RNA secondary structure. J Mol Biol 288:911–940

32. Hagenauer J, Offer E, Papke L (2006) Iterative decoding of binary block and convolutional codes. IEEE Trans Inform Theory 42:429–445

33. Berrou C, Glavieux A, Thitimajshima P (1993) Near Shannon limit error-correcting coding and decoding: Turbo-codes. 1. Technical Program, Conference Record, IEEE International Conference on Communications, 1993. ICC 93. Geneva, vol 2, pp 1064–1070

34. Lu ZJ, Gloor JW, Mathews DH (2009) Improved RNA secondary structure prediction by maximizing expected pair accuracy. RNA 15:1805–1813

35. Do CB, Woods DA, Batzoglou S (2006) CONTRAfold: RNA secondary structure prediction without physics-based models. Bioinformatics 22:e90–e98

36. Knudsen B, Hein J (1999) RNA secondary structure prediction using stochastic context-free grammars and evolutionary history. Bioinformatics 15:446–454

37. Dowell R, Eddy S (2006) Efficient pairwise RNA structure prediction and alignment using sequence alignment constraints. BMC Bioinformatics 7:400

38. Dowell RD, Eddy SR (2004) Evaluation of several lightweight stochastic context-free grammars for RNA secondary structure prediction. BMC Bioinformatics 5:71

39. Do CB, Foo C-S, Batzoglou S (2008) A max-margin model for efficient simultaneous alignment and folding of RNA sequences. Bioinformatics 24:i68–i76

40. Chen J-H, Le S-Y, Maizel JV (2000) Prediction of common secondary structures of RNAs: a genetic algorithm approach. Nucleic Acids Res 28:991–999

Chapter 4

Predicting RNA–RNA Interactions Using RNAstructure

Laura DiChiacchio and David H. Mathews

Abstract

RNA–RNA binding is a required step for many regulatory and catalytic processes in the cell. Identifying RNA–RNA hybridization sites is challenging because of the competition between intramolecular and intermolecular structure formation. A complete picture of RNA–RNA binding includes an understanding of single-stranded folding and binding site accessibility, and is strongly concentration-dependent. This chapter provides guidance for using RNAstructure to predict RNA–RNA binding sites and RNA–RNA structures, utilizing free energy minimization and partition function calculations. RNAstructure is freely available at http://rna.urmc.rochester.edu/RNAstructure.html.

Key words RNA hybridization, RNA Duplex Formation, Bimolecular RNA structure

1 Introduction

RNA has been increasingly recognized as an active player in cellular metabolism, with roles in regulation of gene expression, posttranscriptional editing and splicing, protein localization, and catalysis [1–4]. RNA structure is closely related to function, and determining RNA structure using experimental and computational techniques is an active area of research. RNA secondary structure, i.e., the set of canonical base pairs (AU, GC, GU), forms readily and is highly stable, creating a scaffold on which tertiary interactions occur [5]. Predicting secondary structure is therefore an important step in determining RNA function. One popular computational approach is to compute the minimum free energy structure using a dynamic programming algorithm [6, 7]. This is accomplished using a set of nearest neighbor thermodynamic rules to evaluate folding stability and then the algorithm implicitly considers all possible secondary structures [8, 9]. These algorithms have been expanded to predict suboptimal structures with low folding free energy as alternative possible stable conformations [10, 11]. Partition functions consider the entire ensemble of possible secondary structures, and are used to compute the probability that given base pairs occur based on their prevalence within the

Douglas H. Turner and David H. Mathews (eds.), *RNA Structure Determination: Methods and Protocols*, Methods in Molecular Biology, vol. 1490, DOI 10.1007/978-1-4939-6433-8_4, © Springer Science+Business Media New York 2016

ensemble [12]. These calculations have improved upon secondary
structure prediction and provide a measure of assessment of the likelihood that each base pair in the structure occurs [13]. This chapter
introduces the applications of both free energy minimization and partition function calculations to the more complex problem of predicting RNA–RNA interactions.

1.1 Bifold

The first algorithm available in RNAstructure to predict intermolecular base pairs is Bifold, a free energy minimization algorithm. Bifold
computes the Gibbs free energy change for folding using Turner nearest neighbor parameters for RNA [8, 9] or a recent set of parameters
for DNA [14]. The lower the folding free energy change, the more
stable the structure and the more likely it occurs at equilibrium. Bifold
considers the RNA–RNA interaction problem by concatenating the
two RNA sequences with a virtual linker sequence and predicting the
lowest free energy structure [15]. The free energy contribution of the
linker sequence is handled correctly, i.e., it contributes the correct
bimolecular initiation term and not a loop free energy. It can be used
to predict base pairs that occur both within a strand and between
strands, or can be used to consider only inter-strand structure. This
algorithm is guaranteed to compute the lowest free energy structure
given the energy model, and additionally computes suboptimal structures of low folding free energy to generate alternative hypotheses.

1.2 Bipartition

A second algorithm in RNAstructure is Bipartition, which performs
a bimolecular partition function calculation [13]. The use of a partition function calculation can improve prediction accuracy compared to free energy minimization and give a confidence measure
in an individual predicted pair [16]. Similar to the prediction
scheme in Bifold, Bipartition concatenates the two strands of RNA
with a linker sequence and performs a partition function calculation on this "single" strand [15]. Bipartition, however, does not
predict self-structure within a sequence and therefore considers
only intermolecular base pairs.

The results of partition function calculations can be parsed in
multiple ways, the two most common being thresholding and
maximum expected accuracy (MEA) structure prediction [16].
The partition function outputs the probability that any given base
pair occurs at equilibrium, and highly probable base pairs can be
selected to assemble a probable structure. In thresholding, these
base pairs are selected by setting a minimum probability and
assembling a secondary structure containing only those base pairs
whose probability of occurring exceed this threshold. The probability must be strictly greater than 50 % to avoid predicting multiple pairing partners for a single nucleotide [13]. Alternatively,
the structure can be assembled by MEA. In this scheme, structures are assembled from pairs and unpaired nucleotides, where
the sum of probabilities is maximized.

Table 1
Computational complexity

Program name	Bifold	Bipartition	DuplexFold	AccessFold
Computational complexity	$O((N_1+N_2)^3)$	$O(N_1 N_2 l)$	$O(N_1 N_2 l)$	$O(N_1^3 + N_2^3)$

The computational complexity explains how much time will be required to run a calculation, as the length of the sequences increase in size. Here, N_1 is the length of sequence 1, N_2 is the length of sequence 2, and l is the maximum number of unpaired nucleotides allowed in a loop (the maxloop parameter). For example, Bifold is cubed with N_1+N_2, thus doubling the length of N_1+N_2 would require eight times as much computer time. DuplexFold, however, is linear with N_1, thus doubling the length of N_1 would require only a doubling in the computer time

1.3 DuplexFold

Another program for bimolecular prediction is DuplexFold [17]. This algorithm does not predict intramolecular structure, and is currently available only for command line use. The advantage of DuplexFold is the speed-up in computational time compared to Bifold that results from not predicting intramolecular pairs. Table 1 shows the computational complexity for the algorithms.

1.4 AccessFold

The most recent addition to RNAstructure is AccessFold, which also predicts only intermolecular base pairs [18]. AccessFold uses the partition function, calculated for each sequence separately, to account for accessibility for base pairing to the second sequence [13]. A simple additive model is used to calculate a per nucleotide penalty for interacting with the other strand. In this way, strong intramolecular structure in either strand can alter the choice of pairing regions for the intermolecular structure.

2 Materials

RNAstructure is available with precompiled binaries for Linux, Macintosh OS X, and Microsoft Windows. It is written in C++ and JAVA and should readily compile on other operating systems. RNAstructure is available for free download at http://rna.urmc.rochester.edu/RNAstructure.html.

3 Methods

3.1 Download and Install RNAstructure

Browse to http://rna.urmc.rochester.edu/RNAstructure.html and click on the link entitled "Register to Download". Input your name, institution, and e-mail address to register. The code is provided with the GNU public license, but registration is requested. The registration information is used to track the number of independent downloads of the software and helps make the case for continued funding to support maintenance and development. Click the "Submit Registration" button, and you will be taken to a thank you screen. Click the link entitled "Download page" to continue.

The Graphical User Interfaces (GUIs) and text interfaces are available for download for Windows as a .zip and Linux or Mac as a gzipped tarball. Source code is additionally available for local compilation as a .zip in DOS format and a tarball in UNIX format. A full set of help and installation instructions are available online at: http://rna.urmc.rochester.edu/RNAstructureHelp.html.

For Linux, the RNAstructure package will be downloaded as RNAstructureforLinux.tgz. Extract the software from command line using the command "tar-xvzf RNAstructureforLinux.tgz". This will create a directory called "RNAstructure" containing several subdirectories such as "data_tables", "examples", etc. If Java is not installed, it can be downloaded at http://java.com. To launch the GUI, enter the subdirectory "exe" and run RNAstructureScript.

The installation for Mac works similarly to that described above for Linux. The package will be downloaded as RNAstructureforMac.dmg. Navigate into the RNAstructureForMac folder, and double-click RNAstructure. Be sure that your computer will allow applications to run when downloaded from the internet. To do this, in "System Preferences", choose "Security and Privacy". Then click the lock to make changes, supply your password, and, for "Allow apps downloaded from:", choose "Anywhere".

For Windows, the software package is available as RNAstructure.zip. Run RNAstructure.exe for installation. The Setup Wizard will pop up to step through the installation process. By default, RNAstructure will be installed under "All Programs" on the start menu. The GUI can be launched from there. Alternatively, from the command line, the RNAstructure.bat file can be run from the RNAstructure subdirectory "exe".

3.2 Enter Sequences

Once the GUI is launched, a sequence of interest can be entered by clicking on "New Sequence" under the "File" menu item, or on the toolbar where the blank page icon is located. A title must be entered as well as the sequence. Note that nucleotides in lower case will be single-stranded in the predicted structure. Unknown nucleotides can be entered as "X". To save the sequence file, exit the input box once the information is complete. This will generate a prompt to save the file, in .fasta format by default. Sequence files can be generated without the use of the GUI using a text editor from the command line, and must follow .seq or .fasta format. The file formats used by RNAstructure can be seen at: http://rna.urmc.rochester.edu/Text/File_Formats.html.

3.3 Using Bifold with the GUI

Once RNAstructure is launched, Bifold can be called by selecting "Fold RNA Bimolecular" under the "RNA" menu. This will bring up a dialog box through which the input sequences and structure file name can be specified (Fig. 1). Sample sequences are located in

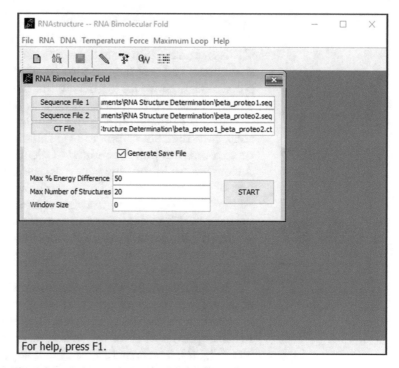

Fig. 1 Sample input window for Bifold. Two sequences have been selected, and the calculation can now be started by clicking "START"

RNAstructure/examples, and are labeled as .seq or .fasta corresponding to the format. Click first on the "Sequence File 1" button to browse for your first sequence file, and then the "Sequence File 2" button. The save file name for the structure file will be automatically generated as <seq1>_<seq2> .ct, but can be manually altered by clicking the ct file button or by typing in the text box. Three parameters will be set to default: "Max % Energy Difference" to 50, "Max Number of Structures" to 20, and "Window Size" to 0. "Max % Energy Difference" specifies the percentage of the minimum free energy by which suboptimal structures can deviate. The larger this value, the less stringent the energetic stability requirements, and the greater the number of potential structures that can be generated. "Max Number of Structures" puts a hard limit on the number of structures to generate within this energy difference. Finally, "Window Size" is a measure for how different the structures need to be from one another to be considered as a distinct structure. The larger the window size, the more diverse the set of suboptimal structures. Each of these parameters can be manually changed by typing directly into the text box. Another user option at this point is to limit the structure prediction to intermolecular base pairs by clicking "Forbid Unimolecular Pairs" under the "Force" menu item. A save file, which will have a .sav extension, can be created by selecting the option "Generate Save File". This can be used to refold the structures in the future without recomputing the energies, particularly if it is necessary to produce multiple or more diverse suboptimal structures. The .sav file can also be used to generate energy dot plots, which show for each pair the lowest folding free energy structure that can be generated for a structure with that pair.

After the inputs, output, and parameters are selected appropriately, click the "Start" box to begin folding the bimolecular structure. A box will pop up entitled "Calculation in Progress...", and the movement of the blue bar across the screen will track the progress of the computation. Once complete, a new box will pop up asking "Do you want to draw structures?" This will provide two options: "OK" to draw structures now and "Cancel". If "Cancel" is selected, RNAstructure will not draw the predicted structures. It will, however, save the .ct structure file and the structures can be drawn from this .ct file at a later time.

By default, when drawing structures, the minimum free energy structure will be depicted. This image will be labeled with the structure number being displayed, the folding free energy of the structure, and a label for the structure, derived from the sequence files (Fig. 2). The structure can be enlarged by clicking "Zoom" under the "Draw" menu item or holding the control key and the

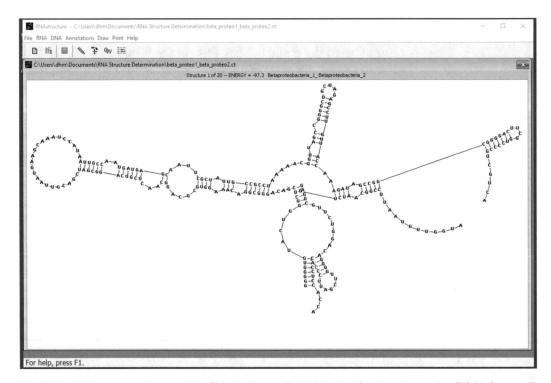

Fig. 2 The RNAstructure draw module. This is the predicted bimolecular structure, using Bifold, for a split tmRNA from *D. aromatica* [24]

right arrow key. Similarly, control and the left arrow key will zoom out. Different suboptimal structures can be drawn by selecting "Draw" and then "Go to Structure" and indicating which suboptimal structure to draw. Alternatively, control-up and control-down will change the currently drawn structure. The lowest free energy structure is structure 1, and then the subsequent structures have increasingly higher folding free energy change.

3.4 Bipartition

The partition function calculation for bimolecular structure can also be computed. As noted in the Introduction, this calculation does not consider intramolecular structure formation. To first compute the probability dotplot, or the probability of base pairing for each possible pair, click "Partition Function RNA Bimolecular" under the "RNA" menu item. A window will pop up through which the two input sequences must be selected. Choose "Sequence File 1" and "Sequence File 2," and note that the name for the partition function save file is automatically generated as <seq1>_<seq2>. This can be modified by typing directly into the text box or by clicking the "Save File" button. Press "Start" to begin computing the partition function. A progress box will pop up as in the folding calculation to indicate the completeness of the calculation. Once this is complete, a probability dotplot will appear (Fig. 3). This is an $n \times m$ matrix of colored dots representing the probability that base pair i–j occurs, where n is the length of sequence 1, m is the length of sequence 2, i is the position of the nucleotide in sequence 1 and j-n-3 is the position of the nucleotide in sequence 2. This computation generates a partition function save file, or .pfs, which can be used to annotate a predicted structure with pairing probabilities. It can be used in the GUI or command line to predict the maximum expected accuracy structure or to generate structures using base pairing thresholds.

The thresholded structure can be generated directly from the .pfs. Upon completion of the bimolecular partition function, the probability dotplot will be displayed and a menu entitled "Output" will be accessible. Under this menu item, select "Output Probable Structure" to display eight structure predictions, containing only those base pairs with greater than or equal to 99%, 97%, 95%, 90%, 80%, 70%, 60%, and strictly greater than 50% probability, respectively.

The bimolecular maximum expected accuracy structure can be predicted by selecting "MaxExpect: Predict RNA MEA Structure" under the "RNA" menu item. On the window that opens, select the partition function save file of choice, and note that the name for the structure file is automatically filled. This can be changed by typing directly into the text box or by clicking the "CT File" button. Suboptimal structure parameters are set to default as in the Folding calculation in Subheading 3.3, and can be changed as desired. One additional parameter, gamma, is set to a default of one.

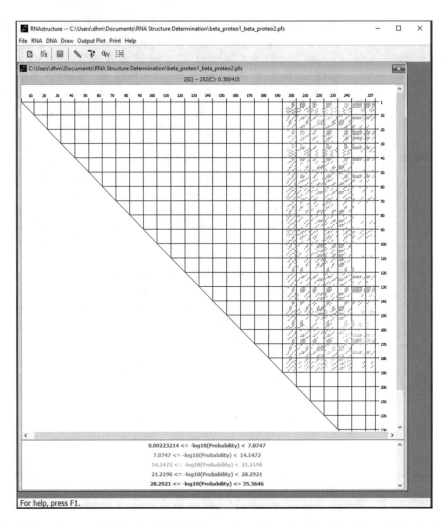

Fig. 3 The RNAstructure probability dot plot. This figure shows the probability dot plot, calculated with a bimolecular partition function, for the split tmRNA from *D. aromatica* [24] as shown in Fig. 2. Note that the first sequence starts at index 1 (along the *right*), and the second sequence starts (along the top) at an index equal to the first sequence length plus 4 (the intermolecular linker that connects the sequences is 3 nucleotides long). By clicking on a dot, the pair identity and log$_{10}$ probability appear above the plot

Gamma controls the balance between the sensitivity and positive predictive value (PPV) of structure prediction. A value of 1 balances sensitivity and PPV, where larger numbers place a higher value on sensitivity and smaller numbers place a higher value on PPV. In other words, higher values of gamma favor the prediction of more base pairs in the structure. Lower values of gamma (between 0 and 1) will predict fewer pairs, but the pairs will more likely be correct predictions. Click "Start" and then "Draw Structures" after the calculation is complete. The drawn structure will be labeled with a structure number, an energy, and a label that derives from the sequence files. The indicated "ENERGY", however, is not the folding free energy, but the expected accuracy score.

These structures can be color annotated to illustrate base pairing probabilities by selecting "Add Color Annotation" under the "Annotations" menu item and selecting the .pfs file corresponding to the folded structure (Fig. 4). At the bottom of the window is a key that displays the corresponding pairing probability range for each color. Table 2 shows the positive predictive value of base pairs for single-stranded folding as a function of base pairing probability threshold. Higher confidence can be placed in highly probable base pairs as compared to pairs with lower estimated pairing probability. It is expected that this trend is the same for bimolecular structure prediction.

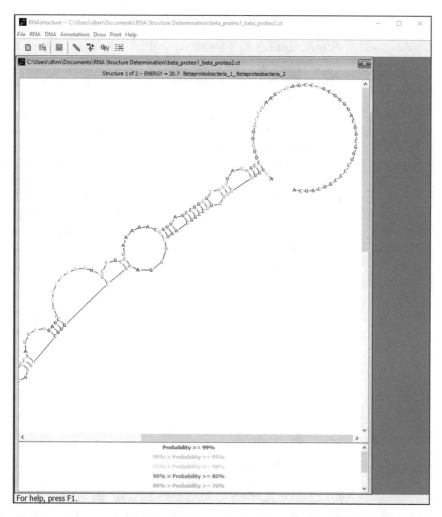

Fig. 4 The MaxExpect structure with probability annotation. This shows the predicted MaxExpect structure, using the bimolecular partition function, for the split tmRNA from *D. aromatica* [24] as shown in Figs. 2 and 3. For clarity, the drawing is zoomed to a portion of the structure. The color key appears below the drawing

Table 2
Accuracy of base pair prediction for pairs exceeding a specified probability threshold

Probability threshold	99%	90%	70%	50%
Average PPV	90.9 ± 6.0	83.0 ± 8.7	75.4 ± 11.0	70.3 ± 11.8
Average sensitivity	24.4 ± 5.8	47.1 ± 7.2	62.1 ± 9.6	70.0 ± 10.0

Positive predictive value (PPV) is the fraction of pairs above the probability threshold that are in the accepted structure. Sensitivity is the fraction of pairs in the accepted structure that exceed that probability threshold. These values are averages for single-stranded structure prediction [13]

3.5 DuplexFold

DuplexFold is available for use on command line. Typing "DuplexFold --help" will display the options for using DuplexFold. A more complete help page for DuplexFold and the other command line interfaces is available at: http://rna.urmc.rochester.edu/Text/index.html.

DuplexFold has a number of adjustable parameters. "Loop" defines the number of nucleotides that are allowed in a single internal loop or bulge, or the number of unpaired nucleotides separating intermolecular structure. The default is set to 6 nucleotides, but can be changed by using the flag "-l" or "--loop" followed by the new number of nucleotides. "Maximum" refers to the maximum number of structures, "percent" to the maximal percent difference in energy between suboptimal structures and the optimal structure, "temperature" to the folding temperature in Kelvin, and "window" to the window size controlling diversity of suboptimal structures. These are set to defaults of 10, 40, 310.15, and 0, respectively, and can be controlled using the -m, -p, -t, and -w flags as in the following example: "DuplexFold -l 30 -m 20 -p 50 -t 315 -w 10 sequence_1.seq sequence_2.seq duplex.ct". This calculation will allow up to 30 unpaired nucleotides between intermolecular base pairs, will generate 20 structures within 50% energy value of the optimal structure, at temperature 315 K and with a window size of 10. The default values are sufficient for most calculations.

DuplexFold does not consider self-structure and predicts only intermolecular pairs. The benefit to using DuplexFold over Bifold with intramolecular structure prediction forbidden is the increase in speed available by using a smaller loop size. Bifold is equivalent to using a loop size of 30. Especially when using long sequences, the ability to limit the search space for base pairs greatly increases computational speed and improves prediction accuracy. Choice of loop size, however, requires intuition about the specific interaction, and using several loop sizes to confirm that the structure prediction is reasonable might be necessary.

3.6 AccessFold

AccessFold is another RNAstructure program that is available on the command line. AccessFold has the same parameters as DuplexFold (Subheading 3.5 above), but also has one additional parameter that can be adjusted. The parameter gamma, default 0.4, scales the cost of opening intramolecular pairs to form a duplex structure. The default has the best average performance, and making gamma larger will tend to disfavor bimolecular pairs. AccessFold has excellent accuracy at predicting bimolecular base pairs between short interacting sequences.

4   Notes

There are a number of diverse examples of RNA–RNA duplexes that serve important functions in the cell, and in this chapter computational approaches to predict the formation of these duplexes are described. The algorithms in this chapter utilize thermodynamic information to predict probable structures at equilibrium. Here, we discussed four approaches to balance the competition between unimolecular and bimolecular base pairs: (1, Bifold) free energy minimization, treating intramolecular and intermolecular pairs equally; (2, bipartition) partition function calculations ignoring intramolecular structure and computing the probability of intermolecular pairs; (3, DuplexFold) free energy minimization that does not allow unimolecular base pairs; and (4, AccessFold) a simple model for predicting bimolecular pairs and accounting for accessibility to intramolecular pairs. The DuplexFold approach is faster than the other approaches for calculations on long sequences, for example, scanning for binding sites in whole viral genomes [17].

These algorithms provide a general prediction method in which the details of the duplex's function do not need to be known to predict the intermolecular structure. These approaches do not make assumptions about patterns of binding, such as algorithms trained to predict a single class of duplex [19–23], and are of great use for developing hypotheses and experiments to test the roles of newly identified duplexes.

Acknowledgement

This protocol was written with the support of National Institutes of Health Grant R01GM076485 to D.H.M.

References

1. Storz G, Gottesman S (2006) Versatile roles of small RNA regulators in bacteria. In: Gesteland RF, Cech TR, Atkins JF (eds) The RNA world, 3rd edn. Cold Spring Harbor Laboratory Press, Cold Spring Harbor, pp 567–594

2. Wu L, Belasco JG (2008) Let me count the ways: mechanisms of gene regulation by miRNAs and siRNAs. Mol Cell 29(1):1–7. doi:10.1016/j.molcel.2007.12.010

3. Walter P, Blobel G (1982) Signal recognition particle contains a 7S RNA essential for protein translocation across the endoplasmic reticulum. Nature 299:691–698

4. Doudna JA, Cech TR (2002) The chemical repertoire of natural ribozymes. Nature 418:222–228

5. Tinoco I Jr, Bustamante C (1999) How RNA folds. J Mol Biol 293(2):271–281

6. Seetin MG, Mathews DH (2012) RNA structure prediction: an overview of methods. Methods Mol Biol 905:99–122. doi:10.1007/978-1-61779-949-5_8

7. Hofacker IL (2014) Energy-directed RNA structure prediction. Methods Mol Biol 1097:71–84. doi:10.1007/978-1-62703-709-9_4

8. Mathews DH, Disney MD, Childs JL, Schroeder SJ, Zuker M, Turner DH (2004) Incorporating chemical modification constraints into a dynamic programming algorithm for prediction of RNA secondary structure. Proc Natl Acad Sci U S A 101:7287–7292

9. Xia T, SantaLucia J Jr, Burkard ME, Kierzek R, Schroeder SJ, Jiao X, Cox C, Turner DH (1998) Thermodynamic parameters for an expanded nearest-neighbor model for formation of RNA duplexes with Watson-Crick pairs. Biochemistry 37:14719–14735

10. Zuker M (1989) On finding all suboptimal foldings of an RNA molecule. Science 244:48–52

11. Steger G, Hofmann H, Fortsch J, Gross HJ, Randles JW, Sanger HL, Riesner D (1984) Conformational transitions in viroids and virusoids: comparison of results from energy minimization algorithm and from experimental data. J Biomol Struct Dyn 2(3):543–571

12. McCaskill JS (1990) The equilibrium partition function and base pair probabilities for RNA secondary structure. Biopolymers 29:1105–1119

13. Mathews DH (2004) Using an RNA secondary structure partition function to determine confidence in base pairs predicted by free energy minimization. RNA 10:1178–1190

14. Reuter JS, Mathews DH (2010) RNAstructure: software for RNA secondary structure prediction and analysis. BMC Bioinformatics 11:129

15. Mathews DH, Burkard ME, Freier SM, Wyatt JR, Turner DH (1999) Predicting oligonucleotide affinity to nucleic acid targets. RNA 5:1458–1469

16. Lu ZJ, Gloor JW, Mathews DH (2009) Improved RNA secondary structure prediction by maximizing expected pair accuracy. RNA 15:1805–1813

17. Piekna-Przybylska D, DiChiacchio L, Mathews DH, Bambara RA (2009) A sequence similar to tRNA3Lys gene is embedded in HIV-1 U3/R and promotes minus strand transfer. Nat Struct Mol Biol 17:83–89

18. DiChiacchio L, Sloma MF, Mathews DH (2016) AccessFold: predicting RNA-RNA interactions with consideration for competing self-structure. Bioinformatics 32:1033–1039. doi:10.1093/bioinformatics/btv682

19. Lu ZJ, Mathews DH (2007) Efficient siRNA selection using hybridization thermodynamics. Nucleic Acids Res 32:640–647, PMC2241856

20. Lu ZJ, Mathews DH (2008) Fundamental differences in the equilibrium considerations for siRNA and antisense oligodeoxynucleotide design. Nucleic Acids Res 36:3738–3745

21. Tafer H, Ameres SL, Obernosterer G, Gebeshuber CA, Schroeder R, Martinez J, Hofacker IL (2008) The impact of target site accessibility on the design of effective siRNAs. Nat Biotechnol 26(5):578–583. doi:10.1038/nbt1404

22. Watanabe Y, Tomita M, Kanai A (2007) Computational methods for microRNA target prediction. Methods Enzymol 427:65–86. doi:10.1016/S0076-6879(07)27004-1

23. Rennie W, Liu C, Carmack CS, Wolenc A, Kanoria S, Lu J, Long D, Ding Y (2014) STarMir: a web server for prediction of microRNA binding sites. Nucleic Acids Res 42(Web Server issue):W114–W118. doi:10.1093/nar/gku376

24. Sharkady SM, Williams KP (2004) A third lineage with two-piece tmRNA. Nucleic Acids Res 32(15):4531–4538. doi:10.1093/nar/gkh795

Chapter 5

A Method to Predict the Structure and Stability of RNA/RNA Complexes

Xiaojun Xu and Shi-Jie Chen

Abstract

RNA/RNA interactions are essential for genomic RNA dimerization and regulation of gene expression. Intermolecular loop–loop base pairing is a widespread and functionally important tertiary structure motif in RNA machinery. However, computational prediction of intermolecular loop–loop base pairing is challenged by the entropy and free energy calculation due to the conformational constraint and the intermolecular interactions. In this chapter, we describe a recently developed statistical mechanics-based method for the prediction of RNA/RNA complex structures and stabilities. The method is based on the virtual bond RNA folding model (Vfold). The main emphasis in the method is placed on the evaluation of the entropy and free energy for the loops, especially tertiary kissing loops. The method also uses recursive partition function calculations and two-step screening algorithm for large, complicated structures of RNA/RNA complexes. As case studies, we use the HIV-1 Mal dimer and the siRNA/HIV-1 mutant (T4) to illustrate the method.

Key words RNA/RNA complex, Tertiary motif entropy, Partition function, Two-step screening

1 Introduction

RNA–RNA interactions play widespread roles in RNA biological functions from mRNA splicing [1–3] and microRNA-target recognition [4–7] to RNA/RNA dimerization [8–10]. RNA folding induced by RNA–RNA binding can be important for RNA-related cellular processes. For example, during the mRNA splicing process, RNA/RNA complexes formed by small nuclear RNAs undergo multiple structural rearrangements in the different steps of splicing [11], microRNAs regulate gene expression by binding to gene targets (at 3′ untranslated regions of target mRNA transcripts) [12], and RNA/RNA dimerization plays essential role in viral replication [13, 14]. Many of the processes of RNA–RNA binding are facilitated by the intermolecular loop–loop interactions between RNA molecules.

Douglas H. Turner and David H. Mathews (eds.), *RNA Structure Determination: Methods and Protocols*, Methods in Molecular Biology, vol. 1490, DOI 10.1007/978-1-4939-6433-8_5, © Springer Science+Business Media New York 2016

Accurate prediction of RNA/RNA complex formation requires a reliable method to treat (1) the change of the conformational statistics in the folding process, (2) interplay between intermolecular and intramolecular base pairing, (3) tertiary interactions, such as kissing-loop interactions and pseudoknotted interactions between two RNAs. Most of the currently available folding algorithms for RNA/RNA complexes can treat intermolecular and intramolecular competitions at the secondary structure level [11, 15–19]. However, many biologically important RNA/RNA complexes involve tertiary (cross-linked) intermolecular contacts. As a result of the cross-linkage between the different loops and between the different loops and helices, the folding free energy of a structure becomes nonadditive, i.e., the total stability of a structure is not the simple additive sum of the stability of each structure subunit. Studies by us and other groups show that a physical entropy model can lead to improvements in the predictions of RNA secondary structures and thermodynamic stabilities [20]. For example, the recently developed models [21, 22], based on the partition function calculations and simplified thermodynamic models for simple kissing interactions can account for complex loop kissing interactions. However, to explicitly account for the nonadditive free energy, especially the entropy for the different loop kissing motifs, we need a new physics-based model.

The recently developed Vfold model is a statistical mechanics-based RNA folding model. The model relies on a coarse-grained (virtual bond) representation for RNA conformation [23–25]. Compared with other free energy-based RNA/RNA complex structure prediction models, the Vfold model computes loop entropy parameters from explicit conformational sampling in three-dimensional space. Furthermore, by enumerating all the possible structures, including tertiary structures containing cross-linked loops, in the partition function calculation, the Vfold model computes the free energy landscape for secondary and simple tertiary structures. The results led to several predictions for RNA mechanisms, such as pseudoknot-involved conformational switch between bistable secondary structures [26], microRNA–gene target interactions [12], and RNA/RNA kissing dimerization in viral replication [13, 14].

2   Tertiary Loop Entropy Calculation

With two virtual bonds per nucleotide to represent the backbone conformation, the Vfold model samples fluctuations of loops/junction conformations in three-dimensional space through conformational enumeration (*see* Fig. 1). By calculating the probability of loop formation, the Vfold model gives the conformational entropy parameters for the formation of the different types of loops

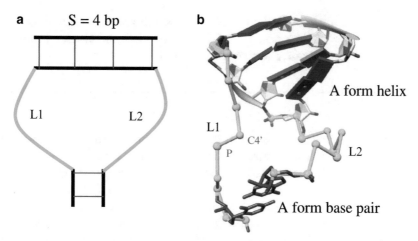

Fig. 1 The Vfold model uses two bonds (P–C4′ and C4′–P) to represent each nucleotide and computes loop entropies by sampling virtual bond conformations in three-dimensional space. (**a**) A tertiary motif which shows a hairpin loop stretched through base pairing with a bound RNA. (**b**) A virtual bond (in *cyan*) backbone conformation of the three-dimensional tertiary structure corresponding to the two-dimensional structure shown in (**a**). In the three-dimensional structure, the two ends of the loops L_1 and L_2 are fitted to the base pairs of A-form helices (in *red*). Starting from an A-form helix with the given number of base pairs, Vfold enumerates loop backbone conformations on a diamond lattice with bond length of 3.9 angstrom, bond angle of ~ 109.5°, and three equiprobable torsional angles (60°, 180°, 300°). From the probability of loop closure, Vfold calculates RNA motif based loop entropies

including pseudoknot loops [27, 28] and hairpin kissing loops [13]. Please check if the edit made to the sentence, "The model is…" is fine. The model is based on the complete conformational ensemble and accounts for the chain connectivity and excluded volume effects. Here we use the a hairpin loop stretched by a bound RNA (Fig. 1) to show the steps of entropy calculation for a kissing loop.

1. We first use A-form helix (*see* **Note 1**) to configure the 4-nt stem in Fig. 1.

2. We then enumerate all the possible virtual bond backbone conformations for a given chain length (*see* **Note 2**) and count the total number Ω_{coil} of the conformations (*see* **Note 3**).

3. From the conformational ensemble above, we identify loop conformations according to the loop closure condition. For the structure in Fig. 1, we fit the two ends of a loop to a base pair configuration in an A-form helix. We generate the virtual bond conformations through self-avoiding random walks and count the total number Ω_{loop} of viable loop conformations.

4. We calculate the loop entropy $\Delta S_{loop} = k_B \ln(\Omega_{loop} / \Omega_{coil})$, where k_B is the Boltzmann constant.

5. The above Vfold-based computation leads to pre-tabulated entropy parameters for hairpin loops [23], internal/bulge

loops [23], H-type pseudoknots with/without inter-helix junction [27, 28], hairpin–hairpin kissing motifs [13], and other tertiary motifs [29].

3   Methods

Partition function is a Boltzmann-weighted sum over all the possible structures. From the partition function, we can compute (a) the base pairing probability for each nucleotide pair, from which we can predict the probable structures, (b) the melting curve, and (c) the other folding thermodynamic properties such as folding free energies. Furthermore, the method can predict not only the global minimum free energy structure but also all the possible alternative structures (local minima on the free energy landscape).

One of the key ingredients in partition function calculation is the enthalpy and entropy parameters for a given structure. In our calculation, the enthalpy and entropy for the canonical and the mismatched base stacks are given by Turner's experimental data [30]. The loop entropies are calculated from the Vfold pretabulated parameters.

3.1   RNA/RNA Complex Structure Prediction Based on Complete Structure Enumeration

1. For given sequences of two interacting RNAs, we insert a three-nucleotide phantom link (*see* **Note 4**) between the RNAs. The three-nucleotide linker transforms the original two-RNA system into an effective one-RNA system (*see* Fig. 2).

2. For each RNA sequence, we first generate the structure ensemble by enumerating all the possible base pair arrangements, including H-type pseudoknots with/without inter-helix loop and other tertiary motifs shown in Fig. 2 (*see* **Note 5**).

3. For each sequence, we compute the partition function by summing over all the structures in the ensemble generated above. We denote the partition functions as Z_1 and Z_2 for the two RNAs, respectively.

4. We repeat the above procedure to calculate the partition function Z_3 for the effective one-RNA system above. Note that Z_3 includes structures with and without inter-molecular base pairs.

5. We calculate the partition function for the complex (structures with intermolecular base pairs) as $Z_{12} = Z_3 - Z_1 \cdot Z_2$.

6. We compute the total partition function $Z(c_s, T)$ for the system: $Z(c_s, T) = Z_1 \bullet Z_2 + \alpha\, e^{-(\Delta G_{init}/k_B T)} Z_{12}$. Here c_s is the RNA strand concentration, T is the temperature, and $\Delta G_{init} = 3.61 + 0.75\, k_B T$ (kcal/mol) (*see* **Note 6**). The parameter α is equal to $c_s/4$ for non-self-complementary strands and c_s for self-complementary strands.

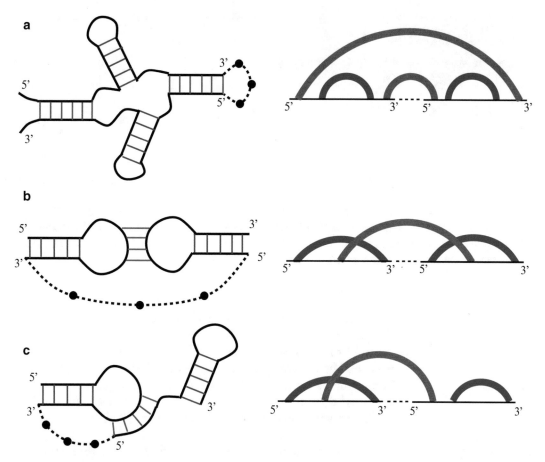

Fig. 2 Examples of intermolecular interactions (base pairing) between two RNAs that can be treated by the current Vfold model. The *thick curved links* in the polymer graph (*right panels*) denote helices. The *straight lines* represent RNA main chain. The *dashed lines* denote the phantom link, which is used to convert the two-RNA system into an effective one-RNA system. The *blue lines* in the *left panels* are intramolecular base pairs and the *red lines* are the intermolecular base pairs. (**a**) The effective one-RNA system containing secondary structures only. (**b**) and (**c**) Tertiary kissing motifs with cross-linked base pairs

7. By following the similar procedure as above, we compute the conditional partition function $Z_{ij}(c_s, T)$ for all the structures that contain the (i, j) base pair (*see* **Note 7**).

8. From the above partition functions, we calculate the probability of finding the (i, j) base pair: $p_{ij}(c_s, T) = Z_{ij}(c_s, T) / Z(c_s, T)$.

9. From the base pairing probability for all the possible (i, j) pairs, we predict the most probable (*see* **Note 8**) as well as alternative structures (*see* **Note 9**).

We use the HIV-1 Mal complex as an example to show how Vfold predicts the RNA/RNA complex structure. Given the 23-nt

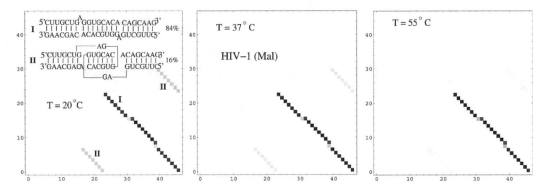

Fig. 3 Density plots for the predicted base pairing probabilities at different temperatures for the HIV-1 Mal dimer. The RNA strand concentration C_s is 150 μM, which is adopted from the experiment [31]. At room temperature, the kissing-loop and the extended-duplex dimer (structures shown in *inset*) coexist. As the temperature increases, the extended-duplex becomes dominant

RNA sequence of the HIV-1 Mal (*see* **Note 10**), Vfold calculates the base pairing probabilities p_{ij} for all the possible base pairs (*see* **Note 7**) for the given temperatures T and RNA strand concentration (*see* Fig. 3). Our prediction indicates that thermal heating can induce the conformational switch from the kissing complex to the extended-duplex dimer for the HIV-1 Mal dimer. The result is consistent with the experimental observation [32].

3.2 Two-Step Screening Method for RNA/RNA Complex Prediction

The partition function method with complete structure enumeration is computationally expensive, especially when the tertiary motifs are included in the conformational ensemble. To treat large and complicate RNA/RNA complexes, we use a two-step screening method to efficiently predict the structure and the folding stability of RNA/RNA complexes. The essence of the model is to parse the structure prediction for the whole system into two steps: we first identify the most probable binding sites (binding mode), we then calculate the base pairing probabilities based on the most probable binding site (binding mode).

1. For the given RNA sequences, we enumerate all the possible binding regions (*see* **Note 11**) between two RNAs (see the red base pairs in Fig. 4a). We call RNA–RNA binding at a given region m as a binding mode.

2. For each binding mode m, we use the nearest-neighbor model to calculate the free energy $\Delta G^{(m)}_{binding\text{-}helix}$ for the intermolecular base pairs: $\Delta G^{(m)}_{binding\text{-}helix} = \sum_{stack} \Delta G_{stack}$, where ΔG_{stack} is the free energy of a constituent base stack in the binding region.

3. For a given binding mode, we enumerate all the possible intramolecular base pairs (*see* **Note 12**), with the condition that the

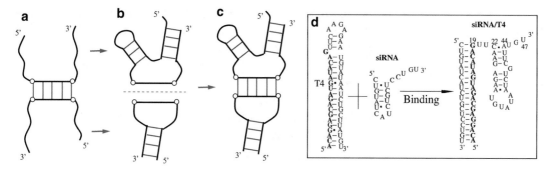

Fig. 4 ((a)–(c)) Enumeration of RNA/RNA complex structures. For a given binding mode (base pairs in *red*), the intramolecular base pairs (shown in *blue*) are enumerated independently for the two RNAs. The final RNA/RNA complex structures are generated by the combination of the different intramolecular base pairs. (**d**) The conformational change caused by the siRNA binding to a HIV-1 mutant (T4). siRNA can induce the complete unzipping of T4, which refolds into a new structure after siRNA binding

nucleotides in the binding region are not allowed to base pair with other nucleotides (see the blue base pairs in Fig. 4b, c).

4. We assign the free energy for each structure in the conformational ensemble: $\Delta G_s^{(m)} = \Delta G_{helix}^{(m)} + \Delta G_{loop}^{(m)}$. Here, $\Delta G_{helix}^{(m)}$ includes the intermolecular helix $\Delta G_{binding\text{-}helix}^{(m)}$ in the binding region and $\Delta G_{loop}^{(m)}$ accounts for the free energy (loop entropic) changes caused by the conformational constraint due to the formation of the loop-kissing interactions (Fig. 2) (*see* **Note 13**).

5. We calculate the total partition function for mode *m* as the sum over all the possible structures:

$$Z_{tot}^{(m)} = \sum_{structures} e^{-\Delta G_s^{(m)}/k_B T}$$

6. By following the similar procedure, we enumerate all the possible binding modes and calculate the partition function $Z_{tot}^{(m)}$ for each binding mode. The most probable binding mode (M) is the one with the maximum total partition function Z_{tot}^{M} (*see* **Note 14**).

7. In the next step, we compute the RNA/RNA complex structure for the most probable binding mode. For the most probable mode *M*, following the above procedure, we compute the partition function Z_{ij}^{M} for all the conformations with base pair (i,j).

8. From the partition functions, we calculate the probability of finding intramolecular base pair (i,j): $p_{ij}^{M} = Z_{ij}^{M} / Z_{tot}^{M}$.

9. For the most probable binding site (M), we predict the intermolecular base pairs by minimizing the free energy for the binding region. We assume that the binding region is a helix stem that can possibly contain at most a bulge loop (*see* **Note 11**).

10. From the base pairing probabilities for all the (i,j) pairs, we predicted the most probable (*see* **Note 8**) as well as the alternative complex structures (*see* **Note 9**).

We use the *siRNA/HIV-1 mutant (T4)* complex (*see* **Note 15**) to illustrate the above two-step screening method. As shown in Fig. 4d, both RNAs can fold into a stem-loop structure. We found [12] a single dominant binding site for the two-RNA system. The stem of T4 is completely disrupted upon siRNA binding at the dominant binding site. Meanwhile, the nucleotides in the 3′ tail of T4 refolds into a new hairpin-like structure after siRNA binding. Since the two RNAs in this case are short (19 nt and 47 nt, respectively), we can also predict its complex structure using the exact structure enumeration as described in the previous section. The two methods give consistent results [12].

It should be noted that depending on the sequences of the two RNAs, we might find multiple dominant binding sites with comparable binding affinities, as the case of the HIV-1 Mal dimer shown in Fig. 3. If there exist multiple most probable binding modes, we need to follow the above procedure for each mode to predict the respective complex structures.

4 Notes

1. The coordinates (r, θ, z) for atoms P and C4′ in the A-form helix are $(8.71\, \mathring{A}, 70.5 + 32.7i, -3.75 + 2.81i)$ and $(9.68\, \mathring{A}, 46.9 + 32.7i, -3.10 + 2.81i)$ $(i = 0, 1, 2, ...)$ [33].

2. A survey of the known structures suggests that the virtual bonds (P–C4′ and C4′–P) have bond length of ~ 3.9 $\mathring{A}$ and bond angle in the range of 90°–120°.

3. An acceptable loop conformation (with virtual bond backbone) is restricted by the chain connectivity, excluded volume effects, and the loop closure condition.

4. The three nucleotides in the phantom linker cannot form base pairs with any other (physical) nucleotides. Moreover, for the effective one-RNA system, no loop parameters will be assigned to any (nonphysical) loops that contain phantom nucleotides.

5. To consider the compatibility for the connection between the different structural subunits, we classify the partition functions into different types (e.g., different types of loops) in our recursive partition function algorithm [11, 13, 23, 27].

6. The physical origin of an additional ΔG_{init} is due to the entropy loss associated with the conversion from two single-stranded RNAs to a single RNA complex.

7. Vfold only calculates conditional partition function $Z_{ij}(c_s, T)$ ($|i - j| > 3$) for A-U, G-C, or G-U base pairs.

8. The predicted most probable structure is formed by the base pairs of the largest base pairing probabilities.

9. We recommend users to also predict the possible alternative structures from the base pairing probability pattern, since many biological functions involve the suboptimal (alternative) structures.

10. The sequence of the HIV-1 Mal is: 5′CUUGCUGAGGU GCACACAGCAAG3′.

11. In the binding region, we assume that the helix has at least two base pairs. We allow the formation of a bulge loop in the inter-molecular helix stem at the binding site.

12. For each binding mode, with the assumption that the intermo-lecular interactions occur only at the predicted binding site, the enumeration of intramolecular base pairs can be performed independently for the two RNAs. This assumption significantly enhances the computational efficiency since the two RNAs are treated independently.

13. We have pre-tabulated parameters for the different types of the loops [13, 23, 27–29].

14. The two-step screening method for RNA/RNA complex structure prediction calculates base pairing probabilities only for the most stable binding modes.

15. The sequence of the siRNA is: 5′CUGUAUCAUCUGCU CCUGU3′. The sequence of the HIV-1 mutant (T4) is: 5′ACAGGAGCAGAUGAUACAGUUCAAGAGAAUGUA UAAUCUGCUUAUGU3′.

5 Acknowledgement

This research was supported by NIH grant GM063732.

References

1. Black DL (2003) Mechanisms of alternative pre-messenger RNA splicing. Annu Rev Biochem 72:291–336

2. Roy SW, Gilbert W (2006) The evolution of spliceosomal introns: patterns, puzzles and progress. Nat Rev Genet 7:211–221

3. Taggart AJ, DeSimone AM, Shih JS, Filloux ME, Fairbrother WG (2012) Large-scale mapping of branchpoints in human pre-mRNA transcripts in vivo. Nat Struct Mol Biol 19:719–721

4. Kertesz M, Iovino N, Unnerstall U, Gaul U, Segal E (2007) The role of site accessibility in

microRNA target recognition. Nat Genet 39:1278–1284

5. Bartel DP (2009) MicroRNAs: target recognition and regulatory functions. Cell 136:215–233

6. Fabian MR, Sonenberg N, Filipowicz W (2010) Regulation of mRNA translation and stability by microRNAs. Annu Rev Biochem 79:351–379

7. Westerhout EM, Berkhout B (2007) A systematic analysis of the effect of target RNA structure on RNA interference. Nucleic Acids Res 35:4322–4330

8. Russell RS, Liang C, Wainberg MA (2004) Is HIV-1 RNA dimerization a prerequisite for packaging? Yes, no, probably? Retrovirology 1:23

9. Lorenz C, Piganeau N, Schroeder R (2006) Stabilities of HIV-1 DIS type RNA loop-loop interactions in vitro and in vivo. Nucleic Acids Res 34:334–342

10. Paillart JC, Shehu-Xhilaga M, Marquet R, Mak J (2004) Dimerization of retroviral RNA genomes: an inseparable pair. Nat Rev Microbiol 2:461–472

11. Cao S, Chen S-J (2006) Free energy landscapes of RNA/RNA complexes: with applications to snRNA complexes in spliceosomes. J Mol Biol 357:292–312

12. Cao S, Chen S-J (2012) Predicting kissing interactions in microRNA-target complex and assessment of microRNA activity. Nucleic Acids Res 40: 4681–4690

13. Cao S, Chen S-J (2011) Structure and stability of RNA/RNA kissing complex: with application to HIV dimerization initiation signal. RNA 17:2130–2143

14. Cao S, Xu X, Chen S-J (2014) Predicting structure and stability for RNA complexes with intermolecular loop-loop base-pairing. RNA 20 835–845

15. Andronescu MS, Zhang ZC, Condon AE (2005) Secondary structure prediction of interacting RNA molecules. J Mol Biol 345:987–1001

16. Bernhart SH, Tafer H, Flamm C, Stadler PF, Hofacker IL (2006) Partition function and base pairing probabilities of RNA heterodimers. Algorithms Mol Biol 1:3

17. Dirks RM, Bois JS, Schaeffer JM, Winfree E, Pierce NA (2007) Thermodynamic analysis of interacting nucleic acid strands. SIAM Rev 49:65–88

18. Dimitrov RA, Zuker M (2004) Prediction of hybridization and melting for double-stranded nucleic acids. Biophys J 87:215–226

19. Mathews DH (2010) Using OligoWalk to identify efficient siRNA sequences. Methods Mol Biol 629:109–121

20. Andronescu MS, Pop C, Condon AE (2010) Improved free energy parameters for RNA pseudoknotted secondary structure prediction. RNA 16:26–42

21. Huang FWD, Qin J, Reidys CM, Stadler PF (2009) Partition function and base pairing probabilities for RNA–RNA interaction prediction. Bioinformatics 25:2646–2654

22. Chitsaz H, Salari R, Sahinalp SC, Backofen R (2009) A partition function algorithm for interacting nucleic acid strands. Bioinformatics 25(12):i365–i373

23. Cao S, Chen S-J (2005) Predicting RNA folding thermodynamics with a reduced chain representation model. RNA 11:1884–1897

24. Chen S-J (2008) RNA folding: conformational statistics, folding kinetics, and ion electrostatics. Annu Rev Biophys 37:197–214

25. Xu X, Zhao P, Chen S-J (2014) Vfold: a web server for RNA structure and folding thermodynamics prediction. PLoS One 9:e107504

26. Xu X, Chen S-J (2012) Kinetic mechanism of conformational switch between bistable RNA hairpins. J Am Chem Soc 134:12499–12507

27. Cao S, Chen S-J (2006) Predicting RNA pseudoknot folding thermodynamics. Nucleic Acids Res 34:2634–2652

28. Cao S, Chen S-J (2009) Predicting structures and stabilities for H-type pseudoknots with inter-helix loop. RNA 15:696–706

29. Cao S, Chen S-J (2012) A domain-based model for predicting large and complex pseudoknotted structures. RNA Biol 9:200–211

30. Turner DH, Mathews DH (2010) NNDB: the nearest neighbor parameter database for predicting stability of nucleic acid secondary structure. Nucleic Acids Res 38:D280–D282

31. Ennifar E, Walter P, Ehresmann B, Ehresmann C, Dumas P (2001) Crystal structures of coaxially stacked kissing complexes of the HIV-1 RNA dimerization initiation site. Nat Struct Biol 8:1064–1068

32. Muriaux D, De Rocquigny H, Roques BP, Paoletti J (1996) NCp7 activates HIV-1Lai RNA dimerization by converting a transient loop-loop complex into a stable dimer. J Biol Chem 271:33686–33692

33. Arnott S, Hukins DW, Dover SD (1972) Optimised parameters for RNA double-helices. Biochem Biophys Res Commun 48:1392–1399

Chapter 6

STarMir Tools for Prediction of microRNA Binding Sites

Shaveta Kanoria, William Rennie, Chaochun Liu, C. Steven Carmack, Jun Lu, and Ye Ding

Abstract

MicroRNAs (miRNAs) are a class of endogenous short noncoding RNAs that regulate gene expression by targeting messenger RNAs (mRNAs), which results in translational repression and/or mRNA degradation. As regulatory molecules, miRNAs are involved in many mammalian biological processes and also in the manifestation of certain human diseases. As miRNAs play central role in the regulation of gene expression, understanding miRNA-binding patterns is essential to gain an insight of miRNA mediated gene regulation and also holds promise for therapeutic applications. Computational prediction of miRNA binding sites on target mRNAs facilitates experimental investigation of miRNA functions. This chapter provides protocols for using the STarMir web server for improved predictions of miRNA binding sites on a target mRNA. As an application module of the Sfold RNA package, the current version of STarMir is an implementation of logistic prediction models developed with high-throughput miRNA binding data from cross-linking immunoprecipitation (CLIP) studies. The models incorporated comprehensive thermodynamic, structural, and sequence features, and were found to make improved predictions of both seed and seedless sites, in comparison to the established algorithms (Liu et al., Nucleic Acids Res 41:e138, 2013). Their broad applicability was indicated by their good performance in cross-species validation. STarMir is freely available at http://sfold.wadsworth.org/starmir.html.

Key words miRNA, CLIP, Target mRNA, RNA secondary structure, miRNA binding site

1 Introduction

MicroRNAs (miRNAs) are a class of naturally occurring, small noncoding RNAs (ncRNAs) of ~21–25 nucleotide (nt) in length. miRNAs have been found in plants, animals, and some viruses. A mature miRNA guides RNA-induced silencing complex (RISC) for target recognition by hybridizing to partially complementary sequences typically in the 3′ untranslated regions (3′ UTRs) of the target mRNAs, leading to translational repression and/or mRNA degradation of the target mRNA [2, 3]. miRNA mediated gene regulation is rather extensive, as one miRNA may regulate hundreds of targets, whereas an individual mRNA can be targeted by multiple miRNAs [4]. miRNAs play important roles in numerous

Douglas H. Turner and David H. Mathews (eds.), *RNA Structure Determination: Methods and Protocols*, Methods in Molecular Biology, vol. 1490, DOI 10.1007/978-1-4939-6433-8_6, © Springer Science+Business Media New York 2016

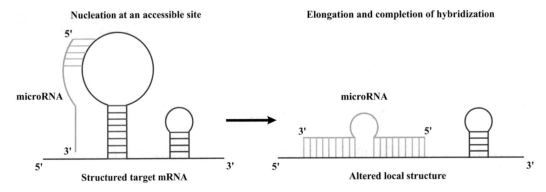

Fig. 1 A two-step hybridization model: nucleation at an accessible target site, followed by hybrid elongation to disrupt local target secondary structure and form the complete microRNA–target duplex [19]

biological processes including development, differentiation, apoptosis, and proliferation [3, 5]. Additionally, misregulation in miRNA activity has been found to be associated with human diseases [6, 7]. However, our current understanding of miRNA functions in physiological processes and diseases is rather limited. Identification of miRNA targets is essential for a full characterization of miRNA functions. For plants, identification of miRNA targets is straightforward, as most miRNAs are perfectly complementary to their target sequences [8]. However, in animals, the complementarity between miRNA and target mRNA is imperfect [9], presenting a challenge for binding site identification. Most of the algorithms for miRNA binding site prediction are based on the seed rule, i.e., the nucleotides of the target site forms Watson–Crick (WC) base pairs with nucleotide 2–7 or 8 of the 5′ end of the miRNA [10]. However, an increasing number of studies show that some miRNA binding sites do not follow the seed rule [11–15]. In addition to seed, several sequence features have been proposed to be important for miRNA target binding. These include sequence conservation, strong base-pairing to the 3′ end of the miRNA, local AU content and location of miRNA binding sites [16]. Based on a two-step model (Fig. 1) for the hybridization between a miRNA and an mRNA with target secondary structure predicted by Sfold [17, 18], the importance of target structure for miRNA target recognition was convincingly demonstrated [19–22]. Another independent mammalian study, established that structure based predictions could be more efficient than seed based predictions [23]. A recent study revealed that genetic variations can influence miRNA–target interactions and alter the structural accessibility of the binding sites as well as the flanking regions [24].

1.1 Identification of miRNA Binding Sites

Most existing algorithms for miRNA target prediction are primarily based on the seed rule. With the development of the CLIP technique [25], it has become possible to identify short AGO cross-linked sequences that contain miRNA binding sites. CLIP involves UV irradiation of tissues, organisms, or cells, to covalently cross-link miRNA targets to the Argonaute (AGO) proteins (the catalytic component of the RISC complex). The cross-linked RNAs are shortened by partial RNase digestion to ~50 nt and further amplified by RT-PCR. The shortened RNA fragments are then sequenced for identification of AGO tags containing miRNA binding sites on the target mRNAs. Numerous CLIP studies have been published in the recent years, including HITS-CLIP for mouse brain [25], PAR-CLIP in human cell lines [26], variants of PAR-CLIP [27], and a study in worm [28]. These CLIP studies generate short target fragments containing miRNA binding sites, thereby providing a genome wide map of miRNA target interactions. The high throughput data from the CLIP studies have been successfully utilized in the development of logistic models for making improved miRNA binding site predictions [1]. These models are based on a comprehensive list of sequence, thermodynamic, and target structure features that were found to be enriched for miRNA binding sites identified by CLIP, and were validated by intra-dataset, inter-dataset as well as cross-species validations [1]. The models have been implemented into the STarMir application module of the Sfold RNA package, which predicts miRNA binding sites on a target mRNA [29]. This chapter describes a detailed protocol for using STarMir web server. STarMir is a free web service available to all without any registration or e-mail requirement.

2   Materials

As an application module of the Sfold RNA package (http://sfold.wadsworth.org), STarMir can be freely accessed at http://sfold.wadsworth.org/starmir.html. Through a web browser such as Safari, Internet Explorer, or Firefox, the user can use the web service by providing either the miRNA ID and RefSeq ID for the mRNA or by submitting their miRNA and the target sequences.

3   Methods

3.1   Web Protocol for Using STarMir

This protocol outlines input and output of STarMir web service, provided through Sfold web server (http://sfold.wadsworth.org). The user can start by pointing a web browser to http://sfold.wadsworth.org/starmir.html.

3.2   STarMir Input Page

Figure 2 illustrates the main page with manual sequence entry option selected for both miRNA and target sequences. The user can input the sequence information for a single or multiple miRNAs and a single target mRNA for predicting miRNA binding

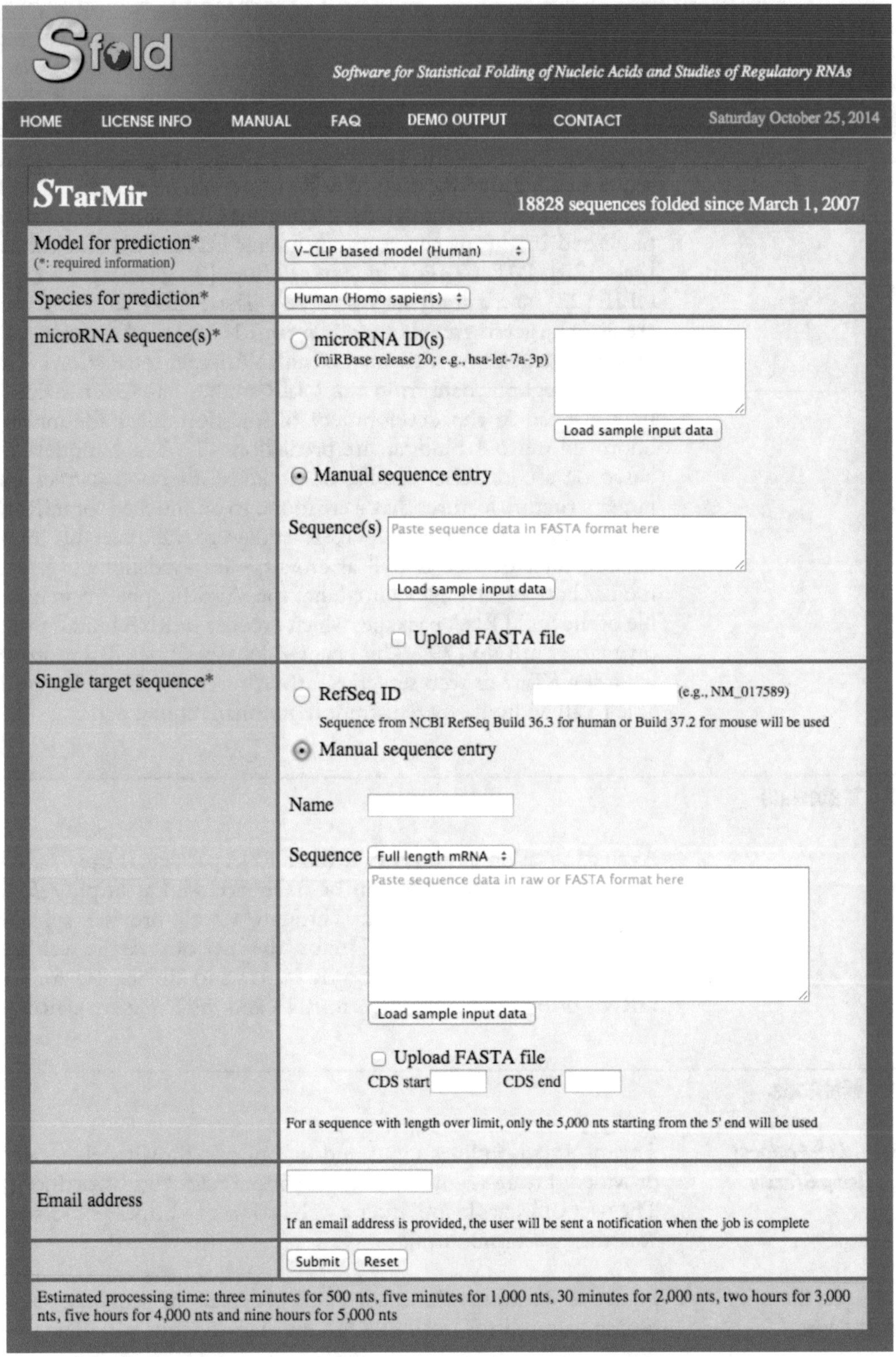

Fig. 2 STarMir input page displaying the input requirements for submitting miRNA and target mRNA sequences

sites. Upon job submission, a link is provided to the user for tracking the progress of the job and to access the prediction results. A detailed description of input is given below.

3.2.1 Model

STaRMir predicts miRNA binding sites based on three models for human, mouse, and worm. These models have been trained on V-CLIP data for human (*Homo sapiens*) [26], HITS-CLIP data for mouse (*Mus musculus*) [25], and ALG-1 CLIP data for worm (*Caenorhabditis elegans*), respectively [28]. The two mammalian models were cross-validated and can be broadly used for other species [1].

3.2.2 Species

The user needs to select a species for prediction. If the user enters the RefSeq ID of the target mRNA and selects one of the three modeling species, the species information will be used for retrieving pre-stored evolutionary conservation information in predictions. If the mRNA sequence information were entered manually, the selection of species would not have any effect on predictions. Furthermore, if "Other" is selected, conservation information cannot be used in predictions by our models.

3.2.3 miRNA

miRNA information can be provided in two ways. For the default option, one or more miRNA IDs can be entered (an example of miRNA ID is shown in Fig. 2), for which the sequences are retrieved from an internal database developed using release 20 of the miRBase [30]. An alternative is to enter one or more miRNA sequences into the input box in FASTA format, or upload a FASTA file (Fig. 2). Although there is no limit on the number of miRNA sequences that can be entered, each sequence must not be longer than 55 nt in length. Any characters other than A, T, G, C, and U in the entered miRNA sequence are removed.

3.2.4 mRNA

The target mRNA information can be entered in three different ways. The default method is to enter the RefSeq ID in the provided input box (Fig. 2), for which the sequence will be retrieved from our internal database of mRNA sequences for human and mouse. If the RefSeq ID of the mRNA is provided, evolutionary conservation information [31] will be used to make more accurate miRNA binding site predictions [1]. Alternatively, by selecting the 'Manual sequence entry' option, one can enter the sequence information in raw or FASTA format or upload a FASTA file. If the sequence is uploaded using a FASTA file, the file must not contain more than one sequence. As in the case of miRNA, any character in the mRNA sequences other than A, T, G, C and U is removed. As the current limit of the web server on the length of the mRNA sequence is 5000 nt, longer sequences will be truncated to 5000 nt starting from the 5′ end.

3.2.5 mRNA Region	For manual sequence entry, the user needs to inform the server if the entered sequence represents an entire mRNA or a single region, i.e., 3′ UTR, CDS or 5′ UTR, through a region dropdown box directly above the sequence input box. In the case of an entire mRNA, the nucleotide positions for the start and end of the coding region must be specified in the boxes shown below the input window (the first nucleotide of an entered sequence is counted as 1).
3.2.6 mRNA Name	If the user provides a RefSeq ID for the mRNA, the CDS start and end would be retrieved from our internal mRNA database and the binding sites will be predicted for all three mRNA regions. RefSeq ID would be considered as the name of the sequence for output. However, for a manually entered sequence, the user can enter the name of the sequence.
3.2.7 Email Address	Provision of an email address is optional. If an email address is provided, the user receives a notification once the job is completed. Alternatively, the user can check for job status using the link provided after job submission.
3.3 STarMir Output	Upon job completion, the results are presented through both an interactive viewer and downloadable files. An illustration of a typical output as an interactive viewer is shown in Fig. 3, with "CDS-seedless" tab and "hsa-let-7a-3p" selected for display. The results are categorized as seed and seedless sites for each of the three target mRNA regions, i.e., 3′ UTR, CDS and 5′ UTR. Each tab represents prediction results for one or all miRNAs, which can be selected from the dropdown menu. The sites are presented in the descending order of their logistic probability scores. The output presents comprehensive sequence, thermodynamic and target structure features including the logistic probability score as the measure of confidence for a predicted site. Additionally, a link is provided to the graphic representation of the hybrid conformation. Hybrid diagrams for a 7mer-m8 seed site and a seedless site are shown in Fig. 4. The PDF of the hybrid diagram is also available for visualization and download. Further, a file providing definitions of the features is available via the link for "Feature definitions" below the result table. The results are also provided as downloadable tab-delimited text files, which present all site features calculated by STarMir. The features marked with an asterisk (*) are the ones that are used in the prediction model. The prediction models are based on the features that were enriched in the CLIP experiments [1]. A text file is provided for each of the six categories, as shown in different tabs. Alternatively, all the results can also be downloaded as a compressed archive, including a text version of the hybrid conformation diagrams for each site and a file showing the probability of each nucleotide in the site to be unpaired or single-stranded.

Sfold — *Software for Statistical Folding of Nucleic Acids and Studies of Regulatory RNAs*

HOME   LICENSE INFO   MANUAL   FAQ   DEMO OUTPUT   CONTACT

Output for STarMir

Interactive site viewer for miRNA: hsa-let-7a-3p **and target: NM_017589**   **Prediction model training data (species): V-CLIP (human)**

3'UTR-seed | 3'UTR-seedless | CDS-seed | CDS-seedless | 5'UTR-seed | 5'UTR-seedless

miRNA	Site_Position	Hybrid Conformation	LogitProb†	3'_bp*	ΔG_{hybrid}	ΔG_{nuc}*	ΔG_{total}*	Site_Access*	Upstream_Access (10nt)*	Dwstream_Access (15nt)*	Upstream_AU (20nt)*	Dwstream_AU (20nt)*	Site_Consv*	Site_Location*
hsa-let-7a-3p	404-417	View	0.778	0	-16.600	-0.745	-3.105	0.261	0.534	0.389	0.700	0.800	0.999	0.326
hsa-let-7a-3p	537-549	View	0.749	0	-16.500	-1.133	-7.715	0.403	0.502	0.322	0.700	0.650	0.997	0.524
hsa-let-7a-3p	537-557	View	0.736	0	-19.100	-1.267	-3.810	0.330	0.502	0.538	0.700	0.700	0.936	0.524
hsa-let-7a-3p	404-423	View	0.666	0	-17.100	-0.285	-2.589	0.390	0.534	0.117	0.700	0.650	0.992	0.326
hsa-let-7a-3p	404-429	View	0.655	0	-17.400	-0.352	-1.880	0.312	0.534	0.291	0.700	0.600	0.955	0.326
hsa-let-7a-3p	455-496	View	0.522	0	-17	-2.892	0.447	0.348	0.228	0.114	0.450	0.600	0.998	0.402
hsa-let-7a-3p	455-490	View	0.513	0	-15.100	-0.326	4.866	0.294	0.228	0.332	0.450	0.600	0.997	0.402
hsa-let-7a-3p	188-230	View	0.503	1	-15.100	-0.484	10.202	0.349	0.538	0.643	0.800	0.750	0.998	0.004

† Logistic probability, our measure of confidence in the predicted site, is used to sort the binding sites in descending order

* Feature included in our prediction model for the selected target region.

Feature definitions

Output for download

Features and predictions for 3'UTR-seed sites	No sites for this case
Features and predictions for 3'UTR-seedless sites	3UTR_seedless_sites.txt
Features and predictions for CDS-seed sites	CDS_seed_sites.txt
Features and predictions for CDS-seedless sites	CDS_seedless_sites.txt
Features and predictions for 5'UTR-seed sites	No sites for this case
Features and predictions for 5'UTR-seedless sites	5UTR_seedless_sites.txt
Predicted conformations for all sites	conformation_all_sites.out
Probabilities for single-stranded bases at target sites	siteprob.out

Download all output files

Choose the file format for archiving and compressing output   zip   Download

Fig. 3 STarMir output page showing the interactive site viewer with "CDS-seedless" tab and 'hsa-let-7a-3p' selected for display. The download links for the text files are also shown

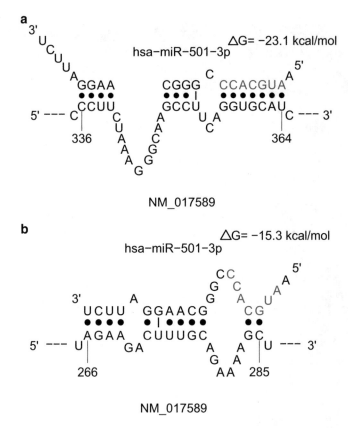

Fig. 4 Schematic representation of the hybrid diagrams for (**a**) a seed site (miRNA seed region (nt 2–7)) and (**b**) a seedless (noncanonical) site. The seed regions are shown in *red*

4   Notes

1. To further assist the users with STarMir input and output features, an online "MANUAL" as well as "DEMO OUTPUT" are provided at the STarMir front page.

2. As described above, the STarMir computes a logistic probability score from a selection of thermodynamic and structure based features. The logistic probability provides the measure of confidence in the predicted miRNA binding site. A site with a probability of 0.5 indicates a good chance of being a true miRNA binding site. Further, higher probability scores, e.g., 0.75 and above, suggests greater likelihood of miRNA binding in vivo.

3. In general, STarMir based predictions are time consuming due to RNA folding. For current Sfold web server, typical processing time is 3 min for 500 nt, 5 min for 1000 nt, 30 min for 2000 nt, 2 h for 3000 nt, 5 h for 4000 nt, and 9 h for 5000 nt.

Before a job submission, the users should first check STarMirDB, a database of precomputed transcriptome-scale prediction results currently available for human, mouse, and worm. STarMirDB complements STarMir, and is available at: http://sfold.wadsworth.org/starmirDB.php.

4. As the underlying models of the STarMir performed very well in cross-species validations, the applications of STarMir are not limited to the species with available CLIP data, but rather can be extended to other species as well.

5. As the CLIP methodology provides information of miRNA binding, the models developed from the CLIP data are efficient for prediction of miRNA binding sites and may not always be extendable to miRNA functions. In other words, these models do not make predictions for the functional outcome of miRNA binding (i.e., target degradation or translational repression) and the extent of regulation on either the mRNA or the protein.

6. A specific database is under development, based on a recent study on genetic variants within and near miRNA binding sites [24]. The database will allow users to search for polymorphisms in the context of miRNA binding sites.

Acknowledgements

The Computational Molecular Biology and Statistics Core at the Wadsworth Center is acknowledged for supporting computing resources for this work. This work is supported in part by the National Science Foundation (DBI-0650991 to Y.D.), National Institutes of Health (GM099811, GM116885 to Y.D. and J.L.).

References

1. Liu C, Mallick B, Long D, Rennie WA, Wolenc A, Carmack CS, Ding Y (2013) CLIP-based prediction of mammalian microRNA binding sites. Nucleic Acids Res 41:e138. doi:10.1093/nar/gkt435

2. Ambros V (2004) The functions of animal microRNAs. Nature 431(7006):350–355. doi:10.1038/nature02871

3. Bartel DP (2004) MicroRNAs: genomics, biogenesis, mechanism, and function. Cell 116(2):281–297

4. Friedman RC, Farh KK, Burge CB, Bartel DP (2009) Most mammalian mRNAs are conserved targets of microRNAs. Genome Res 19(1):92–105. doi:10.1101/gr.082701.108

5. Harfe BD (2005) MicroRNAs in vertebrate development. Curr Opin Genet Dev 15(4):410–415. doi:10.1016/j.gde.2005.06.012

6. Esau CC, Monia BP (2007) Therapeutic potential for microRNAs. Adv Drug Deliv Rev 59(2-3):1–114. doi:10.1016/j.addr.2007.03.007

7. Erson AE, Petty EM (2008) MicroRNAs in development and disease. Clin Genet 74(4):296–306. doi:10.1111/j.1399-0004.2008.01076.x

8. Rhoades MW, Reinhart BJ, Lim LP, Burge CB, Bartel B, Bartel DP (2002) Prediction of plant microRNA targets. Cell 110(4):513–520

9. Lewis BP, Shih IH, Jones-Rhoades MW, Bartel DP, Burge CB (2003) Prediction of mammalian microRNA targets. Cell 115(7):787–798

10. Lewis BP, Burge CB, Bartel DP (2005) Conserved seed pairing, often flanked by adenosines, indicates that thousands of human genes are microRNA targets. Cell 120(1):15–20. doi:10.1016/j.cell.2004.12.035

11. Tay Y, Zhang J, Thomson AM, Lim B, Rigoutsos I (2008) MicroRNAs to Nanog,

Oct4 and Sox2 coding regions modulate embryonic stem cell differentiation. Nature 455(7216):1124–1128.doi:10.1038/nature07299

12. Vella MC, Choi EY, Lin SY, Reinert K, Slack FJ (2004) The C. elegans microRNA let-7 binds to imperfect let-7 complementary sites from the lin-41 3′UTR. In: Genes Dev 18(2):132–137. doi:10.1101/gad.1165404

13. Didiano D, Hobert O (2006) Perfect seed pairing is not a generally reliable predictor for miRNA-target interactions. Nat Struct Mol Biol 13(9):849–851. doi:10.1038/nsmb1138

14. Loeb GB, Khan AA, Canner D, Hiatt JB, Shendure J, Darnell RB, Leslie CS, Rudensky AY (2012) Transcriptome-wide miR-155 binding map reveals widespread noncanonical microRNA targeting. Mol Cell 48(5):760–770. doi:10.1016/j.molcel.2012.10.002

15. Lal A, Navarro F, Maher CA, Maliszewski LE, Yan N, O'Day E, Chowdhury D, Dykxhoorn DM, Tsai P, Hofmann O, Becker KG, Gorospe M, Hide W, Lieberman J (2009) miR-24 Inhibits cell proliferation by targeting E2F2, MYC, and other cell-cycle genes via binding to "seedless" 3′UTR microRNA recognition elements. Mol Cell 35(5):610–625. doi:10.1016/j.molcel.2009.08.020

16. Bartel DP (2009) MicroRNAs: target recognition and regulatory functions. Cell 136(2):215–233. doi:10.1016/j.cell.2009.01.002

17. Ding Y, Lawrence CE (2003) A statistical sampling algorithm for RNA secondary structure prediction. Nucleic Acids Res 31(24):7280–7301

18. Ding Y, Chan CY, Lawrence CE (2004) Sfold web server for statistical folding and rational design of nucleic acids. Nucleic Acids Res 32(Web Server issue):W135–W141. doi:10.1093/nar/gkh449

19. Long D, Lee R, Williams P, Chan CY, Ambros V, Ding Y (2007) Potent effect of target structure on microRNA function. Nat Struct Mol Biol 14(4):287–294. doi:10.1038/nsmb1226

20. Long D, Chan CY, Ding Y (2008) Analysis of microRNA-target interactions by a target structure based hybridization model. Pac Symp Biocomput:64–74

21. Hammell M, Long D, Zhang L, Lee A, Carmack CS, Han M, Ding Y, Ambros V (2008) mir-WIP: microRNA target prediction based on microRNA-containing ribonucleoprotein-enriched transcripts. Nat Methods 5(9):813–819. doi:10.1038/nmeth.1247

22. Liu C, Rennie WA, Mallick B, Kanoria S, Long D, Wolenc A, Carmack CS, Ding Y (2014) MicroRNA binding sites in C. elegans 3′ UTRs. RNA Biol 11(6):693–701

23. Malhas A, Saunders NJ, Vaux DJ (2010) The nuclear envelope can control gene expression and cell cycle progression via miRNA regulation. Cell Cycle 9(3):531–539

24. Liu C, Rennie WA, Carmack CS, Kanoria S, Cheng J, Lu J, Ding Y (2014) Effects of genetic variations on microRNA: target interactions. Nucleic Acids Res 42(15):9543–9552. doi:10.1093/nar/gku675

25. Chi SW, Zang JB, Mele A, Darnell RB (2009) Argonaute HITS-CLIP decodes microRNA-mRNA interaction maps. Nature 460(7254):479–486. doi:10.1038/nature08170

26. Hafner M, Landthaler M, Burger L, Khorshid M, Hausser J, Berninger P, Rothballer A, Ascano M Jr, Jungkamp AC, Munschauer M, Ulrich A, Wardle GS, Dewell S, Zavolan M, Tuschl T (2010) Transcriptome-wide identification of RNA-binding protein and microRNA target sites by PAR-CLIP. Cell 141(1):129–141. doi:10.1016/j.cell.2010.03.009

27. Kishore S, Jaskiewicz L, Burger L, Hausser J, Khorshid M, Zavolan M (2011) A quantitative analysis of CLIP methods for identifying binding sites of RNA-binding proteins. Nat Methods 8(7):559–564. doi:10.1038/nmeth.1608

28. Zisoulis DG, Lovci MT, Wilbert ML, Hutt KR, Liang TY, Pasquinelli AE, Yeo GW (2010) Comprehensive discovery of endogenous Argonaute binding sites in Caenorhabditis elegans. Nat Struct Mol Biol 17(2):173–179. doi:10.1038/nsmb.1745

29. Rennie W, Liu C, Carmack CS, Wolenc A, Kanoria S, Lu J, Long D, Ding Y (2014) STarMir: a web server for prediction of microRNA binding sites. Nucleic Acids Res 42(Web Server issue):W114–W118. doi:10.1093/nar/gku376

30. Kozomara A, Griffiths-Jones S (2014) miRBase: annotating high confidence microRNAs using deep sequencing data. Nucleic Acids Res 42(Database issue):D68–D73. doi:10.1093/nar/gkt1181

31. Siepel A, Bejerano G, Pedersen JS, Hinrichs AS, Hou M, Rosenbloom K, Clawson H, Spieth J, Hillier LW, Richards S, Weinstock GM, Wilson RK, Gibbs RA, Kent WJ, Miller W, Haussler D (2005) Evolutionarily conserved elements in vertebrate, insect, worm, and yeast genomes. Genome Res 15(8):1034–1050. doi:10.1101/gr.3715005

Chapter 7

Traditional Chemical Mapping of RNA Structure In Vitro and In Vivo

Pierre Fechter, Delphine Parmentier, ZongFu Wu, Olivier Fuchsbauer, Pascale Romby, and Stefano Marzi

Abstract

Chemical probing is often used to gain knowledge on the secondary and tertiary structures of RNA molecules either free or engaged in complexes with ligands. The method monitors the reactivity of each nucleotide towards chemicals of various specificities reflecting the hydrogen bonding environment of each nucleotide within the RNA molecule. In addition, information can be obtained on the binding site of a ligand (noncoding RNAs, protein, metabolites), and on RNA conformational changes that accompanied ligand binding or perturbation of the environmental cues. The detection of the modifications can be obtained either by using end-labeled RNA molecules or by primer extension using reverse transcriptase. The goal of this chapter is to provide the reader with an experimental guide to probe the structure of RNA in vitro and in vivo with the most suitable chemical probes.

Key words RNA structure probing, Chemical mapping, Lead(II) induced cleavages

1 Introduction

Despite its chemical simplicity, RNAs fold into intricate three-dimensional structures that are able to recognize a variety of *trans*-acting ligands such as nucleic acids, proteins, and small molecules with high affinity and specificity. Moreover, the ability of RNA molecules to adopt alternative conformations makes them ideal regulators of gene expression (for reviews *see* refs. [1, 2]). For instance, bacterial mRNAs can adopt highly structured domains in their 5′ untranslated regions which serve as genetic switches in response to temperature [3, 4], pH [5], divalent ions [6], and to the intracellular concentration of metabolites [7], uncharged tRNAs [8], RNA-binding proteins [9], noncoding RNAs [10, 11], and foreign DNA [12]. Furthermore, the folding of an RNA molecule is a complex process that occurs during its transcription. Analysis of the transcription speed, pausing properties of RNA polymerase and the effect of the transcriptional complex and

Douglas H. Turner and David H. Mathews (eds.), *RNA Structure Determination: Methods and Protocols*, Methods in Molecular Biology, vol. 1490, DOI 10.1007/978-1-4939-6433-8_7, © Springer Science+Business Media New York 2016

associated factors can reveal insights on the folding pathway of the nascent transcript and on folding intermediates occurring along this pathway [13]. Thus, there is an increasing interest in studying the structural features of RNAs, their plasticity and versatility, and their folding pathways [14], and many of these aspects of RNA biology can be addressed using chemical mapping experiments.

Chemicals have the obvious advantage of probing RNA molecules of any size under a wide range of experimental conditions (i.e., by varying temperature, pH, and the concentration of monovalent and divalent ions). The accessibility or the reactivity of each nucleotide towards chemicals identifies without ambiguity the unpaired regions of RNAs. The combination of dimethylsulfate (DMS), 1-cyclohexyl-3-(2-morpholinoethyl)carbodiimide metho-p-toluene sulfonate (CMCT), and kethoxal provides information on the four bases at one of their Watson–Crick positions. Diethylpyrocarbonate (DEPC) and Nickel-complex map the adenines and guanines, respectively, at their N7-position (Table 1). These two reagents are very sensitive to the stacking of the base rings and attack only these positions within a helix if the deep groove is widened [15]. Besides these base-specific reagents, other probes cleave or modify RNA in a sequence-independent manner. Hydroxyl radicals generated by Fe-EDTA, which cleave the riboses, are useful to map the solvent-accessible surface and divalent ion binding pocket of large and compact RNA structures. This tool has been particularly used in time-resolved probing techniques to follow conformational rearrangements and transient interactions occurring during RNA folding or during the assembly of RNA-ligand complexes [16]. Finally, other approaches such as lead(II)-induced cleavages [17], acylation of ribose 2'-OH functions by 1M7 (SHAPE) [18], and in-line probing [19] are based on differences in the flexibility of individual internucleotide linkages and gave information on unpaired regions regardless of the RNA sequence.

The reactivity of each nucleotide is used as constraints to elaborate reliable RNA secondary structure model inferred from the sequence. This is often obtained by coupling the mapping data with the help of several computer folding programs which are based on energy minimization [20], statistics [21], stochastic simulations [22], nearest-neighbor methods [23], and on phylogenetic and sequence comparison [24]. The latter approach takes into account the base compensatory changes and/or mutations occurring during evolution in addition to the structure probing data. Several programs can also predict long-range interactions like pseudoknots or tertiary structure modules [25–28]. Once the secondary structure has been established, three-dimensional models can be built ab initio or by homology modeling using an RNA motif database (for a review, *see* ref. [29]). The resulting model can be further validated by site-directed mutagenesis studies coupled

Table 1
List of the most commonly used chemicals for probing RNA structure

Probes	Target	Modification	Direct detection	RT detection	In vivo	Comments
Base-specific chemicals						
DMS	A(N1)	**N1**–CH$_3$	–	+	+	• pH 4.5–10
	C(N3)	**N3**–CH$_3$	+^{a}	+	+	• $T°$ 4–90 °C
	G(N7).	**N7**–CH$_3$	+^{a}	+^{a}	+	• Tris should be avoided because DMS reacts with amine groups
DEPC^b	A(N7)	**N7**–CO$_2$H$_2$	+^{a}	+	?	• pH 4.5–10 • $T°$ 4–90 °C • Tris should be avoided because DEPC reacts with amine groups
CMCT	G(N1)	**N1**–C=N–R	–	+	–	• pH 8
	U(N3)	| NH–R′ **N3**–C=N–R | NH–R′	–	+	–	• $T°$ 4–90 °C • Soluble up to 300 mg/mL in water
Kethoxal	G(N1)	**N1**–CH–OH	–	+	+	• pH 8
	G(N2)	| R– C–OH | **N2**–N–H				• Stabilized by borate ions
Ribose specific reagent						
1M7^c	• 2′-OH ribose	O-acylation	–	+	+	• Active under a wide range of conditions
	• Monitor nucleotide flexibility					• Rapidly hydrolyzed in water
Divalent ions and hydrolytic cleavages						
Pb(II) acetate	• Specific binding sites for divalent ions • Unpaired and dynamic regions	…Np (3′p)	+	+	+	• Chloride should be avoided • Reaction is stopped by the addition of EDTA
Ni(II) complex	• Unpaired guanines, G(N7)	Oxidation of guanine	+^{a}	+	?	• Reaction is stopped by the addition of EDTA

(continued)

Table 1
(continued)

Probes	Target	Modification	Direct detection	RT detection	In vivo	Comments
Fe-EDTA (radical hydroxyl)	• Accessible surface of large RNA • Binding sites for divalent ions	• Cleavage at ribose (C1′, C4′)	+	+	?	• Reactivity relatively insensitive to pH, $T°C$ • Only sodium phosphate should be avoided and glycerol (lower than 0.5%)
In-line probing[b]	• Unpaired nt	Phosphate linkage cleavage	+	+	?	• Works under a wide range of conditions: salt and Mg, $T°C$ • Optimal pH 7.5–8 • Long incubation time

DMS dimethylsulfate, *DEPC* diethylpyrocarbonate, *CMCT* 1-cyclohexyl-3-(2-morpholinoethyl) carbodiimide metho-*p*-toluene sulfonate

[a]A chemical treatment is necessary to cleave the ribose–phosphate chain prior to the detection. In vivo mapping: probes, which diffuse efficiently across membranes and cell walls (+), other probes can be used after permeabilization of the cell (–), probes that have not yet been used in vivo (?). Specificity, and products generated by the probe action are indicated. Most of the probes provided information useful to build a secondary structure model and elements of the tertiary folding, and to map the binding sites of RNA ligands

[b]Not appropriate for mapping the binding sites of proteins because DEPC modifies proteins and the time of incubation for in-line probing is quite long

[c]1M7, 1-methyl-7-nitroisatoic anhydride, other derivatives of 1M7 are NMIA (*N*-methylisatoic anhydride) and BzCN (benzoyl cyanide). Detection method: (direct) detection of cleavages on end-labeled RNA molecule; (indirect) detection by primer extension with reverse transcriptase using either ^{32}P-labeled primer or primer labeled at the 5′ end with a fluorophore. (+) The corresponding detection method can be used

Bold characters indicate modified nitrogens, numbered according to standard nucleotide nomenclature

with chemical probing to analyze the effect of mutations on the RNA structure. For instance, compensatory base changes validate the existence of base pairings, and appropriate deletion help to define independent structural domains.

Alternative methods using chemicals have been developed. Chemicals have been extensively used to map the binding site of a specific ligand, to study RNP assembly and the conformational changes of the RNA (for reviews *see* refs. [30, 31]). A complementary approach, the so-called chemical interference, defines a set of nucleotides, which have lost the capability to interact with a ligand when they are modified by a chemical probe. Finally, chemical probes tethered to protein or RNA can provide topographical information on ligand-RNA complexes by inducing site-specific cleavage of a proximal RNA after binding (e.g., [32, 33]).

One of the main concerns is how the RNA can be folded in a more complex environment such as in living cells. Ligand binding may indeed change the RNA folding or stabilize a defined conformation. Structure-specific chemical probes are unique tools to map RNA structure in vivo under different cell growth conditions. The use of probes is however limited by their inability to penetrate the cell wall and membrane due to their size, structure, and/or charge. The reagents that have gained widespread use for in vivo RNA probing are dimethylsulfate (e.g., [34, 35]), to a lesser extent kethoxal [36], lead(II)-induced cleavages [37], and SHAPE [38]. The comparison between in vivo and in vitro probing provides complementary data for determining functional RNA structure. Interestingly, new high-throughput technologies have been recently developed to study RNA structural features within complex RNA populations in vitro where numerous molecules could be probed at once [39]. These techniques combine acylation of ribose 2'-OH with multiplexed paired-end deep sequencing of primer extension products. Due to these major innovations in the detection and analysis of the chemical probing data, a full appreciation of the RNA structure dynamics in living organisms can be reachable in a near future.

Here, we provide an experimental guide of the most commonly used chemical probes and lead(II)-induced cleavages for mapping the structure of a specific RNA in vitro and in vivo.

2 Material

2.1 Equipment

1. Equipment for denaturing PAGE (Model S2, Gibco BRL) is used to size end-labeled RNA products and labeled cDNA fragments.

2. Basic laboratory materials are required such as microcentrifuge, vortex, thermoblock, water bath, radioactivity counter.

3. Eppendorf tubes, tips, and buffers should be sterilized before use.

2.2 RNA Preparation

1. DNA template for in vitro transcription (e.g., a linearized plasmid or a PCR product containing the sequence of interest under the control of a T7 promoter).

2. T7 RNA polymerase 50,000 U/mL (Biolabs) supplied with 10× reaction buffer.

2.3 End Labeling of RNAs and of Oligo-deoxyribonucleotide

1. Safety rules have to be applied for handling radioactive materials (*see* **Note 1**).

2. In vitro transcribed RNA purified and dephosphorylated at its 5' end (around 5 μg).

3. HPLC-purified oligodeoxyribonucleotide, 50 mM in water. Store at −20 °C.

4. T4 polynucleotide kinase (PNK) 10 U/mL (Ambion, Austin, USA).

5. T4 RNA ligase (Ambion, Austin, USA).

6. Radiochemicals: [γ-³²P]ATP (3000 Ci/mmol); [5′-³²P]pCp (3000 Ci/mmol) (Amersham).

7. *RNA elution buffer*: 500 mM ammonium acetate, pH 6.5, 1 mM ethylenediaminetetraacetic acid (EDTA).

8. Phenol saturated with 0.1 M Na-acetate, pH 5.5.

9. Phenol–chloroform–isoamyl alcohol (25:24:1) mixture, pH 5.5.

2.4 Modification Reaction

1. Most of these chemical reagents are potential carcinogens; therefore, until the removal of the first ethanol supernatant, chemical modification procedures are carried out under a fume hood. DMS and kethoxal solutions are discarded in 1 M sodium hydroxide waste and CMCT in 10 % acetic acid waste (*see* **Note 1**).

2. RNA transcripts are synthesized in vitro using T7 RNA polymerase and purified on polyacrylamide gel electrophoresis under denaturing conditions. After elution, the RNA is kept at −20 °C in sterile bi-distilled water and renatured just before use.

3. Buffer N1 5×: 250 mM sodium cacodylate pH 7.5, 25 mM magnesium acetate, 250 mM ammonium chloride.

4. Buffer N2 5×: 250 mM sodium borate pH 8.0, 50 mM magnesium acetate, 250 mM ammonium chloride.

5. Buffer N3 5×: 250 mM Tris acetate pH 7.5, 5 mM magnesium acetate, 100 mM potassium acetate (*see* **Note 2**).

6. Chemical probes: DMS (Aldrich) is diluted 1:30 in 100 % ethanol; CMCT (Aldrich) is dissolved at 100 mg/mL in water, and kethoxal (ICN Biochemicals) is diluted at 40 mg/mL in 20 % ethanol (*see* **Note 3**). DEPC (Sigma-Aldrich) is not diluted before the reaction. The reagents are prepared just before use.

7. Lead(II) acetate purchased from Acros organics is extemporaneously dissolved in sterile bi-distilled water.

8. Total tRNA from yeast is purchased from Sigma.

2.5 Fractionation of End-Labeled RNA Fragments

1. *Buffer T1*: 20 mM sodium citrate pH 4.5, 1 mM EDTA, 7 M urea, 0.02 % xylene cyanol, 0.02 % bromophenol blue.

2. *Ladder Buffer*: 0.1 M Na_2CO_3/0.1 M $NaHCO_3$ pH 9.

3. *RNA loading buffer*: 0.02 % xylene cyanol, 0.02 % bromophenol blue in 8 M urea.

2.6 Detection of Cleavages by Primer Extension

1. 10× *RTB buffer*: 500 mM Tris–HCl pH 8.3, 100 mM $MgCl_2$, 500 mM KCl, 10 mM DTT.

2. Prepare a dNTP mix (2.5 mM of dATP, dGTP, dCTP, dTTP) (Promega).

3. For sequencing reactions, prepare each ddNTP at 5 mM (GE Healthcare Life Sciences).

4. Primer extension is performed with avian myeloblastosis virus reverse transcriptase (AMV RT) purchased from Finnzymes (France) or from Life Sciences (USA).

5. *DNA loading buffer*: 1 mM EDTA, 0.02 % xylene cyanol, 0.02 % bromophenol blue in formamide.

2.7 Fractionation of Cleaved Fragments by Polyacrylamide–Urea Gel Electrophoresis

1. Electrophoresis apparatus for slab gels (30 cm×40 cm, BRL) and generator (2000 V, Bio-Rad) are required for the separation of the end-labeled RNA or cDNA fragments generated after enzymatic hydrolysis on polyacrylamide-urea gel electrophoresis (PAGE).

2. *TBE buffer*: 0.09 M Tris-borate pH 8.3, 1 mM EDTA.

3. Prepare 1 L solution of polyacrylamide 25 % in urea 8 M: dissolve 480 g urea (Merck) in 625 mL Rotiphorese 40 (acrylamide–bis-acrylamide: 19/1, Roth, Karlsruhe, Germany). Complete with bi-distillated water, filtrate the solution.

4. Products for acrylamide polymerization: N,N,N',N'-tetramethyl-ethylenediamine or TEMED (Roth); ammonium persulfate should be prepared as a 10 % (w/v) solution in water.

5. *Gel fixing solution*: 10% ethanol, 6% acetic acid in water. Prepare 2 L before gel fixing.

3 Methods

3.1 Establishing the Protocols

1. To probe the structure of RNAs with different chemicals requires the use of defined buffer conditions (pH, ionic strength, magnesium concentration, temperature). The choice of the buffers will depend on the biological function of the analyzed RNA and will take into account the optimal conditions for the chemical reaction (Table 1). For instance CMCT and kethoxal reactions only work at pH 8.0. Many of the chemicals work in a large range of monovalent and divalent ion concentration and of temperature. Hence, the influence of magnesium can be tested on the RNA folding, and thermal transition of RNAs can be obtained by varying the temperature (*see* **Note 4**). These experiments provide information on the stability of stem-loop structures, and on tertiary elements which are the first to break during the melting of the RNA structure.

2. The chemical reaction is influenced significantly by the electro-static environment of the nucleotides. Hence, the reactivity of a nucleotide does not always reflect the stereochemical accessibility. However, chemical probing is a method of choice to build reliable secondary structure models and to unravel the existence of specific structural modules involving noncanonical base pairs (i.e., Loop C motif in Fig. 1 [40]). In particular, base-specific chemicals easily detect noncanonical base pairs like sheared A-G base pair or reverse Hoogsteen A-U base pair, which are widespread in RNA molecules.

3. The probe:RNA ratio must be adapted so that the experiments are conducted under limited and statistical conditions in order to get less than one modification or cleavage per molecule. For the first experiment, different concentrations of the chemical probe and a time-scale dependence should be performed. Reducing agents (DTT, or ß-mercaptoethanol) should be included in footprinting assays if the RNA ligand is a protein.

4. The protocols have been adapted for the analysis of the *Escherichia coli thrS* mRNA [41]. Typical experiment is shown in Fig. 1.

3.2 Choice of the Detection Method

1. The identification of the cleavages depends on the length of the RNA molecule. The use of end-labeled RNA is limited to molecules containing less than 200 nucleotides, and this method can only detect cleavages. The primer extension approach detects stops of reverse transcription (RT) at the residue preceding a cleavage or a modification at a Watson–Crick position. Modification at the N7 position of adenine by DEPC is sufficiently bulky to arrest reverse transcriptase. However, for modification of the N7 position of guanines by DMS, a specific treatment is required to induce specific cleavage at the modification site. The length of the primer varies from 12 to 18 nucleotides. For long RNA, primers are selected every 200 nucleotides when gel electrophoresis is used for data analysis.

Fig. 1 (continued) of *thrS* mRNA in the presence of increasing concentrations of threonyl-tRNA synthetase (ThrRS) (lane 9, 50 nM; lane 10, 100 nM; lane 11, 250 nM). (Lanes A, G, C, U) sequencing ladders corresponding to the mRNA sequence. (**b**) Structure of the stem-loop located in the 5′ leader of *thrS* mRNA that is specifically recognized by ThrRS. (*Top*) Crystallographic structure of the stem-loop structure according to [47]. Nucleotides reactive towards chemicals are in *grey*. (*Bottom*) Secondary structure model showing the reactivity of nucleotides towards DMS (N1A, N3C) and CMCT (N3U, N1G): *circled* nucleotides are reactive: strong (*black circle*) and weak reactivity (*dashed circle*); no symbol, not reactive. The internal loop, the so-called loop C motif, adopts a particular structure formed by three stacked triple base pairs explaining the weak reactivity of A-20 at N1, and the non reactivity of C-21 at N3 towards DMS while U-43 which is bulging out is highly reactive at N3 towards CMCT. Most of the nucleotides of the apical loop are also highly reactive at one of their Watson–Crick position. This loop is the main binding site of ThrRS as evidenced by the protection observed at N3 positions of U-29, U-31, U-34, and U-35 and N1 position of G-32 while N1 position of G-30 became more reactive upon protein binding. The chemical data were fully correlated with the crystal structure of *thrS* mRNA associated with ThrRS [47]

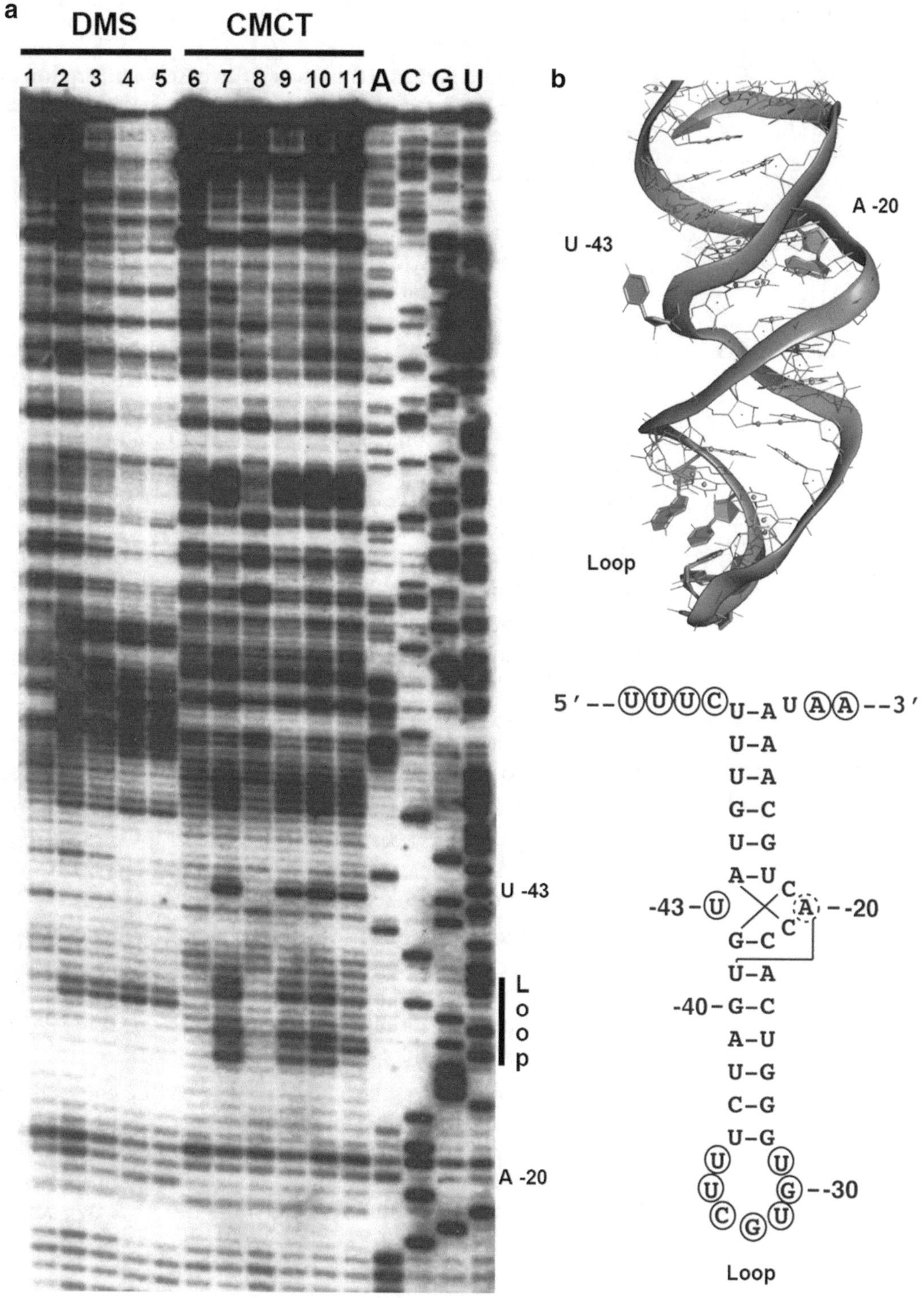

Fig. 1 Chemical probing on *Escherichia coli thrS* mRNA. (**a**) Gel electrophoresis fractionation of products resulting from dimethylsulfate (DMS; N1A≫N3C) and 1-cyclohexyl-3-(2-morpholinoethyl) carbodiimide metho-*p*-toluene sulfonate (CMCT; N3U≫N1G) modifications followed by primer extension analysis. (Lane 1, 6) Incubation controls performed in the absence of DMS or CMCT, respectively; (lanes 2–5) DMS reactions performed with 1 µL of pure DMS (lane 2), 1 µL of DMS diluted in ethanol 1:2 (lane 3), 1:5 (lane 4), or 1:10 (lane 5); (lane 7) CMCT modification of free mRNA in the presence of 4 µL of CMCT 40 mg/mL; (lanes 9–11) CMCT modification

2. Assays should be performed to define the best concentration of the RNA, the choice of the primer sequence, and the hybridization conditions in order to get an efficient primer extension.

3. As an alternative approach, primer extension can be done using fluorescently labeled oligonucleotides and the labeled DNA fragments are sized by capillary electrophoresis. This sensitive method permits an easy quantification of the data using whole-trace Gaussian integration [42].

3.3   RNA Preparation

1. The RNA is transcribed in vitro with T7 RNA polymerase from a plasmid template carrying the T7 promoter fused to the gene of interest. Depending on the size of the RNA, the purification is done by gel filtration column [43], monoQ column [44], or denaturing polyacrylamide-urea gel electrophoresis (PAGE) [45]. Although PAGE is the best method to separate full-length RNA from abortive transcription or cleavage products, the elution process of the RNA from the gel is not highly efficient for rather long RNAs (>500 nts) (*see* **Note 5**).

2. For 5′ end labeling, the RNA is previously dephosphorylated at its 5′ end, and labeled using [γ-^{32}P]ATP (150 μCi) and T4 polynucleotide kinase according to the Ambion protocol (http://www.ambion.com/techlib/misc/RNA5_labeling.html). To avoid the 5′ dephosphorylation of RNA, which is not efficient for structured RNAs, in vitro RNA transcription can be started with ApG (Sigma).

3. The 3′ end labeling is performed with [5′-^{32}P]pCp (150 μCi) and T4 RNA ligase according to the Ambion protocol (http://www.ambion.com/techlib/misc/RNA3_labeling.html).

4. The labeled RNA can be purified by gel filtration. However to get a homogenous RNA, we usually prefer to purify the RNA by electrophoresis on 8 % polyacrylamide (0.5 % bis-acrylamide): 8 M urea slab gels. To the sample, 5 μL of *RNA loading buffer* is added before PAGE loading.

5. After PAGE purification, labeled or cold RNAs are eluted from gel slices covered with the *RNA elution buffer* in the presence of 20 % (vol) phenol, and passive elution is done at 4 °C overnight by gently mixing. After phenol extraction, the RNA is precipitated with 2.5 volumes of cold ethanol. After two washing steps with 200 μL of 70 % cold ethanol, the pellet is vacuum-dried and dissolved in sterile bi-distillated water.

6. Since the RNA is purified under denaturing conditions, it is worth spending effort to carry out a renaturation process before the probing experiments (*see* **Note 6**). One protocol is as follows: the RNA is pre-incubated 1 min at 90 °C in sterile bi-distillated water, quickly cooled on ice (1 min) and brought back (20 min) at 20 °C or at 37 °C in the appropriate buffer containing MgCl$_2$.

3.4 Lead(II)-Induced Cleavages of RNAs In Vitro

1. Labeled mRNA (1 μL, 50,000 cpm) or the cold RNA species (2 pmol, 1 μL) are previously denatured in water (Subheading 3.3, **step 6**) and renatured in the presence of 4 μL of buffer N3 5× at 20 °C (or 37 °C) for 15 min. The reactions are carried out in a total volume of 20 μL.

2. 1 μL of total tRNA (1 μg) is added to all samples.

3. Hydrolysis is initiated with 2.5 μL of different concentrations of lead(II)-acetate from 12 mM, 40 mM, 80 mM to 120 mM for 10 min at 20 °C or 5 min at 37 °C. (The best conditions in our hand is 40 mM.) Mix and centrifuge briefly the samples (*see* **Note 2**).

4. An incubation control is performed in which lead(II)-acetate is replaced by sterile bi-distilled water.

5. The reactions are stopped by adding 5 μL of 0.1 M EDTA.

6. To all samples, 50 μL of 0.3 M sodium acetate pH 5.5 and 150 μL of cold ethanol are added. After a vigorous mix, the samples are transferred to a dry ice–ethanol bath for 10 min and centrifuged ($13,000 \times g$ at 4 °C for 15 min).

7. The supernatant is discarded with caution (if end-labeled RNA is used, check that no radioactivity is present). The pellet is washed with 200 μL of 80% cold ethanol. The samples are centrifuged ($13,000 \times g$ at 4 °C for 5 min), and the supernatants are removed. This step is repeated once.

8. The pellets are vacuum-dried for several seconds and dissolved in either 4 μL of sterile bi-distilled water (for primer extension) or dissolved in 6 μL of *RNA loading buffer* for PAGE analysis.

3.5 Base-Specific Modification of RNA In Vitro

1. We provide here protocols for primer extension of RNAs modified by DMS (N1A, N3C, N7G), CMCT (N1G, N3U), kethoxal (N1, N2G) and DEPC (N7). To visualize methylation of N7 of guanines by DMS, an additional treatment has to be carried out to cleave the ribose–phosphate backbone at the modification sites. For the interpretation of the data, it should be reminded that DMS methylates more strongly N1A than N3C and CMCT modifies more strongly N3U than N1G. Uridines are occasionally stabilized in an enol-tautomer form due to a specific local environment and can be reactive towards DMS at their N3 position. Reactions with CMCT and kethoxal have to be carried out at pH 8.0. In addition kethoxal reacts with the N1 and N2 Watson–Crick positions of guanine, giving a cyclic adduct between these two positions and its two carbonyls, which has to be stabilized by borate ions.

2. All reactions are carried out in a total volume of 20 μL. A control lacking the reagent is incubated in parallel under the same conditions to detect pauses of reverse transcriptase. Unlabeled

mRNA is first heated in sterile bi-distillated water at 90 °C for 1 min, then cooled on ice for 1 min and renatured in the appropriate buffer.

3.5.1 DMS Modification (N3C, N1A)

1. 2 pmol of mRNA (per assay) is renatured by incubation at 37 °C for 5 min in buffer N1 1×.

2. 1 μL of tRNA (2 μg/μL) and 1 μL of pure DMS or 1 μL of DMS freshly diluted in ethanol at 1:2 (vol/vol), 1:5 or 1:10 are added. For the incubation control, DMS is replaced by ethanol. The tubes are gently mixed and rapidly centrifuged. The reaction is performed in a total volume of 20 μL at 37 °C for 5 min. The optimal chemical modification is obtained with DMS diluted at 1:10.

3. The reactions are stopped by ethanol precipitation of the RNA as described above (Subheading 3.4, **steps 6–8**).

3.5.2 DMS Modification (N7G)

1. The same conditions are used as for DMS modifications of N3C and N1A except that the reaction is carried out for 15 min at 37 °C.

2. After ethanol precipitation (*see* Subheading 3.4, **steps 6, 7** and **8**), the pellets are dissolved in 10 μL of 1 M Tris–HCl pH 8.3 and 10 μL of 8 mg/mL sodium borohydrate (dissolved in water extemporaneously). The reaction is carried out in the dark and on ice for 10 min, followed by ethanol precipitation of the modified RNA (Subheading 3.4, **steps 6, 7** and **8**).

3. The RNA pellets are dissolved in 10 μL of aniline (100 μL of bi-distilled aniline (Fluka), 60 μL acetic acid, 930 μL H_2O) and incubated at 60 °C for 10 min in the dark. The reactions are stopped by ethanol precipitation and treated as described above (Subheading 3.4, **steps 6, 7–9**).

3.5.3 CMCT Modification (N3U, N1G)

1. 2 pmol of mRNA (per assay) is first incubated at 37 °C for 10 min in buffer N2 1× in a total volume of 15 μL.

2. 1 μL of tRNA (2 μg/μL) and 4 μL of CMCT (40 or 60 mg/mL dissolved in buffer N2 1× just before use) are added, and the samples are gently mixed. The modification is carried out in a total volume of 20 μL at 37 °C for 10 min or at 20 °C for 20 min. The optimal modification of mRNA is seen with CMCT at 40 mg/mL. The reactions are stopped by ethanol precipitation and treated as described above (Subheading 3.4, **steps 6–8**).

3.5.4 DEPC Carbethoxylation (N7A)

1. 2 pmol of mRNA (per assay) is renatured by incubation at 37 °C for 15 min in buffer N1 1× in a total volume of 15 μL.

2. 1 μL of tRNA (2 μg/μL) and 4 μL of pure DEPC are added, and the tubes are mixed gently. The reaction is carried out at

37 °C for 20 min in a total volume of 20 μL. The reactions are stopped by ethanol precipitation as described above (Subheading 3.4, **steps 6–8**).

3.5.5 Kethoxal Modification (N1,N2G)

1. 2 pmol of mRNA (per assay) is renatured by incubation at 37 °C for 15 min in buffer N3 1× in a total volume of 15 μL.

2. To the samples are added 1 μL of total tRNAs (2 μg/μL) and 1 μL or 2 μL of kethoxal solution (kethoxal is diluted at 40 mg/mL in 20% of ethanol). The reactions are done at 37 °C for 5 min in a total volume of 20 μL. The optimal modification of mRNA is with 2 μL of kethoxal at 40 mg/mL. After the reactions, 10 μL of 100 mM sodium borate pH 8.0 is added (*see* **Note 7**).

3. The reactions are stopped by ethanol precipitation and treated as described above (Subheading 3.4, **steps 7–9**) except that the pellets are dissolved in 4 μL of 100 mM sodium borate pH 8.0 instead of water.

3.6 Fractionation of End-Labeled RNA Fragments

3.6.1 Ladders for Cleavage Assignments

1. RNase T1 ladder: labeled mRNA (25,000 cpm) is pre-incubated at 50 °C for 5 min in 5 μL of *Buffer T1* containing 1 μg total tRNA. The reaction is performed at 50 °C for 10 min in the presence of 1 μL of RNase T1 (0.5 U). The sample is shifted to 4 °C and kept at –20 °C.

2. Alkaline ladder: labeled mRNA (100,000 cpm) is incubated at 90 °C for 3 min in the presence of total tRNA (2 μg) in 5 μL of *ladder buffer*. The sample is shifted to 4 °C and kept at –20 °C.

3.6.2 Purification of End-Labeled RNA Fragments by PAGE

1. The end-labeled RNA fragments are sized by electrophoresis on 15% polyacrylamide (0.5% bis)–8 M urea slab gels (0.35 mm × 30 cm × 40 cm) in 1× TBE.

2. 15% PAGE is prepared as follows: 100 mL of solution containing 60 mL 25% polyacrylamide–8 M urea, 10 mL 10× TBE buffer, 30 mL 8 M urea, TEMED (75 μL), and 10% ammonium persulfate (750 μL) (*see* **Note 8**). The gel solution is poured slowly between two glass plates that are separated by one spacer on each side and placed at the horizontal on the bench. After polymerization (around 30 min), the comb is removed and the wells are washed carefully. Gels are pre-run for 30 min at 75 W.

3. The samples are heated (except the RNase T1 and alkaline ladders) for 3 min at 90 °C, centrifuged briefly and 3 μL is loaded per well. Before loading, be aware that each sample contains the same amount of radioactivity (except for the ladder that should be twice amount).

4. PAGE is run warm (75 W) to avoid band compression. The migration conditions must be adapted to the length of the RNA, knowing that on 15 % PAGE, xylene cyanol migrates as a 39 nucleotide-long RNA and bromophenol blue as 9 nucleotides.

5. At the end of the run, the 15 % PAGE is transferred without drying on an old autoradiography film, and wrapped with a plastic film. Overnight exposure is done at –80 °C using an intensifying screen.

6. Several technical problems might be observed (*see* **Notes 9–14**).

3.7 Detection of Cleavages or Modifications by Primer Extension

3.7.1 Hybridization and Primer Extension

1. To the 4 μL of the modified or cleaved mRNA (2 pmol), 1 μL of 5′ end-labeled DNA primer (around 100,000 cpm) is added. The samples are heated for 1 min at 90 °C, and quickly cooled on ice after a brief centrifugation.

2. RTB buffer 5× (1 μL) is added and the samples are incubated for 15 min at 20 °C.

3. Primer extension is performed in a total volume of 15 μL. To the hybridization mix are added 2 μL of RTB 5×, 2 μL of dNTP mix (2.5 mM of each dNTP), 4 μL sterile H_2O, 1 μL of RT (2 U/μL diluted freshly in the commercial buffer). The samples are incubated for 30 min at 37 °C.

4. To improve the quality of the gels, the RNA template is hydrolyzed by alkaline treatment. Just after primer extension are added 20 μL of the buffer (50 mM Tris–HCl pH 7.5, 7.5 mM EDTA, 0.5 % SDS), and 3.5 μL of 3 M KOH. The samples are heated at 90 °C for 3 min and at 37 °C for at least 1 h. To all samples, 6 μL of 3 M acetic acid, 100 μL 0.3 M sodium acetate pH 5.5, and 300 μL of cold ethanol are added. After precipitation, the pellets are washed twice with 70 % ethanol, vacuum-dried and dissolved in 6 μL of *DNA loading buffer.*

3.7.2 Gel Fractionation of Labeled cDNA Fragments

1. The cleavage positions are identified by running in parallel a sequencing reaction. The elongation step is performed as described above (Subheading 3.7.1, **step 3**) except in the presence of one of the dideoxyribonucleotide ddXTP (2.5 μM), the corresponding deoxyribonucleotide dXTP (25 μM), and the three other desoxyribonucleotides (100 μM).

2. All samples are heated at 90 °C for 3 min, and centrifuged briefly.

3. 3 μL is loaded on 8 % polyacrylamide (0.4 % bis)–8 M urea slab gels in TBE 1× as described above (Subheading 3.6.2). The migration conditions must be adapted to the size of the fragments to be analyzed, knowing that on 8 % PAGE, xylene cyanol migrates to 81 nucleotides and bromophenol blue to 19

nucleotides. After migration, the gels are dried, and exposed at −80 °C with an autoradiography and intensifying screen overnight.

4. Technical problems that are revealed on the autoradiography might occur during the handling process (*see* **Notes 14–16**).

3.8 In Vivo Lead(II)-Induced Cleavages

1. For the first experiment, it is essential to evaluate the quantity of lead(II) required for mild hydrolysis. For this preliminary experiment, total RNAs are prepared and fractionated on agarose gels and the most abundant rRNAs are visualized by ethidium bromide [37]. Upon increasing concentrations of lead(II)-acetate (25–200 mM), the intensities of 16S and 23S rRNAs significantly decreased. Choose a concentration of lead(II)-acetate where significant amount of full-length rRNAs is observed.

2. The protocol described below has been adapted for *E. coli* to map the structure of mRNA and ncRNAs [37] (*see* **Note 17**).

3. Bacteria (20 mL of culture) are grown in LB medium to mid-logarithmic phase at 37 °C (until an OD_{600} of 0.5 has reached) in a Falcon tube.

4. A fresh solution of 1 M lead(II)-acetate in sterile bi-distillated water is extemporaneously prepared (*see* **Note 2**). Then, 2.8 mL of this solution is mixed with 3.2 mL of sterile water and 2 mL of pre-warmed 4× concentrated LB (at 37 °C) to give 8 mL of lead(II)-acetate/LB solution at 350 mM.

5. 8 mL of the lead(II)-acetate/LB solution (350 mM) is then added to 20 mL of cells at mid-logarithmic phase. This gives a final concentration of lead(II)-acetate 100 mM. For the first trials, different concentrations of lead(II)-acetate (50, 100, 150, and 200 mM final concentration) should be used, and the reaction is performed for 5 min at 37 °C with gentle shaking.

6. Incubation control is performed under the same experimental conditions, except that lead(II)-acetate is avoided.

7. The reactions are stopped by addition of 10 mL of cold 0.5 M EDTA (1.5-fold molar excess) and immediately put on ice. The cells are pelleted ($3000 \times g$ for 15 min at 4 °C) and resuspended in 1.5 mL of cold buffer 10 mM Tris–HCl pH 8, 100 mM NaCl, 1 mM EDTA. The cells are transferred in a 1.5 mL microtube and centrifuged ($13,000 \times g$, 15 min at 4 °C).

8. *E. coli* cells are disrupted by adding 200 μL of buffer containing 50 mM Tris–HCl pH 8.0, 8% sucrose, 0.5% Triton, 10 mM EDTA, 4 mg/mL lyzozyme, and incubated 5 min in ice.

9. Total RNAs are prepared by phenol extraction treatment (*see* **Note 18**). To the samples, 200 μL of phenol saturated with 0.1 M sodium acetate pH 5.5 and 10 mM EDTA is added.

Cells are vortexed during 30 sec at high speed under the fume hood. The samples are heated at 65 °C during 15 min and mixed every 5 min.

10. The mixture is cooled on ice and centrifuged (10 min, 13,000×g). The aqueous phases are carefully collected, and the phenol and interface are re-extracted by vortexing the samples with 100 µL 0.1 M sodium acetate pH 5.5.

11. After centrifugation, the aqueous phases are pooled and extracted once with phenol–chloroform previously saturated in sodium acetate 0.1 M pH 5.5, and once with chloroform. Sodium acetate is added to the sample to give a final concentration of 0.3 M and the RNA is then precipitated twice with 3 volumes of cold ethanol.

12. The pellets are washed twice with 200 µL of 80% ethanol, vacuum-dried, and dissolved in a small volume of sterile bi-distillated water. The RNA concentration is measured and 10 µg of material is used for primer extension.

13. Primer hybridization, elongation by reverse transcriptase, and PAGE fractionation are as described (Subheading 3.8), except that primer extension is conducted at 45 °C for 30 min with 5 U of reverse transcriptase.

14. Technical problems might occur during the handling process (*see* **Notes 19** and **20**).

3.9 In Vivo DMS Modification

1. DMS modification can be performed in vivo under different growth conditions (temperature, medium, growth phase). The protocol described below has been adapted for *E. coli* to map the structure of mRNA at 15 and 37 °C [4].

2. Bacteria (15 mL of culture) are grown in LB medium in a 50 mL sterile tube to mid-logarithmic phase at 37 °C (until an OD_{600} of 0.5 has reached).

3. The reactions are performed with 30, 60, or 120 µL of DMS for 3 min at 37 °C, or with 60, 120, and 240 µL of DMS for 3 min at 15 °C after gentle shaking. The best conditions for modifications are with 60 µL of DMS at 37 °C and 120 µL of DMS at 15 °C.

4. The reactions are stopped by adding 75 mL of cold stop buffer containing 100 mM Tris–HCl pH 8, 100 mM ß-mercaptoethanol, 5 mM EDTA.

5. The cells are pelleted (3000×g, 15 min, 4 °C), and dissolved in 1.5 mL of cold buffer 10 mM Tris–HCl pH 8, 100 mM NaCl, 1 mM EDTA. The cells are transferred in a 1.5 mL micro tube and centrifuged (13,000×g, 15 min, 4 °C).

6. Incubation control is performed on cells grown and treated in the same conditions as above but in the absence of DMS. A

stop control is also done to verify that no DMS modification occurred during the RNA extraction. In that control, DMS is added after the addition of the stop buffer.

7. Preparation of total RNAs, primer extension, and PAGE fractionation are as described above (Subheading 3.8, **steps 8–13**).

4 Notes

1. Safety rules. For manipulating radioactivity, work behind a plexiglass screen, and wear glasses and gloves. For phenol extraction, work under a fume hood. Since all the chemicals modify nucleic acids, they are potential carcinogens. It is therefore essential to manipulate the reagents under a fume hood and to wear protective gloves. The reagent solutions, the supernatant derived from the first precipitation step following the RNA modification, and all the tubes that have been in contact with the reagent must be treated as follows: for DMS and kethoxal, all samples are discarded in 1 N sodium hydroxide, and for CMCT all samples are treated in 10 % acetic acid.

2. For lead(II)-induced cleavages, buffers with chloride ions should be avoided as Pb(II) acetate might form precipitates with it. Since Pb^{2+} competes with Mg^{2+} for RNA binding, the efficiency of cleavages will depend on the Pb^{2+}/Mg^{2+} ratio.

3. Kethoxal is a highly viscous solution and should therefore be weighed instead of pipetted. First, tare a micro tube, transfer some kethoxal to the tube with a 200 μL pipettor, and weigh the tube again. The same procedure is done with CMCT.

4. Since the chemical reactions are influenced by the temperature, the experimental conditions have to be adapted for each temperature. For instance, DMS modification at 4 °C is for 20 min with 1 μL of DMS whereas at 50 °C the reaction is for 5 min with 1 μL of DMS diluted 1:16; CMCT modification is at 4 °C for 45 min with 5 μL of CMCT 40 mg/mL and is at 50 °C for 5 min with 5 μL of CMCT 14 mg/mL; kethoxal modification at 4 °C is for 30 min with 5 μL of kethoxal 20 mg/mL and at 50 °C is for 5 min with 1 μL of kethoxal 10 mg/mL.

5. In vitro RNA transcripts generated by T7 RNA polymerase have a heterogenous 3′ end and sometimes at the 5′ end. A solution is to incorporate ribozymes into the transcripts at the 5′- and/or 3′-end of the target RNA sequence [46]. Fractionation of RNA on PAGE remains the method of choice for purification. For long RNA molecules, electro-elution might help to increase the elution efficiency.

6. During PAGE purification, the RNA is denatured, and thus it is essential to design renaturation protocols in order to obtain

homogeneous RNA population and to test whether this conformation is biologically relevant (enzymatic activity for ribozyme, efficient ligand binding). Alternative RNA conformations may coexist and by varying the concentration of $MgCl_2$, one of the two conformers might be stabilized. If the conformers have different electrophoretic mobilities on native polyacrylamide gel, chemical probing can be used to distinguish them. After chemical modification, the coexisting structures are separated on a native polyacrylamide gel, and the modification sites for each conformer are then identified by primer extension.

7. Kethoxal might have a partially denaturing effect on RNA structure even if the reaction is not too strong (all the guanines are modified). Concentration of kethoxal or the incubation time should be reduced in order to get only modifications at guanines located in single-stranded regions.

8. To keep high resolution of the gels, acrylamide, urea solutions, and in particular ammonium persulfate should be prepared freshly.

9. Each experiment should be repeated at least twice, and only the reproducible cleavages/modifications will be considered. As mentioned previously, the elaboration of a reliable secondary structure RNA model requires data from various chemicals.

10. No full-length RNA: the reaction has been too strong (*see* Fig. 1, lanes 4 and 5). Time of the reaction and/or chemical concentrations have to be reduced (Fig. 1, lane 2).

11. Compression of bands due to stable secondary structure (in general rich in G-C base pairs) can be observed using end-labeled RNA. Heat the samples before loading on the gel and the gels should be warm before sample loading and during the migration.

12. Aggregation of end-labeled RNA in the gel pockets and only fragments of small sizes can be visualized. The pellets have not been correctly dried after ethanol precipitation. The data cannot be interpreted.

13. Samples do not migrate correctly during electrophoresis due to the presence of salt. Add several washing steps with ethanol 80 % at the end of the procedure.

14. Appropriate incubation controls are essential to identify cleavages that are induced during the incubation treatments, and the pauses of reverse transcriptase that are due to stable secondary structures or cuts. Nucleotides for which strong bands are visible in the control lanes are not considered for the interpretation. If too many bands occur in the incubation controls of end-labeled RNA, repurify the RNA and prepare new sterile buffers. If too many RT pauses in the incubation controls, it can be due

to RNase contamination, strong secondary structure of RNA (the extension can be done at 42 °C), or to the primer location. AMV (avian myeloblastosis virus) RT should be used rather than MMLV (Moloney murine leukemia virus) RT, the latter being more sensitive to RNA secondary structure.

15. Absence of signal after primer extension: the modified RNA has not efficiently precipitated, the pellet has been lost during the removal of supernatant, and the hybridization conditions need to be optimized. Optimal conditions for primer hybridization should be established in a series of pilot experiments. The optimal temperature for annealing varies from RNA to RNA, depending on the G+C content, the propensity of the RNA to form secondary structure, and the length of the primer.

16. Reverse transcriptase stops at the nucleotide preceding the cleaved nucleotide. Thus, the resulting cDNA is one nucleotide shorter than the cDNA corresponding to the sequencing lane (*see* Fig. 1).

17. Data from in vivo probing are more complex to interpret than the in vitro probing. One of the main reasons is that the studied RNA might be involved simultaneously in several complexes. However, in vivo mapping becomes powerful when it is used in a comparative manner. For example, conformational changes of mRNA induced by a *trans*-acting ligand can be identified upon repression or activation of translation. DMS and lead(II)-induced cleavages can be used to monitor the conformational changes of mRNA under different growth conditions and environmental cues such as temperature [4].

18. Alternative to phenol extraction, other protocols used to extract total RNAs can be used. Reagents combining phenol and guanidine thiocyanate enable a straightforward isolation of total RNAs from samples of human, yeast, bacterial and viral origin. Fastprep instrument and the associated commercial kits (Q-biogen) to lyse the cells and to prepare total RNA extracts is also an efficient method.

19. Weak signals and no-more full-length RNA: incomplete homogenization or lysis of samples, not enough material (increase the quantity of RNA), the reaction has been too strong (reduce either the quantity of the reagent, or/and the time of incubation). Check that the reaction has been efficiently stopped before the extraction of total RNAs.

20. Strong stops in the control lanes: degradation of RNA, pauses of RT due to stable secondary structures, posttranscriptional modifications which stop reverse transcriptase elongation (primer should be changed in order to cover the modified base).

Acknowledgments

We thank all members of the team for helpful discussions, and we are grateful to E. Westhof for his constant support. This work was supported by the Centre National de Recherche (CNRS), the Agence Nationale de la Recherche (ANR-09-BLAN-0024-01; ANR-PATHOGENOMICS-ARMSA). D.P. receives support from the CNRS and the Délégation Générale de l'Armement.

References

1. Lioliou E, Romilly C, Romby P, Fechter P (2010) RNA-mediated regulation in bacteria: from natural to artificial systems. N Biotechnol 27:222–235

2. Bastet L, Dube A, Masse E, Lafontaine DA (2011) New insights into riboswitch regulation mechanisms. Mol Microbiol 80:1148–1154

3. Narberhaus F (2010) Translational control of bacterial heat shock and virulence genes by temperature-sensing mRNAs. RNA Biol 7:84–89

4. Giuliodori AM, Di Pietro F, Marzi S, Masquida B, Wagner R, Romby P, Gualerzi CO, Pon CL (2010) The cspA mRNA is a thermosensor that modulates translation of the cold-shock protein CspA. Mol Cell 37:21–33

5. Nechooshtan G, Elgrably-Weiss M, Sheaffer A, Westhof E, Altuvia S (2009) A pH-responsive riboregulator. Genes Dev 23: 2650–2662

6. Ramesh A, Winkler WC (2010) Magnesium-sensing riboswitches in bacteria. RNA Biol 7:77–83

7. Roth A, Breaker RR (2009) The structural and functional diversity of metabolite-binding riboswitches. Annu Rev Biochem 78:305–334

8. Green NJ, Grundy FJ, Henkin TM (2010) The T box mechanism: tRNA as a regulatory molecule. FEBS Lett 584:318–324

9. Marzi S, Myasnikov AG, Serganov A, Ehresmann C, Romby P, Yusupov M, Klaholz BP (2007) Structured mRNAs regulate translation initiation by binding to the platform of the ribosome. Cell 130:1019–1031

10. Thomason MK, Storz G (2010) Bacterial antisense RNAs: how many are there, and what are they doing? Annu Rev Genet 44:167–188

11. Vogel J (2009) A rough guide to the non-coding RNA world of Salmonella. Mol Microbiol 71:1–11

12. Terns MP, Terns RM (2011) CRISPR-based adaptive immune systems. Curr Opin Microbiol 14:321–327

13. Wong TN, Pan T (2009) RNA folding during transcription: protocols and studies. Methods Enzymol 468:167–193

14. Zemora G, Waldsich C (2010) RNA folding in living cells. RNA Biol 7:634–641

15. Woodson SA, Muller JG, Burrows CJ, Rokita SE (1993) A primer extension assay for modification of guanine by Ni(II) complexes. Nucleic Acids Res 21:5524–5525

16. Ralston CY, Sclavi B, Sullivan M, Deras ML, Woodson SA, Chance MR, Brenowitz M (2000) Time-resolved synchrotron X-ray footprinting and its application to RNA folding. Methods Enzymol 317:353–368

17. Chevalier C, Geissmann T, Helfer AC, Romby P (2009) Probing mRNA structure and sRNA-mRNA interactions in bacteria using enzymes and lead(II). Methods Mol Biol 540:215–232

18. Wilkinson KA, Merino EJ, Weeks KM (2006) Selective 2′-hydroxyl acylation analyzed by primer extension (SHAPE): quantitative RNA structure analysis at single nucleotide resolution. Nat Protoc 1:1610–1616

19. Wakeman CA, Ramesh A, Winkler WC (2009) Multiple metal-binding cores are required for metalloregulation by M-box riboswitch RNAs. J Mol Biol 392:723–735

20. Zuker M (2003) Mfold web server for nucleic acid folding and hybridization prediction. Nucleic Acids Res 31:3406–3415

21. Do CB, Woods DA, Batzoglou S (2006) CONTRAfold: RNA secondary structure prediction without physics-based models. Bioinformatics 22:e90–e98

22. Xayaphoummine A, Bucher T, Isambert H (2005) Kinefold web server for RNA/DNA folding path and structure prediction including pseudoknots and knots. Nucleic Acids Res 33:W605–W610

23. Reuter JS, Mathews DH (2010) RNAstructure: software for RNA secondary structure prediction and analysis. BMC Bioinformatics 11:129

24. Jossinet F, Westhof E (2005) Sequence to Structure (S2S): display, manipulate and interconnect RNA data from sequence to structure. Bioinformatics 21:3320–3321

25. Sato K, Kato Y, Hamada M, Akutsu T, Asai K (2011) IPknot: fast and accurate prediction of RNA secondary structures with pseudoknots using integer programming. Bioinformatics 27:i85–i93

26. Bellaousov S, Mathews DH (2010) ProbKnot: fast prediction of RNA secondary structure including pseudoknots. RNA 16:1870–1880

27. Bindewald E, Kluth T, Shapiro BA (2010) CyloFold: secondary structure prediction including pseudoknots. Nucleic Acids Res 38:W368–W372

28. Cruz JA, Westhof E (2011) Sequence-based identification of 3D structural modules in RNA with RMDetect. Nat Methods 8:513–521

29. Rother M, Rother K, Puton T, Bujnicki JM (2010) ModeRNA: a tool for comparative modeling of RNA 3D structure. Nucleic Acids Res 39:4007–4022

30. Tijerina P, Mohr S, Russell R (2007) DMS footprinting of structured RNAs and RNA-protein complexes. Nat Protoc 2:2608–2623

31. Woodson SA (2011) RNA folding pathways and the self-assembly of ribosomes. Acc Chem Res 44:1312–1319

32. Joseph S, Noller HF (2000) Directed hydroxyl radical probing using iron(II) tethered to RNA. Methods Enzymol 318:175–190

33. Culver GM, Noller HF (2000) Directed hydroxyl radical probing of RNA from iron(II) tethered to proteins in ribonucleoprotein complexes. Methods Enzymol 318:461–475

34. Mayford M, Weisblum B (1989) Conformational alterations in the ermC transcript in vivo during induction. EMBO J 8:4307–4314

35. Altuvia S, Weinstein-Fischer D, Zhang A, Postow L, Storz G (1997) A small, stable RNA induced by oxidative stress: role as a pleiotropic regulator and antimutator. Cell 90:43–53

36. Balzer M, Wagner R (1998) A chemical modification method for the structural analysis of RNA and RNA-protein complexes within living cells. Anal Biochem 256:240–242

37. Lindell M, Romby P, Wagner EG (2002) Lead(II) as a probe for investigating RNA structure in vivo. RNA 8:534–541

38. Wilkinson KA, Vasa SM, Deigan KE, Mortimer SA, Giddings MC, Weeks KM (2009) Influence of nucleotide identity on ribose 2'-hydroxyl reactivity in RNA. RNA 15:1314–1321

39. Lucks JB, Mortimer SA, Trapnell C, Luo S, Aviran S, Schroth GP, Pachter L, Doudna JA, Arkin AP (2011) Multiplexed RNA structure characterization with selective 2'-hydroxyl acylation analyzed by primer extension sequencing (SHAPE-Seq). Proc Natl Acad Sci U S A 108:11063–11068

40. Leontis NB, Lescoute A, Westhof E (2006) The building blocks and motifs of RNA architecture. Curr Opin Struct Biol 16:279–287

41. Romby P, Caillet J, Ebel C, Sacerdot C, Graffe M, Eyermann F, Brunel C, Moine H, Ehresmann C, Ehresmann B, Springer M (1996) The expression of E.coli threonyl-tRNA synthetase is regulated at the translational level by symmetrical operator-repressor interactions. EMBO J 15:5976–5987

42. Mortimer SA, Weeks KM (2009) Time-resolved RNA SHAPE chemistry: quantitative RNA structure analysis in one-second snapshots and at single-nucleotide resolution. Nat Protoc 4:1413–1421

43. Romaniuk PJ, de Stevenson IL, Wong HH (1987) Defining the binding site of Xenopus transcription factor IIIA on 5S RNA using truncated and chimeric 5S RNA molecules. Nucleic Acids Res 15:2737–2755

44. Jahn MJ, Jahn D, Kumar AM, Soll D (1991) Mono Q chromatography permits recycling of DNA template and purification of RNA transcripts after T7 RNA polymerase reaction. Nucleic Acids Res 19:2786

45. Milligan JF, Uhlenbeck OC (1989) Synthesis of small RNAs using T7 RNA polymerase. Methods Enzymol 180:51–62

46. Walker SC, Avis JM, Conn GL (2003) General plasmids for producing RNA in vitro transcripts with homogeneous ends. Nucleic Acids Res 31:e82

47. Torres-Larios A, Dock-Bregeon AC, Romby P, Rees B, Sankaranarayanan R, Caillet J, Springer M, Ehresmann C, Ehresmann B, Moras D (2002) Structural basis of translational control by Escherichia coli threonyl tRNA synthetase. Nat Struct Biol 9:343–347

Chapter 8

High-Throughput Nuclease Probing of RNA Structures Using FragSeq

Andrew V. Uzilov and Jason G. Underwood

Abstract

High-throughput sequencing of cDNA (RNA-Seq) can be used to generate nuclease accessibility data for many distinct transcripts in the same mixture simultaneously. Such assays accelerate RNA structure analysis and provide researchers with new technologies to tackle biological questions on a transcriptome-wide scale. FragSeq is an experimental assay for transcriptome-wide RNA structure probing using RNA-Seq, coupled with data analysis tools that allow quantitative determination of nuclease accessibility at single-base resolution. We provide a practical guide to designing and carrying out FragSeq experiments and data analysis.

Key words RNA structure prediction, FragSeq, RNA-Seq, Transcriptome, Nuclease probing, Nuclease accessibility, RNA structure probing, Bioinformatics

1 Introduction

Enzymatic or chemical probing of RNA in solution provides informative data from which a structure model can be constructed. Probing agents are used to cleave the phosphate backbone or modify nucleotides in a way that provides structure information due to solvent accessibility of reactive functional groups and their structural context. Traditionally, in order to recover this information, direct end-labeling of the probed RNA or primer extension with labeled primers is used, after which the length of labeled products is inferred by means of high-resolution denaturing gel electrophoresis. A significant amount of work has gone into the development and refinement of such probing approaches over the past four decades [1, 2]. While these techniques are extremely useful and informative, the rate at which structure data can be acquired with them is slowed because they require purification of the RNA of interest or custom primer design, and at least one electrophoresis step must be done.

Over the past few years, several groups [3, 4] have adopted various RNA-Seq protocols to replace electrophoresis with high-throughput sequencing by modifying and extending existing

Douglas H. Turner and David H. Mathews (eds.), *RNA Structure Determination: Methods and Protocols*, Methods in Molecular Biology, vol. 1490, DOI 10.1007/978-1-4939-6433-8_8, © Springer Science+Business Media New York 2016

enzymatic [5–8] or chemical [9–20] structure probing approaches, thus allowing interrogation of complex mixtures of hundreds to thousands of different RNAs in a single reaction. Once calibrated, these methods allow probing of an entire transcriptome at single-nucleotide resolution in one experiment without requiring custom primer design or labeling of one specific RNA of interest; prior knowledge of sequences of the RNAs being probed is not necessary. The scale of information gained allows researchers to tackle scientific questions that were simply not possible to address with classic techniques.

FragSeq is a high-throughput enzymatic probing method that measures accessibility of RNA sites (*see* **Note 1**) to an endonuclease [5]. A complex RNA mixture (i.e., containing many different transcripts at various abundances) is subjected to partial nuclease digestion; a control sample from the same RNA mixture is prepared in parallel in the same manner except without nuclease digestion. RNA fragments in the two samples are reverse transcribed to make cDNA libraries, which are then sequenced to produce reads spanning some or all of the length of each cDNA. Reads are mapped to the reference genome or RNA sequences of interest, and the resulting mapping coordinates are input to our command-line tool to produce cutting scores, which describe nuclease accessibility at each RNA site; other useful statistics are also output. This data can be visualized in VARNA software [21] to examine it in a secondary structure context or in a genome browser to examine it in a genomic context (Fig. 1); additionally, it can be used to guide computational predictions of RNA structure (Fig. 2).

The library preparation strategy employed in ref. 5 is shown in Fig. 3. In that protocol, the P1 nuclease was used, which is specific for single-stranded RNA (ssRNA) and produces fragments with 5′ PO_4 and 3′ OH end chemistry after cleavage. Adapter ligation to ends of RNA fragments containing specifically those end chemistries allowed us to clone them and thus enrich for products of nuclease cleavage, selecting against nonspecific degradation that leaves 5′ OH and 2′,3′-cyclic phosphate. However, other nucleases can be used (Subheading 1.1). Also, although we used Applied Biosystems SOLiD sequencing in the original study, FragSeq does not require this specific sequencing technology because the key informative step is the ligation of adapters to fragment ends during sequencing library preparation; compatible library protocols for Illumina and Ion Torrent sequencing are given in Subheading 3.3. Our command-line tool can be configured to process data from alternative preparation schemes.

The FragSeq computational pipeline is outlined in Fig. 4, with real data at each step shown in Fig. 1 for mouse spliceosomal (sn)

Fig. 1 (continued) similar: undifferentiated embryonic stem cells (UESC) and day 5 neural precursor cells. Other tracks show UESC data only. *SL* stem-loop, *IL* interior loop, *MBL* multibranch loop. Figure is modified from ref. 5

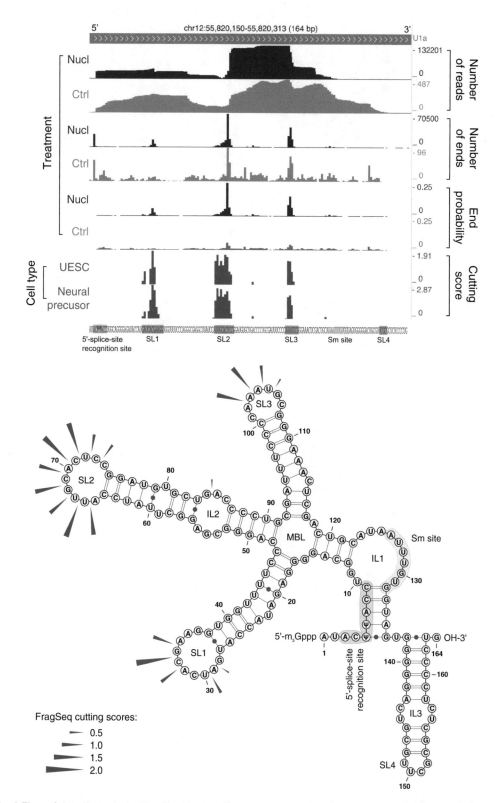

Fig. 1 Flow of data through the FragSeq pipeline (from *top* to *bottom*), displayed in the UCSC Genome Browser [37] (*top* panels) and in VARNA secondary structure viewer [21] (*bottom* panel), for mouse spliceosomal (sn)RNA U1a. Pipeline steps correspond to those shown in Fig. 4. "Cutting score" genome browser tracks compare results obtained from parallel FragSeq experiments on two cell lines where structure of this RNA ought to be

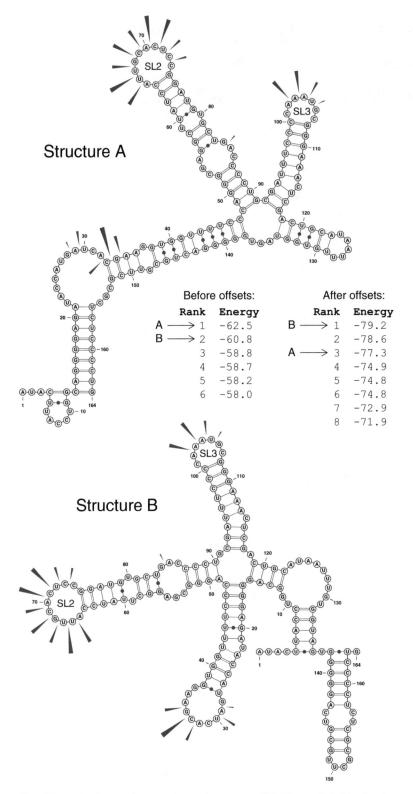

Structure A

Structure B

	Before offsets:			After offsets:	
	Rank	Energy		Rank	Energy
A →	1	-62.5	B →	1	-79.2
B →	2	-60.8		2	-78.6
	3	-58.8	A →	3	-77.3
	4	-58.7		4	-74.9
	5	-58.2		5	-74.8
	6	-58.0		6	-74.8
				7	-72.9
				8	-71.9

Fig. 2 Top-ranked secondary structures of mouse snRNA U1a predicted by the program Fold in the RNAstructure package [25] with (Structure B) and without (Structure A) FragSeq-derived offsets. Tables show energies (standard Gibbs free energy of folding or ΔG°, units of kcal/mol) for the total set of predicted structures, ranked from most to least favorable (lower energies are more favorable); positions of Structures A and B within the ranked list is indicated. Energies are proportional to the natural log of the equilibrium constant between folded and unfolded states.

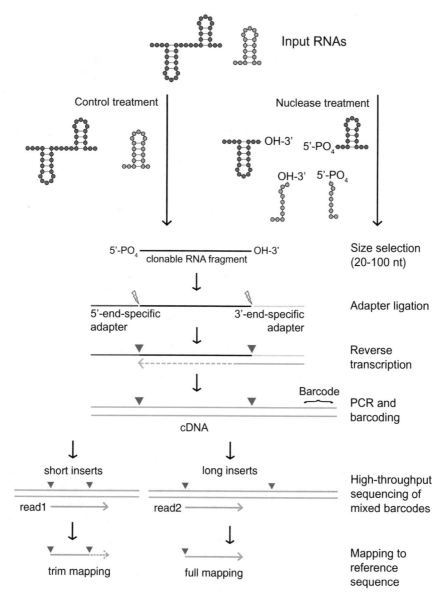

Fig. 3 Library preparation, sequencing, and read mapping strategy employed in ref. 5, which used the Applied Biosystems SOLiD Small RNA Expression Kit (SREK) for the Applied Biosystems SOLiD 3 platform. *Lightning bolts* denote ligation junctions. *Triangles* show sites that are *relevant* (*see* **Note 14**) because they correspond to ligation-competent 5′ and 3′ ends of the original RNA fragment which, in this protocol, yield structure data. An "insert" is the part of a cDNA whose sequence corresponds to the original RNA fragment. If an insert is short, a read can sequence into the opposite adapter; during mapping, adapter sequence was removed ("trimmed," dotted part of read1), producing two relevant mapping ends. If an insert is long, we could only use the 5′ end of a mapping. In this protocol, sequencing of double-stranded cDNA was initiated only from the 5′ adapter end, but sequencing can also be initiated from the 3′ end, or from both ends in two passes (paired-end sequencing), depending on the method. Figure modified from ref. 5

Fig. 2 (continued) The same cutting scores are plotted on top of both structures (*blue arrows*); these are the same as in Fig. 1, which also shows the known U1a structure. These cutting scores are linearly transformed into offsets using a slope of −1 and intercept of 0 (however, multiple slopes work in this specific case), then given to Fold using the -SSO option (other options were kept at default). Offsets lower the energy of all predicted structures because they contain correct folding of SL2 and SL3, with which cutting scores agree; the change in ranking comes from the small number of bases (C33 and G34) with which cutting scores disagree in Structure A

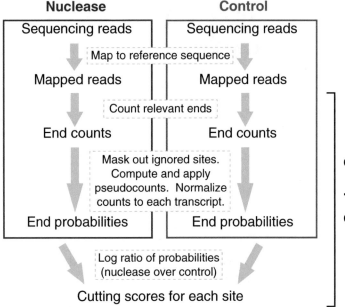

Fig. 4 The FragSeq computational pipeline. Steps carried out by the FragSeq algorithm are indicated. Key pipeline steps are in *dashed boxes*. Figure modified from ref. 5

RNA U1a. The final product is cutting scores, which indicate sites that are more susceptible to the nuclease used (*see* **Note 2**). Importantly, the normalization strategy requires that the researcher identify the RNA loci of interest and their coordinates ahead of time, as that information is input to our command-line tool (*see* **Note 3**).

Some key features distinguish FragSeq from other high-throughput enzymatic probing RNA-Seq methods. First, like in Parallel Analysis of RNA Structure (PARS) [6], FragSeq gets structure information by sequencing at or across the site where adapter ligated to the end(s) of RNA fragments, meaning the read *ends* are important (Fig. 3); in contrast, dsRNA-seq and ssRNA-seq [7] look at coverage by bases in the *body* of reads after enriching for dsRNA or ssRNA fragments. Second, FragSeq requires an explicit no-nuclease control sample for every nuclease used; in contrast, PARS compares samples digested by two different nucleases directly, without a control (*see* **Note 4**). Lastly, the FragSeq pipeline is different from PARS with respect to read count normalization (*see* **Note 3**); also, special attention is paid to dealing with missing and unreliable data so that accuracy on RNAs with lower coverage is not compromised.

In addition to this chapter, readers are encouraged to study the detailed computational and bioinformatics methods from other high-throughput RNA structure probing protocols [22, 23] for insight on experiment and pipeline design.

1.1 Considerations in Designing a FragSeq Experiment

FragSeq aims to probe a complex RNA mixture. This mixture can be total RNA purified from cells (*see* **Note 5**) or may be enriched for a specific RNA population of interest, such as by subcellular fractionation, size-selection, or using immobilized antisense oligonucleotides directed against the RNA of interest. Mixtures of in vitro-transcribed RNAs or synthetic oligonucleotides, or even a single transcript, can also be probed, as long as care is taken to make sure that all sequencing reads can be unambiguously mapped to a specific RNA in the pool (Subheadings 3.5.1 and 3.5.2). In principle, FragSeq nuclease probing can also be carried out on partially purified RNA, such as intact RNPs (more mildly extracted from in vivo or assembled in vitro), or on RNA incubated with a specific protein, ligand, or other RNA(s). These approaches would require modifications to the given sample preparation protocol, but our command-line tool can still be used to infer cutting scores.

We recommend using endonucleases that leave the 5′ PO_4 and 3′ OH end chemistry after cleavage (nucleases P1 or S1, and RNase V1), because those end chemistries are more favorable for adapter ligation and therefore allow enrichment for RNA fragments produced by the nuclease. Our command-line tool can be configured to use data from either the 5′ or the 3′ end of reads or some combination of both. Nucleases leaving other end chemistries, followed by repair to make ligation-competent ends (see below), are possible to use, though that may produce more noise. The key is to always sequence a no-nuclease control sample to control for non-nuclease-specific cleavage or degradation.

It is important to understand how enzyme treatments affect end chemistries in both nuclease and control samples, as comparison of ends between those samples is the most important aspect of the FragSeq method. The ends in the input RNA may or may not be available during subsequent adapter ligation strategies. For example, a capped, polyadenylated Pol II transcript from a eukaryotic cell would not have an available 5′ PO_4 end for ligation due to the 7-methyl guanosine cap, but it would have a free 3′ OH group available for 3′ end ligation. Similarly, an RNA produced by bacteriophage T7 transcription would have 5′ triphosphate and 3′ OH ends. Also of note should be the ends generated by cleavage of RNA by a number of common RNases (e.g., A, T1) and random base-catalyzed hydrolysis. These termini (5′ OH and 2′,3′-cyclic-phosphate), will not be captured by most ligation strategies. If information about these termini is desired, an enzymatic treatment with T4 polynucleotide kinase and ATP can generate the necessary 5′ PO_4 and 3′ OH [5, 24].

We find that cutting scores are more reliable if based on higher quantities of mapped reads. Therefore, it is important to design an experiment that maximizes the number of reads derived from RNAs of interest, which can be done by an enrichment or depletion step or by using fewer barcodes (Subheading 3.3). The length of reads is not important, as long as reads are long enough so that they are accurately mappable to the reference sequence. Rather, it is the *count* of mapped read ends (not the mean per-base coverage) that should be maximized. We have found that we can obtain believable cutting scores for RNAs with mean mapped read ends per site as low as ~2.5 in the nuclease sample and almost no reads in the control sample. However, this number is an average over all sites as the mapped ends are not uniformly distributed (they tend to cluster near ssRNA). So, this is a very coarse estimate of the lower bound on amount of data, and we recommend aiming for at least an order of magnitude greater counts.

To assess whether the assay is producing cutting scores that are reasonable, cutting scores of RNAs with known structures should be examined. Also, it is desirable to add to the complex mixture in vitro-transcribed control RNAs whose structure is already known and preferably for which probing data is available with the specific nuclease used in the high-throughput assay. If resources are available, the different control RNAs should span a range of abundances to identify the number of mapped read ends below which data for an RNA locus becomes unreliable.

The 20–100 nucleotide (nt) size selection step employed in our study [5] is not a requirement of a FragSeq assay—that size selection was performed because that was the optimal cDNA library size for the SOLiD 3 sequencing platform. Larger sizes can be used, and current paired-end sequencing technologies can accommodate longer fragments. Alternatively, a PARS-like approach can be used to randomly shatter long nuclease-digested RNA fragments (producing 5′ OH and 2′,3′-cyclic phosphate end chemistry) so that they fall into sequencing range, followed by end-repair of only one RNA end, so that the other end is used as the tag indicating nuclease cleavage.

2   Materials

2.1 Purification of Complex RNA Mixture for Probing

Refer to the TRIzol manual for specific guidelines for the sample of interest.

1. TRIzol reagent (Sigma-Aldrich or Life Technologies).

2. Chloroform (multiple sources; molecular biology/nucleic acid extraction grade).

3. RNase-free water (multiple sources).

4. 100 % isopropanol, molecular biology grade.

5. 75 % ethanol, molecular biology grade.

6. Acid phenol–chloroform–isoamyl alcohol (125:24:1; Ambion; pH 4.5).

7. RNase-free DNase I and 10× digestion buffer (Ambion).

8. For resuspending the RNA: 10 mM Tris–HCl pH 8.0, 0.1 mM EDTA pH 8.0.

2.2 Nuclease Calibration and Digestion of RNA with Nuclease P1

1. P1 nuclease (Sigma-Aldrich 200U vial; dissolve vial of lyophilized powder into 250 μL of 50 mM Tris base pH 7.0, 1 mM $Zn(OAc)_2$, 50% glycerol; flash-freeze small aliquots and store at –80 °C).

2. 10× P1 nuclease digestion buffer (quasi-physiological conditions): 500 mM Tris–HCl pH 7.5, 1.5 M $NaCl_2$, 50 mM $MgCl_2$, 0.10 mM $Zn(OAc)_2$.

3. Acid phenol–chloroform–isoamyl alcohol (125:24:1; Ambion; pH 4.5).

4. Denaturing loading buffer: 95% formamide, 10 mM Tris–HCl pH 8.0, 10 mM EDTA pH 8.0, 0.1% bromophenol blue.

5. 5 M ammonium acetate (Ambion).

6. 0.5 M EDTA pH 8.0 (Ambion).

7. P1 nuclease stop solution: 10 mM Tris–HCl pH 8.0, 1 M ammonium acetate, 10 mM EDTA pH 8.0.

8. Glycogen (5 mg/mL; Ambion, molecular biology grade).

9. 100% ethanol, molecular biology grade.

10. FlashPAGE gel supplies (Ambion) or other conventional apparatus for urea–polyacrylamide gel electrophoresis.

2.3 Bioinformatics Analysis

1. Software for mapping sequencing reads to reference sequence.

2. FragSeq code version 0.2.0 (https://bitbucket.org/andrewuzilov/fragseq).

3. Python version 2.7.x, or a later 2.x version (http://python.org).

4. Cython version 0.15.x or later (http://cython.org).

5. Compiler for C and C++.

6. Optional: Java virtual machine version 1.5 or later (http://www.java.com).

7. Optional: RNAstructure [25] version 5.3 or later (http://rna.urmc.rochester.edu/RNAstructure.html).

3 Methods

3.1 Calibration of P1 Nuclease for Probing a Complex RNA Mixture

Prior to partially digesting an RNA sample for RNA-Seq library preparation (Subheading 3.2), one must carefully calibrate the properties of the digestion reaction by the nuclease. In this protocol, nuclease P1 is used, but other nucleases are applicable as well (Subheadings 1.1 and 3.3). To do this, a radioactively end-labeled homogenous RNA sample is used, which we will refer to as a "spike-in" RNA. This can be produced by in vitro transcription or by synthesis; the spike-in RNA should be one that has known structural features under probing conditions used (temperature, buffer, etc.). For each spike-in, probing must be carried out in two parallel samples: on the spike-in radiolabeled RNA by itself and a similar reaction on the spike-in radiolabeled RNA in the unlabeled complex mixture of RNA to be used for experimental FragSeq probing. The goal is to assure that digestion of spike-in RNA(s) is the same in the complex mixture as it is by themselves, which shows that the complexity of the RNA mixture does not interfere with obtaining good probing data and that *trans* interactions are not occurring. An example of these experiments is shown in Fig. 5.

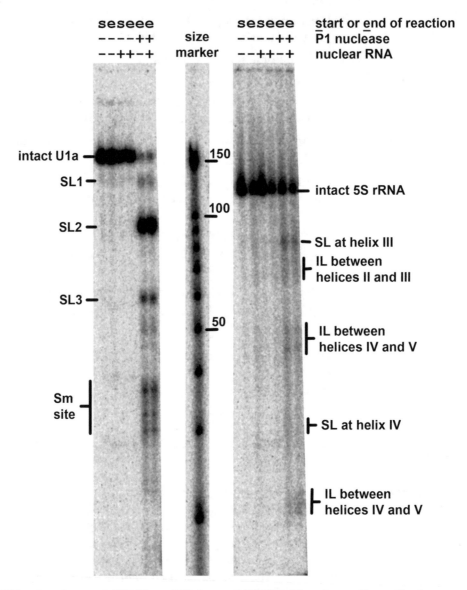

Fig. 5 Digestion of mouse snRNA U1a and 5S ribosomal (r)RNA by P1 nuclease with or without mouse nuclear RNA present. 3′-radiolabeled, in vitro-transcribed RNA was used. Lanes showing RNA at start and end of reaction without nuclease are controls for nonspecific degradation. Size markers are Ambion Decade markers; sizes of 150, 100, and 50 nt are indicated. U1a labeling is as in Fig. 1. 5S rRNA structure and helix numbers are from [46]. Figure and caption are from supplementary material in ref. 5

RNA structure probing is generally carried out under conditions that provide "single-hit kinetics" or "statistical probing"—that is, probing is carried out such that each RNA molecule is exposed to the probing agent at most once, as the first reaction of an RNA molecule may alter its structure and make subsequent reactions less informative [26]. To achieve this, probing conditions must be calibrated such that most RNAs in a sample are not cleaved by the nuclease. Therefore, the small fraction of RNAs that are cleaved will likely be cleaved only once per molecule.

Due to the PCR cycles used when amplifying a sequencing library, even a small number of non-single-hit cleavages can be observed. For certain RNAs where neither end is endogenously ligation-competent (e.g., U6, which contains a 5′ monomethyl phosphate and a 2′,3′-cyclic phosphate [27, 28]), two cleavages are required in order to produce an RNA fragment that can be cloned and amplified. While this is a violation of single-hit kinetics, we find that it tends to be a common case in our sequencing prep and that it yields useful structure information.

Spike-in RNAs should be selected so that their size is in the size range of the RNAs (or RNA domains) that one is interested in probing in the high-throughput assay, because single-hit kinetics will be calibrated for that size range. The size of the full-length RNAs being probed in the complex mixture may be larger, but structured domains of interest may fall within the calibration size range. For example, structured RNA regions in bacterial mRNAs (such as riboswitches and other regulatory elements) tend to be smaller than 200 nt. So although one would probe total, unfragmented mRNA in a FragSeq experiment, single-hit kinetics would be optimized towards domains of size 100–200 nt.

Once a suitable structured spike-in RNA has been identified, an unlabeled in vitro transcript can be produced in bulk from a PCR or plasmid template. It is recommended that this RNA be gel-purified to make sure that all of the material is full length transcript. A small amount of this purified RNA can then be radiolabeled for the calibration experiments.

If 5′ end-labeling of a transcript is desired, the RNA must be dephosphorylated to remove the triphosphate terminus by treatment with alkaline phosphatase, then kinase-labeled with γ-^{32}P-ATP and T4 polynucleotide kinase via standard methods (Sections 10.59–10.67, 11.31–11.33 in ref. 29).

For 3′ end-labeling, the RNA can be used directly after transcription and purification. There are two common methods for 3′ end-labeling with commercially available enzymes and ^{32}P nucleotides:

1. Addition of a single radioactive adenosine base to the 3′ end of the RNA by polyA polymerase and α-^{32}P-cordycepin triphosphate (3′-deoxy-ATP) [30].

2. Addition of a single radioactive cytosine base to the 3′ end of the RNA by T4 RNA ligase and 5′-^{32}P-pCp [31].

If the nuclease properties permit it, digestion conditions should be calibrated at conditions as close to physiological for the species of interest. In the protocol below, conditions are given for physiological conditions for mammalian cells. Nuclease P1 is not especially active at these conditions, but this is a desirable property in the quest for single-hit kinetics.

3.1.1 Calibration Experimental Workflow

1. For each spike-in RNA, prepare two parallel samples: 100 ng of unlabeled spike-in RNA ("homogeneous reaction") and 100 ng of unlabeled complex RNA mixture ("heterogeneous reaction"). Dilute each amount of RNA into 89 μL of water and add 10 μL of 10× P1 nuclease digestion buffer.

2. Dilute trace amount (~0.1 ng or 100,000 cpm of ^{32}P) of 5′ or 3′ end-labeled spike-in RNA into each of the two samples.

3. Heat the RNA at 55 °C for 5 min, then 37 °C for 10 min. This denatures and refolds the RNA to its lowest energy state, so that RNA structures are more consistent.

4. At this point, remove 20 μL of the reaction to serve as an "input" no-nuclease control.

5. Add 1 μL of P1 nuclease to each tube (*see* **Note 6**).

6. Incubate the tube at the desired probing temperature (for mammalian RNAs, we utilized 37 °C).

7. Remove 20 μL aliquots at desired times for optimization. We recommend 5, 15, 30, and 60 min time points for this buffer and temperature combination.

8. As each aliquot is removed, stop the reaction by bringing it to a final volume of 400 μL with P1 nuclease stop solution.

9. Add an equal volume of acid phenol–chloroform to each tube.

10. Once all of the time points are ready, process each extraction carefully and in a fume hood due to both the presence of isotope and phenol–chloroform. Transfer the aqueous portion to a fresh 1.5 mL microfuge tube. Dispose of the radioactive phenol–chloroform waste appropriately per institutional environmental health and safety regulations.

11. Add 4 μL (20 μg) glycogen to each tube.

12. Precipitate by adding 1 mL of 100% ethanol and centrifugation at $14,000 \times g$ at 4 °C.

13. Resuspend and heat each sample to 95 °C in denaturing loading buffer for 5 min, then resolve in parallel lanes on a medium sized (e.g., 15×17 cm) denaturing PAGE gel (*see* **Note 7**). 8 M urea, 8% 19:1 acrylamide–*bis* is applicable for 100–500 nt RNAs.

14. The gel should be dried and imaged with a PhosphorImager plate for analysis.

*3.1.2 Choosing
a Nuclease Condition*

Using the calibration assays with the spike-in RNA, one can determine the digestion parameters to be used for complex mixture probing. For true single-hit kinetics, a condition should be chosen where most of the full length molecule is still intact. One should also note if there are differences between the spike-in RNA probed on its own versus in a complex mixture, since any *trans* interactions will complicate later analysis and make using FragSeq data for guiding RNA structure prediction difficult.

The easiest parameters to alter during this calibration series include: the identity of the spike-in RNA, enzyme concentration, incubation temperature, pH, salt, and time of incubation. Nuclease P1 is a relatively thermostable enzyme, so higher temperatures (up to 70 °C) are possible, but may cause unfolding of the RNA. Increased salt will increase the stability of RNA secondary structures, but may decrease the efficiency of the nuclease. Finally, nuclease P1 is stable at pH 5–8 and shows higher activity at lower pH. As with raising temperature, this higher activity could cause over-digestion, so enzyme dilution for digestion at this pH is recommended.

**3.2 Digestion
of a Complex RNA
Mixture with Nuclease
P1**

This protocol produces RNA fragments for downstream library preparation for high-throughput sequencing.

1. Suspend complex RNA mixture at 1 ng/μL concentration in P1 nuclease digestion buffer. A reaction in the range of 100–500 μL is usually applicable.

2. Separate the above master mix into two equal volumes: "nuclease" sample and "control" sample (*see* **Note 8**).

3. Heat both samples at 55 °C for 5 min, then 37 °C for 10 min.

4. Add the predetermined concentration of P1 per unit volume to the nuclease sample and incubate for the predetermined time (*see* **Note 9**). Keep the control sample at the same temperature and for the same time as the nuclease sample.

5. Stop the nuclease and control reactions at the same time by adding 1/10th of the reaction volume of 0.5 M EDTA pH 8.0 and 1/5th volume of 5 M ammonium acetate.

6. Purify the RNA in the nuclease and control reactions by acid phenol–chloroform extraction and ethanol precipitation as detailed in **steps 9** through **12** in Subheading 3.1.1 (scale up the volume of ethanol used in **step 12** per your reaction volume).

7. For both samples in parallel, select the RNA size fraction required for the specific cDNA library prep and sequencing technology. For this, we recommend the Ambion FlashPAGE system or another small PAGE system. For FlashPage, heat the samples in the included sample loading buffer and carry out initial electrophoresis per manufacturer instructions, collecting the smaller-than-desired RNA fraction in the anode cup. Then, carry out electrophoresis again to collect RNA in the desired

size fraction. We found that 30 min of this second electrophoresis step to be applicable to the 20–100 nt RNA size range (*see* **Notes 10** and **11**).

8. Recover the collected RNAs from the FlashPAGE cup by ethanol precipitation with glycogen. For a PAGE gel, the area of interest can be localized by using radiolabeled markers in parallel lanes and subsequently eluted from the gel overnight with P1 nuclease stop solution, then ethanol precipitated with glycogen. Suspend the RNA pellet at the volume and in the buffer of choice for the downstream library preparation protocol, such as 10 mM Tris–HCl pH 8.0.

3.3 Ligation and Library Prep from Nuclease and Control RNA Samples

The FragSeq methodology and command-line tool can be adapted to a variety of sequencing platforms. Since sequencing technology evolves at an astonishing rate, any specific kit recommendations made in this chapter may rapidly become obsolete. For example, the Applied Biosystems SOLiD Small RNA Expression Kit (SREK) used in ref. 5 is no longer available, though the following currently available kits may be substituted because they use the same approach of ligating to both RNA fragment ends simultaneously using adapters containing overhangs:

- SOLiD Total RNA-Seq Kit (catalog number 4445374, Applied Biosystems).

- Ion Total RNA-Seq Kit v2 (catalog number 4475936 and 4479789, Life Technologies).

Other kits that ligate to both ends of the RNA fragment using different approaches are available:

- TruSeq Small RNA Library Preparation Kit (catalog number RS-200-0012, Illumina).

- NEBNext Small RNA Library Prep Set for Illumina (catalog number E7330S or E7330L, New England Biolabs).

As kit availability and designs change, use the following guidelines when selecting a library preparation method:

1. It is critical to ligate a defined adapter sequence onto the cleaved sites within the RNA such that a sequencing read begins at or crosses the junction between that adapter and the fragment from the probed RNA. Determining the precise identity of this junction is essential for the single-base-resolution.

2. Ligation of defined sequences to *both* ends of an RNA fragment is necessary for PCR amplification. In ref. 5, end-specific adapters were ligated to both ends of RNA simultaneously using SREK. This kit, developed for miRNA and siRNA characterization, can only ligate adapters onto RNA molecules that possess a 5′ PO_4 and 3′ OH, so this was ideal as nuclease P1

cleavage produces these end chemistries. The adapter ligation strategy can be tailored to fit the nucleases of interest and also the possible products of random hydrolysis.

3. Alternately, pre-adenylated adapters can be added to the 3′ end of the RNAs, selecting for 3′-OH ends, followed by reverse transcription primed by an oligonucleotide complementary to the adapter [32]. Then, cDNA 3′ ends can be tagged with another known adapter sequence [33, 34]. The ligation efficiency of pre-adenylated adapter as given above has been criticized as having sequence bias [35]; it may be possible to work around the biases by using NEXTflex Illumina Small RNA Sequencing Kit v2 (catalog number 5132-03 or 5132-04, Bioo Scientific). However, the FragSeq algorithm normalization procedure should ameliorate the ligation bias (*see* **Note 2**) even if the method from ref. 32 is used because cutting scores are based on comparing the *same* site between two conditions.

4. Reverse transcription and PCR are used to convert the adapter-ligated RNA pool into double-stranded DNA molecules applicable to high-throughput sequencing. Barcodes can also be added during this step if desired. Barcoding is a common way to divide up a sequencing run and this is highly recommended for FragSeq methodologies since libraries from control and nuclease conditions can be multiplexed and sequenced simultaneously (e.g., on the same lane of an Illumina instrument), reducing batch effects.

3.4 Summary of Steps in the Bioinformatics Analysis Pipeline

The steps in running a computational FragSeq analysis are:

1. Prepare input files:

   (a) Identify RNA loci for which obtaining structure data is desired.

   (b) Map sequencing reads to reference sequence (Subheading 3.5).

   (c) Put coordinates of RNA loci from **step 1(a)** in a BED file (Subheading 3.6.2).

2. Write configuration file(s) that tell FragSeq command-line tool (readsToStruct.py) what to do (Subheading 3.6.3).

3. Run the FragSeq command-line tool (readsToStruct.py, *see* **Note 12**).

4. Examine the output:

   (a) Examine read mapping end counts, probabilities, and cutting scores for each RNA locus of interest (Subheading 3.7).

   (b) Upload wiggle tracks containing the above data to a genome browser to examine them in genomic context (Subheading 3.7.2).

(c) For RNAs for which secondary structure model(s) are available, use VARNA to plot FragSeq probing data on each structure. If no structure is available, use RNAstructure with constraints derived from cutting scores to predict secondary structures (Subheading 3.7.3).

3.5 Mapping Sequencing Reads to Reference Sequence

Sequencing reads from the cDNA library prepared in Subheading 3.3 must be mapped to a reference sequence so that we can determine which read ends correspond to which sites in our RNAs of interest. The reference sequence can be the genome assembly (e.g., hg38 for human or mm10 for mouse) or a set of RNA sequences (*see* **Note 13**), in which case `readsToStruct.py` must be run in "local" mode. We use this chapter to explain the important properties of an alignment pipeline so that the user can make their own decision in selecting the right tool, as there has been a dramatic proliferation in various alignment tools over the past few years [36] (*see* also: http://www.ebi.ac.uk/~nf/hts_mappers/).

A sequencing read is generally a tag (subsequence) of a cDNA amplicon of an RNA fragment (Fig. 3). In FragSeq, unlike in many other RNA-Seq bioinformatics analyses, we care about the *ends* of RNA fragments because those correspond to sites where the parent RNA was specifically cleaved by a nuclease or nonspecifically broke. Care must be taken that we only use reads whose *relevant* ends (Fig. 3, *see* **Note 14**) align well to reference sequence (Fig. 6). If a mapping tool fails to align the relevant ends of a read, we must not use that read for FragSeq analysis.

Reads may contain adapter sequence (*see* read1 in Fig. 3). It is very important that any such adapter sequences are stripped from the reads *before* aligning reads to reference sequence; otherwise, bases in adapter may be erroneously aligned as if they were part of the insert (*see* **Note 16**). Because single-base resolution at read ends is crucial for accuracy in FragSeq, the erroneous addition of even one or two adapter bases could distort the signal in a way to which the FragSeq algorithm is not robust.

3.5.1 Special Considerations for Spliced or Overlapping RNAs

If a read originates from an exon that occurs in multiple isoforms of a spliced RNA, it is not clear to which isoform the read should be assigned. For example, `read3` in Fig. 7 cannot be unambiguously assigned to either `isoformA` or `isoformB` based on genomic annotations alone. The same issue occurs when assigning reads to *any* RNA loci whose coordinates in the reference sequence overlap. A read can map to a unique position in a reference sequence, but that position has more than one RNA locus annotation. The user must determine which reads belong to which locus; `readsToStruct.py`, although it can load reads and loci containing introns, cannot make this determination.

A simple way to partition ambiguous reads (e.g., `read3` in Fig. 7) amongst multiple loci is to randomly assign them to loci according

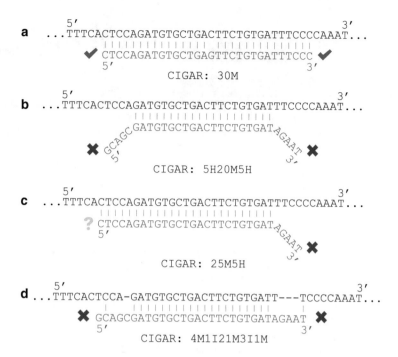

Fig. 6 Example alignments of read sequences (*bottom*) to reference sequence (*top*) illustrating cases when read mapping ends are (*checkmark icon*) and are not (*cross icon*) appropriate to consider by the FragSeq algorithm. To simplify the example, reads are 30 bases long and we assume that 5′ and 3′ ends are relevant (*see* **Note 14**), i.e., the reverse transcriptase copied the RNA fragment to cDNA in its entirety and adapter sequence is trimmed, like read1 in Fig. 3; these assumptions are not valid for all cDNA library preparation strategies. CIGAR alignment strings are shown (*see* **Note 21**). *Vertical lines* denote a sequence match. (**a**) A good alignment that includes both read ends. The single sequence mismatch occurs far away from the ends, so the ends are still useful for FragSeq. (**b**) The alignment algorithm was unable to align read ends, rendering them useless for FragSeq; however, the *middle* of the read is well-aligned and potentially useful for other bioinformatics analyses. This may occur if adapter sequence has been stripped incompletely, if the read is chimeric, or if the read is mapped to the wrong locus (can occur if part of the locus is a repetitive element). (**c**) Only the 5′ end of the read is reliably aligned. Although the lack of alignment at the 3′ end makes the entire mapping suspect, the aligned 5′ end may still be useful for FragSeq (*see* **Note 22**). (**d**) Neither read end is reliably aligned. Such alignments should be discarded prior to input to readsToStruct.py (*see* **Note 12**)

to read density observed for *unambiguous* reads (e.g., read1 and read2 in Fig. 7). For example, if isoformA has twice as many unambiguous reads mapped to it as isoformB, it will randomly get twice as many ambiguous reads. For splicing, a more powerful approach is to use one of several read mapping tools that have been developed specifically for dealing with multiple splicing isoforms

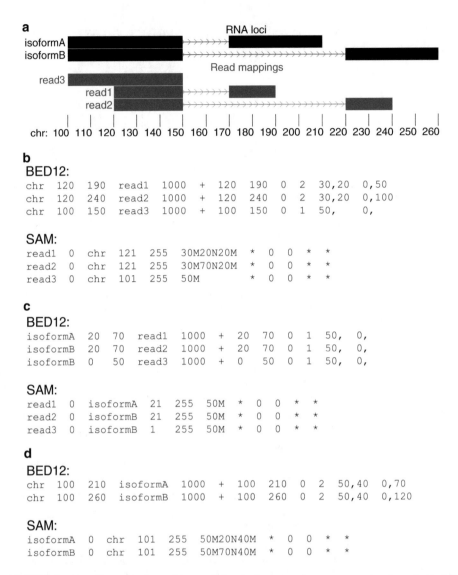

Fig. 7 (**a**) UCSC Genome Browser view of two splicing isoforms and genome-mapped reads that illustrate issues in assignment of reads to isoforms. chr is the name of the genomic reference sequence. (**b**) Alignments of reads using chr as the reference sequence (global mode), in BED12 and SAM formats (*see* **Note 21**). (**c**) Alignments of reads using spliced isoform sequence as the reference sequence (local mode), in BED12 and SAM formats. In this case, we arbitrarily assign read3 to isoformB. (**d**) Annotations of isoforms using chr as the reference sequence, in BED12 and SAM formats

(*see* the "RNA mappers" list on http://www.ebi.ac.uk/~nf/hts_mappers/). For eukaryotic analysis, this would also have the advantage that the alignment algorithms are designed for aligning short reads across large introns that occur in eukaryotic genomes.

If partitioning reads, readsToStruct.py must be told explicitly which read mappings are assigned to which locus. To do this, mapping coordinates must be saved in "local" mode and the configuration file (Subheading 3.6.3) must have the `input.reads.local` setting enabled. We define "local" coordinates to be within the coordinate system of the locus to which a read is mapped (which has introns removed, if there are any; *see* also **Note 13**), as opposed to "global" coordinates within a genomic reference sequence such as chromosomes (which still contain introns). The distinction between local and global coordinates is shown in Fig. 7 (panels c versus d) using commonly used file formats for representing coordinates. The most important point is that the reference sequence (column 1 of BED12 format and column 3 for SAM format) for local coordinates specifies the name of a locus, so `readsToStruct.py` can unambiguously know which read belongs to which locus.

3.5.2 Special Considerations for Multi-copy or Repetitive RNAs

Certain RNAs (such as snRNA in eukaryotes) exist in multiple copies in a genome or have several paralogs whose sequences are similar. This can create issues when mapping reads directly to genomic reference sequence because a read may map to multiple loci equally well. Some mapping tools may discard reads that have too many multiple mappings or may assign such mappings a very low score, which causes them to fall below a cutoff threshold and become discarded. This would result in abundant RNAs having seemingly very little data. For reads that are not discarded, it is ambiguous how they should be partitioned among the multiple matching loci.

For RNAs whose sequence is multi-copy in its entirety (e.g., snRNA), we recommend creating a set of reference sequences where each multi-copy RNA occurs once and initially mapping reads to that, then mapping remaining reads to the genome. This may erroneously over-map some reads to the multi-copy RNAs, but the FragSeq algorithm is somewhat tolerant of that (*see* **Note 2**). Mappings will have to be saved in local coordinates (Subheading 3.5.1).

For RNAs where only a subsequence is multi-copy, we recommend assigning multiply mapping reads according to the number of uniquely mapping reads in the same RNA, similarly to Subheading 3.5.1.

3.6 Running the FragSeq Command-Line Tool (`reads ToStruct.py`)

3.6.1 Overview

The command-line tool `readsToStruct.py` transforms read mappings from the nuclease and control RNA-Seq samples into cutting scores and other informative data, much of which can be uploaded to the UCSC Genome Browser [37] or other tools (*see* **Note 17**) or visualized in a secondary structure context using VARNA software [21] (Subheading 3.7).

These computational methods sections are written for FragSeq version 0.2.0, which has several improvements from version 0.0.1 used for ref. 5, primarily:

- Read mappings can now be input and output in SAM/BAM format.

- Reduced RAM usage.
- Improved configuration file syntax.
- Spliced input can now be handled.

FragSeq version 0.2.0 has been tested on Linux and Mac OS X operating systems. It is written in a portable way using only portable libraries and therefore should, in theory, also work on Windows operating systems; however, this has not been explicitly tested at the time of this writing.

3.6.2 Input Files

As required input, `readsToStruct.py` takes three files: coordinates of read mappings from the nuclease and control samples (Subheading 3.5) and coordinates of RNA loci for which the analysis is desired (*see* **Note 3**). The RNA loci file must be in BED format (*see* **Note 18**; http://genome.ucsc.edu/FAQ/FAQformat). Several variations of the BED file format exist; at a minimum, we require the six-column format (BED6) because the strand information in the sixth column is essential. RNA loci can be spliced, in which case the BED12 (12-column) format must be used, which gives the positions of introns or exons. A set of loci annotations from existing tracks in the UCSC Genome Browser can be downloaded using its Table Browser feature. Likewise, loci can be uploaded as a custom track to the UCSC Genome Browser for viewing (*see* **Note 17**). Read mappings are now encouraged to be in either SAM or BAM format (https://github.com/samtools/hts-specs), which are currently the de facto standard for storing sequencing read data; BED format is discouraged (*see* **Note 15**).

The RNA loci file is used by `readsToStruct.py` to figure out which reads came from which RNA, an important step because the assignment of reads to correct RNAs is crucial for normalization (*see* **Note 3**). If no RNA loci overlap, assigning reads is trivial—if a read overlaps a locus in their common coordinate space, the read is assigned to that locus (*see* **Note 19**). If RNA loci overlap, this simple procedure cannot be used, so the user must provide the reads in local mode (Subheading 3.5.1). In local mode, the assignment of reads to loci is simple and unambiguous—the algorithm just looks at the name of a read's reference sequence and looks it up in the list of RNA loci already given.

3.6.3 Configuration Files

`readsToStruct.py` is controlled by a configuration file that specifies the input files, output files, and the behavior of the algorithm. A very minimal example configuration file is given in Fig. 8; a more complex configuration file example, included with FragSeq code (Subheading 2.3), contains the exact configuration to reproduce our analysis in ref. 5.

The user must write the configuration file and feed it to `readsToStruct.py` (*see* **Note 12**); optionally, the configuration can be spread across several files, which is useful if the same piece

```
%YAML 1.1
---
###############################################################
# A simple FragSeq configuration file.
###############################################################

define:
    IN_DIR: path/to/some/input/directory
    OUT_DIR: path/to/some/output/directory

input:
    reads:
        nucl: IN_DIR/reads.nucl.bam
        ctrl: IN_DIR/reads.ctrl.bam
        type: bam
        local: False
    loci: IN_DIR/knownRnas.bed

output:
    config: OUT_DIR/analysis_log.conf.yaml
    cutscores:
        listfile: OUT_DIR/%.cutscores.list

algorithm:
    numEndSitesToIgnore: 3
    noiseCutoff: 10
```

Fig. 8 A minimal configuration file for `readsToStruct.py`. An analysis run using this file will produce only cutting scores text files and a configuration/analysis log

of configuration is reused in several analyses. You can also define variables in configuration files, which is useful if the same piece of text (e.g., a directory path) is reused several times.

All configuration settings can be saved to a log file before the analysis begins so that there is an automatic record of all parameters of an analysis (the setting `output.config` in Fig. 8). This is done after all input configuration files are merged, all defaults are applied, and all variable substitution is done. So, the saved configuration may contain settings that the user did not specify explicitly (the defaults). The saved configuration file is a valid configuration file itself that can be input to run an analysis.

3.7 Working with the Output of `readsToStruct.py`

Output files fall into two categories: per-locus and per-analysis. For per-locus files, the output file name/path in the configuration file must have a wildcard (%) character, which will be replaced with the name of the RNA locus from the input BED file of loci (Subheading 3.6.2; *see* **Note 18**; Fig. 8). Per-analysis files may not contain wildcards. If a setting is not provided in the configuration file for output of a certain type, then it will simply be skipped.

3.7.1 Interpretation of Cutting Scores

A cutting score for a site indicates how likely we are to observe read mapping end counts in the nuclease sample versus the control sample relative to other sites in that RNA, in those samples. Cutting scores are log ratios (natural log) of read mapping end probabilities in the nuclease sample to the control sample. A positive value at a site indicates it is more likely to have relevant ends at it in the nuclease sample than control, relative to other ends in that RNA in those samples. Magnitudes of scores zero or below are not informative and are therefore filtered out (although this can be turned off for debugging) and replaced with none in text output.

When reviewing cutting scores, it is important to distinguish between "ignored" and "non-ignored" sites. Ignored sites either were masked out by the user (*see* **Note 20**) or had too little data in nuclease and control samples to be included in cutting score calculation (the end count threshold controlling this is tunable by the user via the `algorithm.noiseCutoff` configuration setting). Ignored sites will never have cutting scores, by definition. RNAs with less read mappings tend to have more ignored sites. Ignored sites are identified prior to the normalization step; in Fig. 1, the "number of ends" track shows values for all sites, but the "end probability" and "cutting scores" tracks only show values for non-ignored sites. Sites that are ignored and non-ignored, as well as how many are in each category, are logged to the per-locus stats output files (`output.stats` configuration setting).

A higher cutting score means the site is more susceptible to the nuclease, but the reverse is not true. If the site has no cutting score and is marked non-ignored (or the cutting score is small), it should *not* be interpreted as lacking susceptibility to the nuclease (put another way, absence of evidence is not evidence of absence). This could occur due to artifacts in the algorithm or the experimental method. However, when present and large, cutting scores tend to be accurate.

Moderate to high cutting score magnitudes seem to correlate with susceptibility to probing agents from other studies [5], but we find it is only possible to compare magnitudes of cutting scores between sites in the same RNA, in the same sample. For example, Fig. 1 shows that although the relative magnitudes of cutting scores in UESC and Neural Precursor samples follow the same pattern, their absolute magnitudes are different (maxima of 1.91 and 2.87, respectively).

3.7.2 Genome Browser Output

Data at every step in the FragSeq pipeline (Fig. 4) can be output in plain text wiggle format, which can be uploaded to the UCSC Genome Browser as a custom track (Fig. 1), thus allowing the user to view structure probing data in a genomic context alongside annotations that are already present in the browser or annotations that the user can upload (*see* **Note 17**).

Uncompressed, whole-transcriptome wiggle files can be tens to hundreds of megabytes in size for eukaryotic genomes and therefore may be size-prohibitive for upload to UCSC servers as custom wiggle tracks. Also, custom tracks are not guaranteed to be retained by UCSC for a long time. Lastly, uploaded wiggle data is compressed in a lossy way on UCSC servers, meaning the data values displayed in the browser will not be exactly equal to the data uploaded. All of these issues can be circumvented if the user converts the output wiggle data to bigWig format, which is a terse, indexed, binary format storing the same information. A detailed tutorial on how to do this conversion exists (http://genome.ucsc.edu/goldenPath/help/bigWig.html; download the program `wigToBigWig`).

bigWig-format files are significantly smaller in size than wiggle files storing equivalent data, but they are required to be stored on the *user's* server—the user uploads to the UCSC Genome Browser only a track header containing an URL that points to the file on the user's server, and the browser fetches only the necessary pieces of the file as they are viewed by a user. This is more efficient than keeping all the wiggle data on UCSC servers and it is also not necessary to upload the complete data set to UCSC servers, thus circumventing the file size problem. Using the -unc flag to the `wigToBigWig` program ensures that the data is not compressed, so exact values can be seen; even without compression, there is a significant size reduction when converting wiggle to bigWig.

When input read mappings are in local coordinates (Subheading 3.5.1), output wiggle files will be in the wrong (global) coordinate system and cannot be directly uploaded to the UCSC Genome Browser. The user must write code to convert the coordinates to the genomic coordinate system before upload.

3.7.3 Output for RNA Structure Analysis

To use FragSeq data for RNA secondary structure analysis, two things can be done:

1. A secondary structure can be displayed in Varna [21], with cutting scores plotted on top of it, also highlighting non-ignored sites (Fig. 9). This is useful for evaluating secondary structure models (including comparing several models for a single RNA), producing a publication figure, seeing how well experimental results agree with a known model, etc. Raw end counts and probabilities can be displayed as well, which may be useful for troubleshooting.

2. A secondary structure can be predicted using RNAstructure software [25], using cutting scores as offsets that guide structure prediction.

The command-line version of `RNAstructure` software can predict minimum free energy (MFE) RNA secondary structures using a set of offsets provided by the user (Fig. 2). Offsets are pseudo-free-energies in units of kcal/mol; they can be ssRNA or double-stranded (ds)RNA offsets. If a base has a negative (favorable) offset, and the folding algorithm considers a structure containing that base in the corresponding configuration (i.e., base is ssRNA for an ssRNA offset or dsRNA for a dsRNA offset), the offset value is applied as a reward—the offset value is added to the

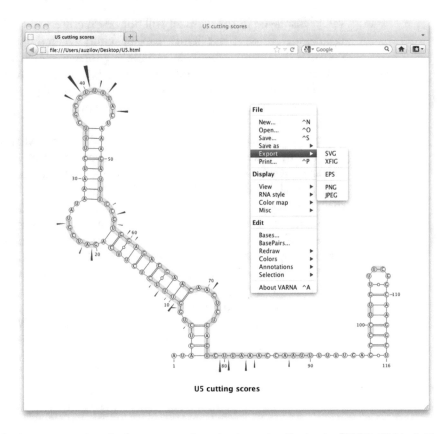

Fig. 9 Cutting scores on top of a known secondary structure, visualized using VARNA. Right-clicking opens a menu (shown) containing many useful options, such as exporting the visualization in various formats, as well as annotating the structure. *Shaded* sites are non-ignored sites

folding free energy change ($\Delta G°$) of that structure, which makes it more likely that the structure containing that base configuration will be the MFE structure.

Cutting scores can be converted to offsets using a simple linear transformation, as has been done with SHAPE probing data [38]. Positive cutting scores must be converted to negative offsets because negative free energies are favorable. Optionally, cutting scores can be filtered to remove all scores below a certain threshold, as low cutting scores may be noise (Subheading 3.7.1).

The choice of slope, intercept, and threshold has a major impact on the predicted secondary structure. In practice, we find that there is no single slope, intercept, and threshold that can be applied uniformly to improve structure prediction for all RNAs, but that is likely due to lack of robust benchmark data, as there have not been enough FragSeq experiments done at this time. In practice, we advise that the user try several slopes, intercepts, and thresholds and compare the resulting structures in VARNA. Superimposing probing data on both "before offsets" and "after offsets" structures allows one to examine how much the structures are changing as a function of these perturbations (e.g., *see* Fig. 2). It is not guaranteed that applying offsets will improve structure prediction in every case; the user must review plots of various secondary structures with probing data superimposed on them and making a judgment based on that and other forms of evidence to derive the best structure model.

4 Notes

1. We define a *site* as a position between two adjacent bases in any sequence (cDNA, RNA, sequencing read, reference sequence, etc.). In RNA, a site is the region between two bases where cleavage of the phosphate backbone could occur. End positions of read mappings are more conveniently described using site coordinates than base coordinates. For ease of algorithm implementation, native (i.e., pre-cleavage) 5′ and 3′ ends of transcripts are also considered sites.

2. Because cutting scores are log-ratios of per-site data between two samples, they are in theory somewhat tolerant of some experimental and computational biases and artifacts. For example, artifacts due to ligation bias at a site or multiple mappings of a read are a function of the reference sequence, so for any given locus they may affect the nuclease and control samples similarly and thus may cancel out. Adapter ligation bias may cancel out for the same reason. However, this robustness has not been rigorously assessed.

3. In FragSeq, read mapping end counts are normalized at each RNA locus independently, using only data for that locus. This normalization procedure is the reason why the user is required to identify coordinates of RNA loci to input to our tool. For each locus, normalization produces a discrete probability distribution of observing an end at a site, specifically in that transcript, in that sample. We chose this normalization strategy because it makes inference of cutting scores for a transcript independent from abundance of other transcripts—the relative probabilities of ends within one gene are not affected by the abundance of other genes. This is especially suitable when read coverage of genes relative to each other varies between the nuclease and control samples. For example, in ref. 5, the control sample was dominated by C/D box snoRNA reads because those RNAs have endogenous 5′ PO_4 and 3′ OH end chemistry which was ligation-competent and many fell within the size selection range; allocation of reads to these RNAs made other RNAs seem less abundant by comparison (an artifact), but the normalization procedure removed that effect.

4. We, as well as others [39], have observed that V1 also tends to cleave at ssRNA positions (including positions cleaved by

ssRNA nucleases); the mechanism of V1 recognition is believed to be stacked bases [26, 40], which can occur in ssRNA. Stacked ssRNA could be cleaved by both ssRNA nucleases and V1; additionally, there may be a substrate length requirement for V1 cleavage [40, 41] that may be different from the ssRNA nuclease requirement. It would therefore be difficult to interpret a scoring scheme based on a ratio of ssRNA-specific nuclease activity to V1 activity. This is why we prefer to base scores on activity of a nuclease with respect to its own control sample. The control sample allows us to get an estimate of ligation-competent RNA fragments that were not specifically produced by the desired nuclease.

5. A common method for purifying RNA from cells without selection for any specific type of RNA is guanidinium isothiocyanate–phenol–chloroform extraction, commonly referred to by the trade name TRIzol extraction [42]. This method is useful for RNA isolation from nearly all specimens (bacteria, archaea, yeast, plant, animal, etc.), although the volumes may need to be scaled to obtain the desired quantity of RNA. Refer to the manual that accompanies the TRIzol reagent for guidance on proper volumes for a particular project of interest. After purification with TRIzol, we recommend a subsequent treatment by DNase I to remove any retained DNA, followed by an acid phenol–chloroform extraction to obtain pure RNA.

6. This is a starting recommendation for enzyme that was diluted and flash-frozen in aliquots as indicated in Subheading 2.2, but this is a parameter than can and should be optimized per batch of P1. A fresh aliquot should be thawed and used each time that a probing experiment is performed to maintain consistency.

7. A size ladder can be produced by making a "G-ladder" by partial RNase T1 digestion of the spike-in radiolabeled RNA. Alternatively, many commercial RNA or DNA ladders can be easily radiolabeled with T4 polynucleotide kinase.

8. Note that a parallel reaction pair with added radiolabeled spike-in RNAs can also be performed if the researcher wants to monitor the digestion by gel in parallel. Keeping this monitoring reaction separate makes sure that radioactivity is not carried forward in sequencing library preparation.

9. These parameters were optimized in Subheading 3.1 for a 100 μL reaction, so scale up in a linear fashion if a larger reaction is desired.

10. Alternatively, a standard urea-PAGE can be used to size-select the desired RNAs.

11. Cleavage by nuclease P1 will leave a 5′ PO_4 and 3′ OH. If one desires smaller overall fragment sizes after nuclease P1 hydro-

lysis, a random hydrolysis ("RNA shattering") by magnesium, heat and alkaline pH can be utilized. This will generate $2',3'$-cyclic phosphates which cannot accept an adapter by T4 RNA ligase. These ends can be either ligated with a tRNA ligase [43] or by converting these cyclic phosphates to $3'$ OH with T4 polynucleotide kinase in the absence of ATP [24].

12. It is space-prohibitive to discuss the `readsToStruct.py` configuration file in this chapter. Therefore, this chapter focuses on explaining the concepts, whereas the README file in the FragSeq source code repository (Subheading 2.3) explains the command-line usage and the configuration file syntax.

13. When aligning to RNA sequences directly, you must align to the sense strand, i.e., the reference sequence index for your alignment tool must be built from FASTA sequences of the sense strand, *not* the genomic plus strand.

14. "Relevant" sites (whether in cDNA, reads, mappings, etc.; *see* **Note 1**) are those sites that correspond to "relevant" RNA fragments ends, which are the fragment ends that yield nuclease accessibility data in the nuclease sample (or the corresponding data in the control sample). Not every RNA fragment end is relevant—this depends on the experiment design and library preparation protocol. For example, in ref. 5, both RNA *fragment* ends are relevant, but for *mappings*, only the $5'$ ends are relevant in *every* mapping (the $3'$ end is relevant only for trim mappings, Fig. 3). To exclude native RNA ends from the relevant end pool, *see* **Note 20**.

15. Support for BED is retained for backwards compatibility with FragSeq version 0.0.1 used in ref. 5.

16. For trimming adapter sequence from paired-end reads, we recommend SeqPrep (https://github.com/jstjohn/SeqPrep) as it takes advantage of the fact that if a read from one end sequences into the opposing adapter, its sequence will overlap the read from the other end and they can be aligned to each other to accurately identify the adapter position; however, a wide variety of other adapter trimming tools also exist.

17. Many file formats suitable for upload to the UCSC Genome Browser are also accepted by other genome browsers. If the researcher is setting up their own genome browser for data viewing, we recommend using JBrowse [44], as it is easy to set up by users themselves and does not require running a web-server, whereas the UCSC Genome Browser aims to provide a centralized data access service managed by UCSC.

18. Names of RNA loci (fourth column in the input BED file) must follow two rules. First, names must be unique—no name can be used more than once in the file. Second, names must contain only printable, non-whitespace ASCII characters. This

is because names of RNA loci will be used to create names of output files, so to avoid issues, we are restricting the set of valid name characters to a small core set. However, there are no restrictions on names of read mappings.

19. It is only useful to input reads that are already known to overlap RNA of interest, otherwise there will be a performance cost—readsToStruct.py will spend a lot of time parsing read data and discarding it if it does not overlap any input RNA loci. Loading read data from disk is currently the rate-limiting step. The samtools package [45] has a feature to do this filtering in a faster way (samtools view -L command-line invocation) than readsToStruct.py.

20. We found that for analysis of mouse nuclear RNA in ref. 5, masking out the first five and last five sites in each known RNA locus (using the configuration setting algorithm.numEnd-SitesToIgnore) was beneficial, especially for RNAs whose mature forms have endogenous 5′ PO_4 and 3′ OH end chemistries that are ligation-competent, such as C/D box snoRNA. This setting excludes the first and last N sites from consideration by adding them to the set of ignored sites, thus excluding counts from native 5′ and 3′ ends of an RNA; only counts from presumed phosphate backbone cleavage are considered. The value of 5 was chosen to provide padding, as transcription data did not perfectly agree with RNA locus annotation boundaries. However, this means that no cutting scores will be produced for the first and last five sites of each RNA. Users are advised to adjust this option to fit their protocol and RNA locus annotations.

21. CIGAR strings are a terse way of describing alignment of two sequences. For an explanation of CIGAR strings, consult the SAM/BAM format specification (https://github.com/samtools/hts-specs). Different alignment tools may use different CIGAR operations to describe the same alignment. Some tools may use = or X to specify sequence match or mismatch, respectively, instead of the more ambiguous M (alignment match). Operation D may be used instead of N to specify introns in reads. Soft clipping (S) operations may be used instead of hard clipping (H). These alternative ways are correctly interpreted by readsToStruct.py.

22. Whether a mapping end should be considered for FragSeq if the other end is misaligned dependents on the cDNA library preparation protocol and the sequencing technology error modes. For example, because base call quality may decrease at one end of a read, misalignment of the low-quality end is more of a concern than the high-quality end. We recommend users try several strategies for filtering ambiguous mappings and examine the effect on cutting score accuracy on spike-in controls or other RNAs of known structure.

Acknowledgements

We thank David H. Mathews for the invitation to write this chapter. We also thank John St. John, Yann Ponty, and Lukasz J. Kielpinski for helpful discussions.

References

1. Wurst RM, Vournakis JN, Maxam AM (1978) Structure mapping of 5′-32P-labeled RNA with S1 nuclease. Biochemistry 17:4493–4499. doi: 10.1021/bi00614a021

2. Weeks KM (2010) Advances in RNA structure analysis by chemical probing. Curr Opin Struct Biol 20:295–304. doi:10.1016/j.sbi.2010.04.001

3. Mortimer SA, Kidwell MA, Doudna JA (2014) Insights into RNA structure and function from genome-wide studies. Nat Rev Genet 15:469–479. doi:10.1038/nrg3681

4. Kwok CK, Tang Y, Assmann SM, Bevilacqua PC (2015) The RNA structurome: transcriptome-wide structure probing with next-generation sequencing. Trends Biochem Sci 40:221–232. doi:10.1016/j.tibs.2015.02.005

5. Underwood JG, Uzilov AV, Katzman S et al (2010) FragSeq: transcriptome-wide RNA structure probing using high-throughput sequencing. Nat Methods 7:995–1001. doi:10.1038/nmeth.1529

6. Kertesz M, Wan Y, Mazor E et al (2010) Probing RNA structure genome-wide using high throughput sequencing. Protoc Exch. doi:10.1038/nprot.2010.152

7. Li F, Zheng Q, Ryvkin P et al (2012) Global analysis of RNA secondary structure in two metazoans. Cell Rep 1:69–82. doi:10.1016/j.celrep.2011.10.002

8. Sugimoto Y, Vigilante A, Darbo E et al (2015) {hiCLIP} reveals the in vivo atlas of {mRNA} secondary structures recognized by Staufen 1. Nature 519:491–494. doi:10.1038/nature14280

9. Lucks JB, Mortimer SA, Trapnell C et al (2011) Multiplexed RNA structure characterization with selective 2′-hydroxyl acylation analyzed by primer extension sequencing (SHAPE-Seq). Proc Natl Acad Sci U S A 108:11063–11068. doi:10.1073/pnas.1106501108

10. Seetin MG, Kladwang W, Bida JP, Das R (2014) Massively parallel RNA chemical mapping with a reduced bias MAP-seq protocol. In: Waldsich C (ed) Methods Mol Biol. Humana, New York, pp 95–117

11. Spitale RC, Flynn RA, Zhang QC et al (2015) Structural imprints in vivo decode RNA regulatory mechanisms. Nature 519:486–490. doi:10.1038/nature14263

12. Talkish J, May G, Lin Y et al (2014) Mod-seq: high-throughput sequencing for chemical probing of RNA structure. RNA 20:713–720. doi:10.1261/rna.042218.113

13. Incarnato D, Neri F, Anselmi F, Oliviero S (2014) Genome-wide profiling of mouse RNA secondary structures reveals key features of the mammalian transcriptome. Genome Biol 15:491. doi:10.1186/s13059-014-0491-2

14. Siegfried NA, Busan S, Rice GM et al (2014) RNA motif discovery by SHAPE and mutational profiling (SHAPE-MaP). Nat Methods 11:959–965. doi:10.1038/nmeth.3029

15. Homan PJ, Favorov OV, Lavender CA et al (2014) Single-molecule correlated chemical probing of RNA. Proc Natl Acad Sci U S A 111:13858–13863. doi:10.1073/pnas.1407306111

16. Hector RD, Burlacu E, Aitken S et al (2014) Snapshots of pre-rRNA structural flexibility reveal eukaryotic 40S assembly dynamics at nucleotide resolution. Nucleic Acids Res 42:12138–12154. doi:10.1093/nar/gku815

17. Poulsen LD, Kielpinski LJ, Salama SR et al (2015) SHAPE Selection (SHAPES) enrich for RNA structure signal in SHAPE sequencing-based probing data. RNA 21:1042–1052. doi:10.1261/rna.047068.114

18. Rouskin S, Zubradt M, Washietl S et al (2013) Genome-wide probing of RNA structure reveals active unfolding of mRNA structures in vivo. Nature 505:701–705. doi:10.1038/nature12894

19. Ding Y, Tang Y, Kwok CK et al (2013) In vivo genome-wide profiling of RNA secondary structure reveals novel regulatory features. Nature 505:696–700. doi:10.1038/nature12756

20. Kielpinski LJ, Vinther J (2014) Massive parallel-sequencing-based hydroxyl radical probing of RNA accessibility. Nucleic Acids Res 42:e70. doi:10.1093/nar/gku167

21. Darty K, Denise A, Ponty Y (2009) VARNA: interactive drawing and editing of the RNA secondary structure. Bioinformatics 25:1974–1975. doi:10.1093/bioinformatics/btp250

22. Kielpinski LJ, Boyd M, Sandelin A, Vinther J (2013) Detection of reverse transcriptase termination sites using cDNA ligation and massive parallel sequencing. In: Shomron N (ed) Methods Mol Biol. Humana, New York, pp 213–231

23. Kielpinski LJ, Sidiropoulos N, Vinther J (2015) Reproducible analysis of sequencing-based RNA structure-probing data with user-friendly tools. Methods Enzymol 558:153–180

24. Cameron V, Uhlenbeck OC (1977) 3′-Phosphatase activity in T4 polynucleotide kinase. Biochemistry 16:5120–5126. doi:10.1021/bi00642a027

25. Reuter JS, Mathews DH (2010) RNAstructure: software for RNA secondary structure prediction and analysis. BMC Bioinformatics 11:129. doi:10.1186/1471-2105-11-129

26. Ehresmann C, Baudin F, Mougel M et al (1987) Probing the structure of RNAs in solution. Nucleic Acids Res 15:9109–9128

27. Gesteland R, Cech T, Atkins J (2005) The RNA World, 3rd edn. Cold Spring Harbor Laboratory Press, Cold Spring Harbor

28. Singh R, Reddy R (1989) Gamma-monomethyl phosphate: a cap structure in spliceosomal U6 small nuclear RNA. Proc Natl Acad Sci U S A 86:8280–8283

29. Sambrook J, Fritsch EF, Maniatis T (1989) Molecular cloning: a laboratory manual, 2nd edn. Cold Spring Harbor Laboratory Press, Cold Spring Harbor

30. Lingner J, Keller W (1993) 3′-End labeling of RNA with recombinant yeast poly(A) polymerase. Nucleic Acids Res 21:2917–2920

31. Bruce AG, Uhlenbeck OC (1978) Reactions at the termini of tRNA with T4 RNA ligase. Nucleic Acids Res 5:3665–3677. doi:10.1093/nar/5.10.366

32. Malone C, Brennecke J, Czech B et al (2012) Preparation of small RNA libraries for high-throughput sequencing. Cold Spring Harb Protoc 2012:1067–1077. doi:10.1101/pdb.prot071431

33. Pak J, Fire A (2007) Distinct populations of primary and secondary effectors during RNAi in C. elegans. Science 315(5809):241–244. doi:10.1126/science.1132839

34. Li TW, Weeks KM (2006) Structure-independent and quantitative ligation of single-stranded DNA. Anal Biochem 349:242–246. doi:10.1016/j.ab.2005.11.002

35. Jayaprakash AD, Jabado O, Brown BD, Sachidanandam R (2011) Identification and remediation of biases in the activity of RNA ligases in small-RNA deep sequencing. Nucleic Acids Res 39:1–12. doi:10.1093/nar/gkr693

36. Fonseca NA, Rung J, Brazma A, Marioni JC (2012) Tools for mapping high-throughput sequencing data. Bioinformatics 28:3169–3177. doi:10.1093/bioinformatics/bts605

37. Kent WJ, Sugnet CW, Furey TS et al (2002) The human genome browser at UCSC. Genome Res 12:996–1006. doi:10.1101/gr.229102

38. Deigan KE, Li TW, Mathews DH, Weeks KM (2009) Accurate SHAPE-directed RNA structure determination. Proc Natl Acad Sci U S A 106:97–102. doi:10.1073/pnas.0806929106

39. Sobczak K, Michlewski G, de Mezer M et al (2010) Trinucleotide repeat system for sequence specificity analysis of RNA structure probing reagents. Anal Biochem 402:40–46. doi:10.1016/j.ab.2010.03.021

40. Lowman HB, Draper DE (1986) On the recognition of helical RNA by cobra venom V1 nuclease. J Biol Chem 261:5396–5403

41. Auron PE, Weber LD, Rich A (1982) Comparison of transfer ribonucleic acid structures using cobra venom and S1 endonucleases. Biochemistry 21:4700–4706. doi:10.1021/bi00262a028

42. Chomczynski P, Sacchi N (1987) Single-step method of RNA isolation by acid guanidinium thiocyanate-phenol-chloroform extraction. Anal Biochem 162:156–159. doi:10.1006/abio.1987.9999

43. Schutz K, Hesselberth JR, Fields S (2010) Capture and sequence analysis of RNAs with terminal 2′,3′-cyclic phosphates. RNA 16:621–631. doi:10.1261/rna.1934910

44. Skinner ME, Uzilov AV, Stein LD et al (2009) JBrowse: a next-generation genome browser. Genome Res 19:1630–1638. doi:10.1101/gr.094607.109

45. Li H, Handsaker B, Wysoker A et al (2009) The sequence alignment/map format and SAMtools. Bioinformatics 25:2078–2079. doi:10.1093/bioinformatics/btp352

46. Luehrsen KR, Fox GE (1981) Secondary structure of eukaryotic cytoplasmic 5S ribosomal RNA. Proc Natl Acad Sci U S A 78:2150–2154

Chapter 9

Mapping RNA Structure In Vitro with SHAPE Chemistry and Next-Generation Sequencing (SHAPE-Seq)

Kyle E. Watters and Julius B. Lucks

Abstract

Mapping RNA structure with selective 2′-hydroxyl acylation analyzed by primer extension (SHAPE) chemistry has proven to be a versatile method for characterizing RNA structure in a variety of contexts. SHAPE reagents covalently modify RNAs in a structure-dependent manner to create adducts at the 2′-OH group of the ribose backbone at nucleotides that are structurally flexible. The positions of these adducts are detected using reverse transcriptase (RT) primer extension, which stops one nucleotide before the modification, to create a pool of cDNAs whose lengths reflect the location of SHAPE modification. Quantification of the cDNA pools is used to estimate the "reactivity" of each nucleotide in an RNA molecule to the SHAPE reagent. High reactivities indicate nucleotides that are structurally flexible, while low reactivities indicate nucleotides that are inflexible. These SHAPE reactivities can then be used to infer RNA structures by restraining RNA structure prediction algorithms. Here, we provide a state-of-the-art protocol describing how to perform in vitro RNA structure probing with SHAPE chemistry using next-generation sequencing to quantify cDNA pools and estimate reactivities (SHAPE-Seq). The use of next-generation sequencing allows for higher throughput, more consistent data analysis, and multiplexing capabilities. The technique described herein, SHAPE-Seq v2.0, uses a universal reverse transcription priming site that is ligated to the RNA after SHAPE modification. The introduced priming site allows for the structural analysis of an RNA independent of its sequence.

Key words SHAPE, SHAPE-Seq, RNA, RNA structure probing, RNA structure mapping, Next-generation sequencing, RNA structure, RNA folding

1 Introduction

Mapping RNA structure with chemical probes has become a powerful technique for uncovering RNA structure–function relationships in a broad array of contexts [1]. Chemical probing experiments use reagents that covalently modify RNAs in a structure-dependent fashion, allowing structural properties of an RNA under study to be inferred once the locations of the modifications are determined. Although chemical probing structural information is lower resolution than that achievable with biophysical methods such as X-ray crystallography and NMR [1, 2], the experimental speed, flexibility,

Douglas H. Turner and David H. Mathews (eds.), *RNA Structure Determination: Methods and Protocols*, Methods in Molecular Biology, vol. 1490, DOI 10.1007/978-1-4939-6433-8_9, © Springer Science+Business Media New York 2016

and accessibility of RNA chemical probing experiments have made them amenable to an increasing number of innovative RNA structural biology studies. In recent years, chemical probing techniques have become powerful and have been extended to investigate a variety of topics including: long-range RNA–RNA interactions [3], ribosomal assembly [4], genome-wide RNA structures inside cells [5–7], viral genome organization [8], and high-resolution structure prediction and modeling [9, 10].

RNA structure probing experiments consist of several distinct steps: preparation and folding of an RNA of interest, structure-dependent covalent modification of the RNA at the nucleotide level, and determination of the modification locations [1]. Since many chemical probes preferentially modify nucleotides that are unstructured, a higher frequency of modification in specific regions can be used to infer the presence of single stranded regions, loops, or bulges (Fig. 1) [14–16]. While there are a wide variety of chemicals that can be used to probe RNA structure [1, 14, 16, 17], here we will focus on the SHAPE class of chemical probes [1, 18, 19]. SHAPE (selective 2′-hydroxyl acylation analyzed by primer extension) reagents react with the 2′-OH group of the ribose backbone of an RNA to form covalent adducts at nucleotides that are structurally flexible [15, 20]. The positions of these adducts are then detected with reverse transcriptase (RT) primer extension, which stops one nucleotide before the modification, to create a pool of cDNAs whose lengths reflect the location of SHAPE modification (+ channel) [21]. A control RT primer extension on an unmodified RNA (– channel) is also performed to identify locations where the RT has a natural propensity to abort extension and "drop off". The (+) and (–) channel cDNAs can then be used to estimate a "reactivity" for each nucleotide in the RNA, where "reactivity" represents the likelihood that a given nucleotide within an RNA sequence will be modified by the SHAPE reagent [22, 23]. High SHAPE reactivities correspond to nucleotides that are unstructured, and are more likely to occur in single-stranded regions, loops, or bulges (Fig. 1). Conversely, low reactivities can correspond to constrained nucleotides located in double-stranded helices, bound to a protein or ligand, or involved in a noncanonical base pair, stacking, or tertiary interaction [24]. In addition to qualitative interpretation, SHAPE reactivity data can also be used quantitatively to restrain secondary structure prediction algorithms to generate RNA structure models that are more consistent with experimental measurements [25, 26].

To estimate SHAPE reactivities, the location and frequency of SHAPE modifications and natural RT drop off sites need to be determined from the cDNA pools. Originally, this was done using gel electrophoresis with radiolabeled primers [21]. A sequencing ladder was used to map the location of the 3′ end of the cDNAs in the (+) and (–) channels, and a comparison of the band intensities

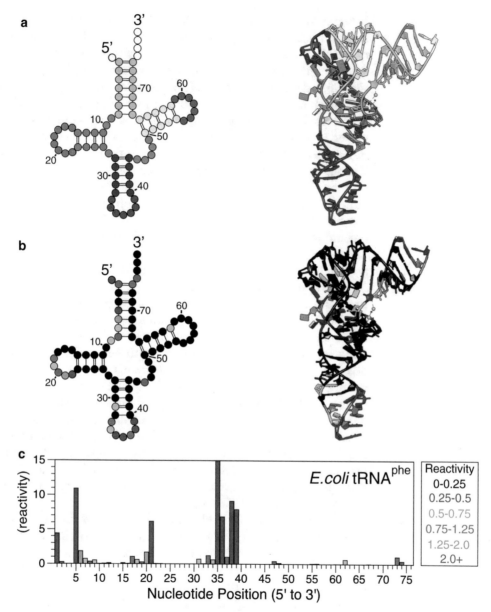

Fig. 1 Secondary and tertiary structures of *E. coli* tRNA^{phe}. (**a**) Secondary structure model of *E. coli* tRNA^{phe} (*left*) colored to show features of the tertiary structure of tRNA^{phe} (*right*, PDB: 3L0U) [11]. Note that the secondary structure image does not capture the tertiary interaction between the hairpin 1 (*orange*) and hairpin 3 (*magenta*) loops. (**b**) Secondary and tertiary structures of tRNA^{phe} colored to show SHAPE-Seq reactivity intensity (ρ) according to the bar chart in (**c**). Also note that the nucleotides involved in the tertiary interaction between hairpins 1 and 3 have low reactivities even though they occur in loops. (**c**) Bar chart showing a representative reactivity spectrum from SHAPE-Seq v2.0 for the unmodified tRNA^{phe} from *E. coli*, colored to show degrees of reactivity intensity. Reactivity data from Loughrey et al. [12] (RMDB ID [13]: TRNAPH_1M7_0002)

between the channels provided the relative frequency of modification at each nucleotide [20]. Fluorescently labeled primers were introduced later as an alternate readout method, which improved throughput with the use of capillary electrophoresis (CE) [18] and simplified data analysis with the ShapeFinder software, which assists with peak intensity quantification and reactivity calculation [27]. However, both methods are limited in that they cannot be multiplexed and suffer from the noise associated with integrating analog signals to determine the abundance of each cDNA length. Ultimately, these problems were solved by coupling the chemical modification step to next-generation sequencing (NGS) to determine the modification and natural RT drop off positions, creating the SHAPE-Seq method [28, 29]. In SHAPE-Seq, and related techniques, cDNA sequences are bioinformatically aligned to determine the precise location of (+) and (−) channel cDNA ends, providing a "digital" read out of this important information.

NGS provides a number of advantages to mapping RNA structure with chemical probes. The digital output of raw counts of modification and RT drop off positions for each nucleotide allows for a more accurate determination of reactivities without having to integrate peak or band intensities as with gel or CE-based methods. This allows for convenient implementation of algorithms that can automatically correct for signal decay due to the unidirectional nature of the RT process [22, 23]. In addition, with NGS any incorrect sequences within the cDNA sequencing reads can be filtered out, such as those that occur from off-target priming during the RT step. Finally, the automation and multiplexing afforded by the increasingly powerful NGS platforms allows for higher throughput, increased accuracy, and the ability to perform experiments on a mixture of RNAs [12, 28].

Here we describe SHAPE-Seq v2.0, which combines the innovations of the original SHAPE-Seq (v1.0) protocol [28, 29] with a number of advances to increase the flexibility and accuracy of the SHAPE-Seq technique. In SHAPE-Seq v2.0, a ssDNA linker is ligated to the 3′ end of the RNA after chemical modification to provide an RT priming site (Fig. 2) [12]. The introduced priming site is "universal", requiring only one RT primer sequence for any SHAPE-Seq v2.0 experiment, regardless of the RNA(s) being studied. Universal priming also removes the requirement of older versions of SHAPE-Seq to contain extra RNA sequences, or structure cassettes, to act as an RT priming site, which had the potential to interfere with RNA folding (Fig. 2) [12, 28]. SHAPE-Seq v2.0 also uses internal barcodes to increase the multiplexing capabilities of SHAPE-Seq and allows more experiments to be sequenced within a single NGS lane [12]. Lastly, an updated set of parameters have been determined with SHAPE-Seq v2.0 for use with RNAstructure [25] to generate experimentally restrained secondary structure models of the probed RNAs [12].

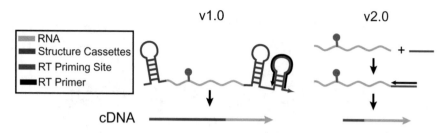

Fig. 2 Comparison of the original SHAPE/SHAPE-Seq vs. SHAPE-Seq v2.0 reverse transcription strategies. The structure cassettes are RNA hairpins added to both ends of an RNA of interest and are designed to fold independently of the desired RNA sequence under study. They were originally designed to mask signal noise that occurs at the 5′ and 3′ ends when capillary or gel electrophoresis is used to quantify the (+) and (−) channel cDNA distributions. The original SHAPE-Seq v1.0 strategy [28] used these structure cassette flanking sequences to provide a reverse transcription priming site. In SHAPE-Seq v2.0, a linker sequence is added to the RNA post-modification, which serves as a priming site for reverse transcription without the need for the structure cassettes [12]. Reproduced from Loughrey et al. 2014 by permission of Oxford University Press [12]

The SHAPE-Seq v2.0 protocol proceeds through the following steps: chemical modification with a SHAPE reagent, linker ligation, reverse transcription, ssDNA adapter ligation and PCR (for NGS library preparation), NGS, and data analysis (Fig. 3) [12]. After library preparation, NGS is performed using paired-end sequencing. Each paired-end sequence contains two reads. One read determines where the RT priming site was, while the other read indicates where the RT stop occurred (the modification site) within a given RNA sequence or set of RNA targets [29]. Data analysis is performed using Spats (http://github.com/LucksLab/spats), which separates sequencing reads into (+) and (−) channels before bioinformatically aligning the reads in each channel to the target sequence(s) to determine the (+) and (−) channel RT stop distributions. Using these distributions, Spats then applies a maximum likelihood estimation procedure to determine the reactivity values for each nucleotide in each RNA of the experiment. The reactivities are reported as θ values, where θ is the probability that a modification occurs at a particular nucleotide within a given RNA sequence [22, 23]. After normalization, the final result is a set of reactivities for each RNA analyzed that indicates the "flexibility" of each nucleotide. These reactivities can then be qualitatively interpreted or used to restrain secondary structure folding algorithms to generate experimentally guided RNA structure models [12, 25].

2   Materials

Prepare all solutions and buffers with RNase-free water. Necessary components and equipment are listed for each section of the protocol for clarity, thus, some components are repeated if needed

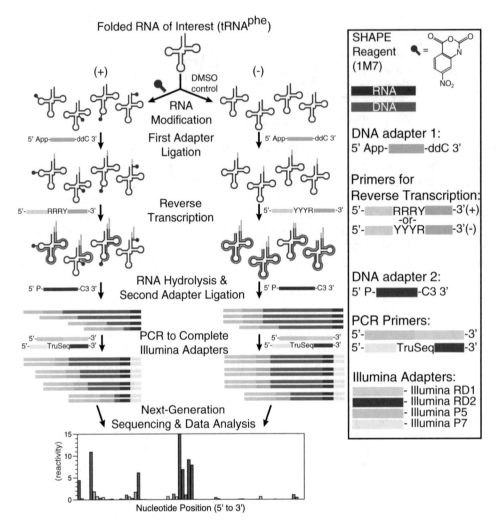

Fig. 3 SHAPE-Seq v2.0 method overview with tRNA[phe] from *E. coli* as an example. In SHAPE-Seq v2.0, RNAs are modified with a SHAPE reagent (+), such as 1M7 [18], in a structure-dependent manner. Less structured nucleotides are more likely to be modified. DNA adapter 1 is then ligated to the RNA to provide a reverse transcription (RT) priming site. Since reverse transcriptase is blocked by SHAPE modifications, RT is used to determine the RNA modification positions by creating a pool of complementary DNAs (cDNAs) whose length distribution reflects the distribution of modification positions. Control reactions (–) are performed to account for the propensity of natural RT drop off from factors other than SHAPE modification. RT primer tails contain an indexing handle that distinguishes between the (+) and (–) channels and a portion of one of the required Illumina sequencing adapters (*see* **Note 14**). The other Illumina sequencing adapter is added to the 3′ end of each cDNA through a single-stranded DNA ligation. A limited number of PCR cycles are used to both amplify the library and add the rest of the required adapters prior to sequencing. A freely available bioinformatic pipeline, Spats (http://github.com/LucksLab/spats), is then used to align sequencing reads, correct for biases due to RT-based signal decay, and calculate reactivity values

in multiple sections. Also, perform all steps in an RNase-free area. We suggest cleaning pipettes and surfaces with RNaseZap (Life Technologies), or a similar RNase-removing solution. This method assumes that a purified RNA (or set of RNAs) of interest has already been generated using in vitro transcription followed by gel purification, or similar methods.

2.1 RNA Modification Components

1. 20 pmol purified RNA of interest (*see* **Note 1**) with a free 2′-OH on the 3′ end (*see* **Note 2**).

2. 1 M HEPES buffer, pH 8.0: Add 4.7 g HEPES to 20 mL H_2O, adjust pH to 8.0 with NaOH.

3. 5 M NaCl.

4. 1 M $MgCl_2$.

5. Anhydrous dimethyl sulfoxide (DMSO).

6. 3.33× folding buffer: 333 mM HEPES, 333 mM NaCl, 33 mM $MgCl_2$, pH 8.0. Combine 333 μL 1 M HEPES, 66.6 μL 5 M NaCl, 33 μL 1 M $MgCl_2$, and 576.4 μL H_2O (*see* **Note 3**).

7. 1-methyl-7-nitroisatoic anhydride (1M7) (*see* **Note 4**): Make a 65 mM solution by weighing out 1 mg of 1M7 and dissolving in 69.3 μL anhydrous DMSO (*see* **Note 5**).

8. Thermal cycler.

9. 0.5 mL microcentrifuge tubes or thin-walled PCR tubes (*see* **Note 6**).

2.2 RNA Ligation Components

1. SuperaseIN RNase Inhibitor (Life Technologies).

2. T4 RNA ligase 2, truncated KQ (New England BioLabs).

3. 10× T4 RNA ligase buffer (*see* **Note 7**): 50 mM Tris–HCl, 10 mM $MgCl_2$, 1 mM DTT, pH 7.5. To 600 μL H_2O, add 7.88 mg Tris–HCl, 10 μL of 1 M $MgCl_2$ stock solution, and 10 μL of 100 mM DTT solution. Adjust to pH 7.5 with NaOH and bring to 1 mL with H_2O. Store at –20 °C.

4. 50% PEG 8000 solution (*see* **Note 7**): Slowly dissolve 1 g of PEG 8000 in 1 mL RNase-free H_2O. May require heat. Store at –20 °C.

5. IDT miRNA cloning linker 2 (DNA adapter 1): /5rApp/ CACTCGGGCACCAAGGA/3ddC/. /5rApp/ indicates an adenylation modification and /3ddC/ is a dideoxycytidine modification. Rehydrate to a final concentration of 20 μM (Integrated DNA Technologies).

6. Ethanol (EtOH), absolute.

7. Glycogen, 20 mg/mL.

8. 3 M NaOAc, pH 5.5.

9. 70% EtOH solution: Dilute 7 mL absolute EtOH by adding 3 mL RNase-free H_2O.

10. Refrigerated microcentrifuge.

2.3 Reverse Transcription (RT) Components

1. RT primers: Both sequences are DNA oligonucleotides. Neither requires any special purification. The (+) sample RT primer sequence is: 5′-CTTTCCCTACACGACGCTCTTC CGATCTRRRYxxTCCTTGGTGCCCGAGTG-3′ and the (−) sample RT primer sequence is: CTTTCCCTACACGACG CTCTTCCGATCTYYYRxxTCCTTGGTGCCCGAGTG (*see* **Note 8**). The "**xx**" sequences can be replaced with internal barcodes or deleted if desired (*see* **Note 9**). Make dilutions of 0.5 μM for both (*see* **Note 1**).

2. 10 mM deoxyribonucleotide triphosphates (dNTPs): Solution of 10 mM each ATP, CTP, GTP, and TTP.

3. SuperScript III (SSIII) reverse transcriptase (Life Technologies).

4. SSIII storage buffer: 20 mM Tris–HCl, 100 mM NaCl, 1 mM DTT, 1 mM EDTA, 0.01% Triton, 50% glycerol, pH 7.5. To 3 mL of H_2O, add 31.5 mg Tris–HCl, 58.4 mg NaCl, 1.54 mg DTT, 2.92 mg EDTA, 10 μL 1% Triton X-100, and 5 mL glycerol. Adjust to pH 7.5 with NaOH. Add H_2O to 10 mL. Store at −20 °C.

5. 100 mM dithiothreitol (DTT) (*see* **Note 10**). Store at −20 °C.

6. 5× SSIII first strand buffer (*see* **Note 10**): 250 mM Tris–HCl, 375 mM KCl, 15 mM $MgCl_2$, pH 8.3. In 500 μL H_2O, dissolve 39.4 mg Tris–HCl, 28.0 mg KCl, and 1.43 mg $MgCl_2$. Adjust to pH 8.3 with NaOH. Add H_2O to 1 mL final volume. Store at −20 °C.

7. RT master mix: Mix 4 volumes of 5× SSIII First Strand Buffer, 1 volume of 100 mM DTT, and 1 volume of 10 mM dNTPs. Store at −20 °C, 100 μL aliquots recommended.

8. 0.5× SSIII: Combine equal parts SSIII storage buffer and SSIII reverse transcriptase. Mix well and store at −20 °C until needed.

9. 4 M NaOH solution.

10. 1 M HCl solution.

11. Thermal cycler.

12. Ethanol, absolute.

13. Glycogen, 20 mg/mL.

14. 3 M NaOAc, pH 5.5.

15. 70% EtOH solution: Dilute 7 mL absolute EtOH by adding 3 mL RNase-free H_2O.

16. Refrigerated microcentrifuge.

2.4 ssDNA Ligation and Quality Analysis (QA) Components

1. DNA adapter 2: PAGE-purified DNA oligonucleotide with sequence 5′-/5Phos/AGATCGGAAGAGCACACGTCTGA ACTCCAGTCAC/3SpC3/-3′. /5Phos/ indicates a phosphate modification and /3SpC3/ is a three-carbon spacer modification. Dilute to 100 μM for use.

2. CircLigase I ssDNA ligase (Epicentre).

3. 10× CircLigase I reaction buffer (*see* **Note 11**): 0.5 M MOPS, 0.1 M KCl, 50 mM MgCl$_2$, and 10 mM DTT, pH 7.5. In 500 μL H$_2$O, dissolve 104.6 mg MOPS salts, 7.46 mg KCl, 4.76 mg MgCl$_2$, and 1.54 mg DTT. Adjust pH to 7.5 with NaOH. Add H$_2$O to a final volume of 1 mL. Store at −20 °C.

4. 1 mM adenosine triphosphate solution (ATP) (*see* **Note 11**).

5. 50 mM MnCl$_2$ solution (*see* **Note 11**).

6. Glycogen, 20 mg/mL.

7. 3 M NaOAc, pH 5.5.

8. Ethanol, absolute.

9. Refrigerated microcentrifuge.

10. Agencourt AMPure XP beads (Beckman Coulter).

11. Magnetic stand for 96-well plate or microcentrifuge tubes.

12. TE Buffer: 10 mM Tris–HCl, 1 mM EDTA, pH 7.5. In 5 mL H$_2$O, dissolve 15.8 mg Tris–HCl and 2.92 mg EDTA. Adjust pH to 7.5 with NaOH, then add H$_2$O to a final volume of 10 mL.

13. Phusion DNA polymerase, supplied with 5× reaction buffer (New England BioLabs).

14. 10 mM dNTPs: Solution of 10 mM each ATP, CTP, GTP, and TTP.

15. 1.5 mL microcentrifuge tubes.

16. QA_R primers: Two fluorescently labeled DNA oligonucleotides are used. No special purification is necessary. The (+) primer is 5′-VIC-GTGACTGGAGTTCAGACGTGTGCTC-3′ and the (-) primer is 5′ NED-GTGACTGGAGTTCAGACGTGTGCTC-3′ (Life Technologies) (*see* **Note 12**).

17. QA_F: DNA oligonucleotide with sequence 5′-CCCTACAC GACGCTCTTCCGATC-3′. No purification is necessary. Make a 1 μM dilution.

18. GeneScan 500 LIZ standard (Applied Biosystems).

19. Deionized formamide.

20. ABI 3730xl DNA Analyzer, or similar DNA analyzer (Applied Biosystems).

21. ShapeFinder software [27] or other program for viewing capillary electrophoresis traces.

22. (Optional) BioAnalyzer and dsDNA high sensitivity chips (*see* **Note 13**) (Applied Biosystems).

2.5 Library
Construction
Components

1. Thin-walled PCR tubes or 96-well reaction plate.

2. Thermal cycler.

3. Phusion DNA polymerase, supplied with 5× reaction buffer.

4. 10 mM dNTPs: Solution of 10 mM each ATP, CTP, GTP, and TTP.

5. PE_F: HPLC-purified DNA oligonucleotide with sequence 5′-AATGATACGGCGACCAC CGAGATCTACACTCTTTC CCTACACGACGCTCTTCCGATCT-3′. Dilute to 100 μM. (Oligonucleotide sequence © 2007–2013 Illumina, Inc. All rights reserved.)

6. Indexing PCR primers: PAGE-purified DNA oligonu cleotide with sequences 5′-CAAGCAGAAGACGGCATACGAGAT **XXXXXX**GTGACTGGAGTTCAGACGTGTGCTC-3′. Replace "XXXXXX" with indexes for Illumina sequencing, as shown in Table 1 for indexes 1–6. Dilute to 100 μM for use (*see* **Note 14**). (Oligonucleotide sequences © 2007–2013 Illumina, Inc. All rights reserved.)

7. Exonuclease I (ExoI).

8. Agencourt AMPure XP beads.

9. Magnetic stand for 96-well plate or microcentrifuge tubes.

10. TE Buffer: 10 mM Tris–HCl, 1 mM EDTA, pH 7.5. In 5 mL H$_2$O, dissolve 15.8 mg Tris–HCl and 2.92 mg EDTA. Adjust pH to 7.5 with NaOH, then add H$_2$O to a final volume of 10 mL.

11. Qubit Fluorometer High Sensitivity dsDNA kit (recommended; Life Technologies) or NanoDrop.

Table 1
Example oligonucleotides for Illumina barcoding, indexes 1–6

Illumina Index #1	CAAGCAGAAGACGGCATACGAGAT**CGTGAT**GTGACT GGAGTTCAGACGTGTGCTC
Illumina Index #2	CAAGCAGAAGACGGCATACGAGAT**ACATCG**GTGAC TGGAGTTCAGACGTGTGCTC
Illumina Index #3	CAAGCAGAAGACGGCATACGAGAT**GCCTAA**GTGACT GGAGTTCAGACGTGTGCTC
Illumina Index #4	CAAGCAGAAGACGGCATACGAGAT**TGGTCA**GTGACT GGAGTTCAGACGTGTGCTC
Illumina Index #5	CAAGCAGAAGACGGCATACGAGAT**CACTGT**GTGACT GGAGTTCAGACGTGTGCTC
Illumina Index #6	CAAGCAGAAGACGGCATACGAGAT**ATTGGC**GTGACT GGAGTTCAGACGTGTGCTC

Sequences are reverse complements of TrueSeq adapter sequences (Oligonucleotide sequences © 2007–2013 Illumina, Inc. All rights reserved)

2.6 NGS and Data Analysis	1. Illumina Sequencing Platform (MiSeq or HiSeq).
	2. Unix, Linux, or Mac OS X equipped system.
	3. Spats, v1.0.0, installed (*see* **Note 15**).

3 Methods

3.1 RNA Modification	1. Dilute 20 pmol of RNA in 12 µL RNase-free H_2O in a 0.5 mL microcentrifuge tube or thin-walled PCR tube.
	2. Prepare fresh 65 mM 1 M7 solution. To a fresh tube, add 1 µL of recently prepared 65 mM 1 M7 and mark as "+". To another fresh tube, add 1 µL of anhydrous DMSO (*see* **Note 16**) and mark as "–". Set both tubes aside until **step 6** (*see* **Note 17**).
	3. Incubate the tube from **step 1** at 95 °C for 2 min to denature the RNA (*see* **Note 18**).
	4. Snap cool the RNA by incubating on ice for 1 min, then add 6 µL of 3.3× folding buffer and mix well. There should now be 18 µL of diluted RNA.
	5. Incubate the RNA at 37 °C for 20 min (*see* **Note 19**).
	6. Add 9 µL of the RNA solution to the "–" tube and the other 9 µL to the "+" tube and mix well. Incubate the "+" and "–" tubes for 2 min (*see* **Note 4**) at 37 °C (*see* **Note 20**), then transfer to ice (*see* **Note 21**). Discard the now empty tube containing the original RNA dilution.

3.2 RNA Ligation	1. Warm 50 % PEG 8000 to room temperature to ease pipetting (*see* **Note 22**).
	2. Add the following reagents in order to each "+" and "–" tube of RNA from Subheading 3.1, **step 6** according to Table 2 (*see* **Note 23**).
	3. Vortex to mix well and incubate overnight (≥8 h) at room temperature.
	4. If using PCR tubes, transfer to 0.5 mL microcentrifuge tubes. Add 130 µL RNase-free H_2O, 1 µL 20 mg/mL glycogen, 15 µL 3 M NaOAc solution, and 450 µL of ice-cold absolute EtOH to both tubes and mix well.
	5. Incubate at –80 °C for 30 min, then spin on a chilled microcentrifuge at maximum speed for 30 min to pellet the RNA. This step can be paused by leaving the precipitations in the freezer until ready to continue.
	6. Aspirate the supernatant (*see* **Note 24**), then add 200 µL of 70 % EtOH and gently shake the tube to wash the pellet. Respin briefly (30 s to 2 min) and aspirate the EtOH wash. Repeat the brief spin and remove any remaining traces of EtOH (*see* **Note 25**), then dissolve each pellet in 10 µL of RNase-free H_2O.

Table 2
DNA adapter 1 ligation reaction components

10 µL	Modified RNA from Subheading 3.1, **step 6**
0.5 µL	SuperaseIn RNase inhibitor
6 µL	50% PEG 8000
2 µL	10× T4 RNA ligase buffer
1 µL	IDT miRNA cloning linker 2 (DNA adapter 1; 20 µM)
0.5 µL	T4 RNA ligase, truncated KQ (200 U/µL)
20 µL	Total volume

3.3 Reverse Transcription

1. Add 3 µL of 0.5 µM (+) RT primer to the "+" tube and 3 µL of 0.5 µM (−) RT primer to the "−" tube (*see* **Note 26**).

2. Incubate both tubes at 95 °C for 2 min, then 65 °C for 5 min to denature the RNA. During this step, mix the SSIII master mix by combining 12 µL of RT master mix with 2 µL 0.5× SSIII and leave on ice until the next step.

3. Snap cool the "−" and "+" tubes by incubating on ice for 30 s, then add 7 µL of SSIII master mix to each tube, mixing well and being sure to knock down any condensation from the tube walls.

4. Incubate at 45 °C for 1 min, then incubate at 52 °C for 25 min.

5. Incubate at 65 °C for 5 min.

6. Add 1 µL of 4 M NaOH solution to each tube and incubate at 95 °C for 5 min to hydrolyze the RNA.

7. Allow the tubes to cool to room temperature (*see* **Note 27**), then add 2 µL of 1 M HCl solution to partially neutralize the base (*see* **Note 28**).

8. Add 69 µL of ice-cold absolute EtOH and incubate at −80 °C for 15 min, followed by centrifugation at 15 min at maximum speed in a chilled microcentrifuge. This will pellet the cDNA. This step can be paused by leaving the precipitations in the freezer until ready to continue.

9. Aspirate the supernatant (*see* **Note 24**), then add 500 µL of 70% EtOH and gently shake the tube to wash the pellet (*see* **Note 29**). Respin briefly (30 s to 2 min) and aspirate the EtOH wash. Repeat the brief spin and remove any remaining traces of EtOH, then dissolve each pellet in 22.5 µL of RNase-free H_2O.

3.4 ssDNA Ligation and Quality Analysis

1. Add the reagents from Table 3 in order to each "+" and "−" tube of RNA from Subheading 3.3, **step 9** and mix well.

2. Incubate at 60 °C for 2 h and then 80 °C for 10 min to heat deactivate CircLigase I.

3. Add 70 μL of H_2O, 1 μL of 20 mg/mL glycogen, 10 μL 3 M NaOAc, and 300 μL ice-cold absolute EtOH to each tube.

4. Incubate at −80 °C for 30 min, then spin on a chilled microcentrifuge at maximum speed for 30 min to pellet the DNA (*see* **Note 30**). This step can be paused by leaving the precipitations in the freezer until ready to continue.

5. Aspirate the supernatant (*see* **Note 24**), then respin briefly (30 s to 2 min) and aspirate any remaining traces of EtOH. Dissolve each pellet in 20 μL of nuclease-free H_2O.

6. Purify the ssDNA libraries with Agencourt AMPure XP beads (*see* **Note 31**). To do this, make sure the beads are well suspended by swirling the bottle, then add 36 μL of the beads to each "+" and "−" tube and mix well. Incubate at room temperature for 5 min. Carefully place the tubes on a magnetic stand and let the beads separate for 2 min. Use 5 min if using a 96-well format (*see* **Note 32**). Aspirate the supernatant. While the tubes are still on the stand, gently wash with 200 μL of 70 % EtOH. Incubate for 30 s before aspirating and discarding the EtOH (*see* **Note 33**). Repeat the wash and aspiration, then let the beads air dry for 3 min (*see* **Note 34**). Remove tubes from the magnetic stand and resuspend the beads in 20 μL of TE buffer. Then, place the tubes/plate back on the magnetic stand and let the beads separate for 1 min. Transfer the supernatant, which contains the ssDNA libraries, to fresh, labeled tubes. Store libraries at −20 °C when not in use.

7. To perform quality analysis two PCRs will be set up, one for the "+" sample and one for the "−" sample (*see* **Note 35**). To do

Table 3
DNA adapter 2 ligation reaction components

22.5 μL	cDNA from Subheading 3.3, **step 9**
3 μL	10× CircLigase I ligation buffer
1.5 μL	$MnCl_2$ solution (50 mM)
1.5 μL	ATP solution (1 mM)
0.5 μL	DNA adapter 2 (100 μM)
1 μL	CircLigase I ssDNA ligase (100 U/μL)
30 μL	Total

this, first set up the "+" reaction by adding the following reagents from Table 4 in order and mixing well. Similarly, set up a "−" reaction by replacing the (+) QA_R primer with the (−) QA_R primer and using the "−" ssDNA library instead of the "+" library. Mix well.

8. Run the following thermal cycler protocol: 98 °C for 30 s, 98 °C for 10 s, 65 °C for 30 s, 72 °C for 30 s, repeat the previous three steps 11 times, 72 °C for 5 min.

9. Combine the "+" and "−" samples in a 1.5 mL microcentrifuge tube and add 50 μL H$_2$O, 10 μL 3 M NaOAc, and 300 μL ice-cold absolute EtOH.

10. Incubate at −80 °C for 15 min, then spin on a chilled microcentrifuge at maximum speed for 15 min to pellet the DNA (*see* **Note 36**).

11. Aspirate the supernatant (*see* **Note 24**), then respin briefly (30 s to 2 min) and aspirate any remaining traces of EtOH. Dissolve each pellet in 10 μL of deionized formamide, incubating at 95 °C to aid dissolution.

12. Add 0.25 μL GeneScan 500 LIZ standard to the dissolved QA DNA and run on ABI 3730xl DNA Analyzer (or similar capillary electrophoresis machine).

13. Open the resulting .fsa files generated by the DNA Analyzer with ShapeFinder [27] (*see* **Note 37**) and use the LIZ standard to identify peak lengths (*see* **Note 38**). There should be a full-length peak clearly visible at a position equal to the number of nucleotides of the RNA + 80 nt (for the Illumina adapters) (Fig. 4). Peaks at 80 nt are indicative of side product dimers that form between unextended RT primer and DNA adapter 2 and are amplified by PCR. A good library trace should show

Table 4
Reaction components for generating QA libraries

14.75 μL	Nuclease-free H$_2$O
5 μL	5× Phusion buffer
0.5 μL	dNTPs solution (10 mM)
1.5 μL	QA_F primer (1 μM)
1.5 μL	(+) QA_R primer (1 μM)
1.5 μL	"+" ssDNA library from Subheading 3.4, **step 6**
0.25 μL	Phusion DNA polymerase (2 U/μL)
25 μL	Total

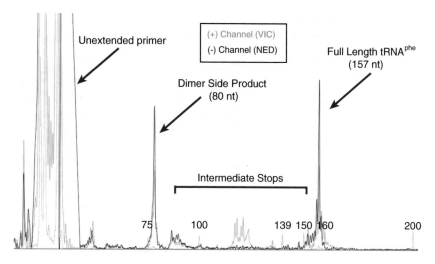

Fig. 4 Quality analysis (QA) example with an *E. coli* tRNA^{phe} dsDNA library viewed with ShapeFinder [27]. The "+" and "−" samples are visualized with the VIC (*green*) and NED (*black*) fluorophores, respectively. Unextended reverse transcription primer (Subheading 3.3) can ligate to DNA adapter 2 (Subheading 3.4) and create an unwanted dimer side product 80 nucleotides (nt) long after PCR amplification. The fully extended cDNA is observed as a large peak at 157 nt for the RNA length (77 nt for tRNA^{phe}) plus 80 nt for the partially added Illumina adapter sequences. Intermediate stops between 80 nt and 157 nt suggest either premature reverse transcriptase drop off or modified positions ("+" sample only). Unextended, fluorescently labeled QA_R primers from the QA library construction step are visible as short fragments on the *left* as indicated. This QA trace falls within our guidelines for a "good" library and was sequenced to produce the data shown in Figs. 1 and 3. Peaks for the LIZ standard (*cyan*) are annotated according to their size distribution (*see* **Note 38**)

considerable peak height and a good full length–side product ratio, with minor peaks between the full length and side product peaks. The minor peaks where the (+) channel exceeds the (−) channel are indicative of RT stops due to SHAPE modifications (*see* **Note 39**). If both the (+) and (−) channels look good, continue to Subheading 3.5, otherwise this procedure should be repeated.

3.5 Library Construction

1. To build the SHAPE-Seq libraries that will be sequenced on the Illumina platform, mix two 50 μL PCRs, one for the "+" sample and one for the "−" sample. Combine the reagents from Table 5, in order, for the "+" and "−" samples separately using the same Illumina index for both. Mix well.

2. Run the following thermal cycler protocol: 98 °C for 30 s, 98 °C for 10 s, 65 °C for 30 s, 72 °C for 30 s, repeat the previous three steps eight times, 72 °C for 5 min (*see* **Note 40**).

3. Incubate at 4 °C for 5 min (*see* **Note 41**), then add 5 U of Exonuclease I to each reaction and incubate at 37 °C for 30 min. This will remove excess primer from the libraries (*see* **Note 42**).

Table 5
Reaction components to create libraries for Illumina sequencing

35.5 μL	Nuclease-free H_2O
10 μL	5× Phusion buffer
0.5 μL	dNTPs solution (10 mM)
0.25 μL	PE_F (100 μM)
0.25 μL	Illumina Index Primer (100 μM)
3 μL	ssDNA library
0.5 μL	Phusion DNA polymerase (2 U/μL)
50 μL	Total

4. Bead purify the dsDNA libraries according to Subheading 3.4, **step 6**, except use 90 μL beads instead of 36 μL. Elute in 20 μL of TE buffer (*see* **Note 43**).

5. Use the Qubit dsDNA High Sensitivity kit or NanoDrop to measure the mass concentration of each library. Any measurable quantity can be sequenced, but a minimal target concentration of 2 ng/μL is sought after (*see* **Note 44**).

3.6 NGS and Data Analysis

1. Determine which SHAPE-Seq dsDNA libraries are to be sequenced (*see* **Note 45**). Then, use the quality analysis traces from Subheading 3.4, **step 13** to determine the average lengths of the "+" and "−" dsDNA libraries (*see* **Note 46**). Use the formula $\dfrac{1000 \times x}{(L+64) \times 607.4 + 157.9}$ to calculate the average micromolar concentration (μM) of each library, where L is the average length of the dsDNA library and x is the mass concentration (ng/μL) measured in Subheading 3.5, **step 5** (*see* **Note 47**). Do this for both the "+" and "−" dsDNA libraries separately, and for all dsDNA libraries being sequenced together (multiplexed).

2. Use the molar concentrations determined in **step 1** to balance all of the dsDNA libraries being sequenced such that they all have the same fmol of library (typically 10–30 fmol) in the final mixture, which should have a total final volume between 10 and 30 μL. Pipette all of the libraries together and measure the mass concentration of the final mixture to be sequenced with the Qubit dsDNA High Sensitivity kit or NanoDrop.

3. Sequence the mixture on the Illumina platform, using 2×35 bp paired end reads. The concentration of the mixture and the average length will be required to properly dilute the sample for sequencing. The MiSeq works well for 20 library pairs ("+"

and "–") or fewer, while the HiSeq is better for a larger number of SHAPE-Seq libraries (*see* **Note 48**). Both platforms will require at least 5 % PhiX DNA included as a control (*see* **Note 49**). Reads longer than 35 bp are not necessary (*see* **Note 50**).

4. Obtain the sequencing data from a local storage drive, sequencing facility, or BaseSpace (www.basespace.com) on a Linux, Unix, or Mac OS X capable computer and unzip the files to extract the *.fastq.gz files. There should be two files present for each Illumina index sequenced, one for read 1 (R1) and one for read 2 (R2) of the paired end reads. Then, use gunzip to decompress these files to the *.fastq format (*see* **Note 51**).

5. Create a fasta (.fa) formatted targets file Include the linker sequence and internal barcodes (if present) (*see* **Note 52**). For each *.fastq pair (R1 and R2), there should only be one *.fa file, that contains all of the target RNAs within that library.

6. Run `adapter_trimmer.py` with the following command: `adapter_trimmer.py <R1_seq.fastq> <R2_seq.fastq> <targets.fa>`, where `<R1_seq.fastq>` and `<R2_seq.fastq>` are the Illumina *.fastq files for R1 and R2, respectively, and `<targets.fa>` is the fasta-formatted targets file created in **step 5** (*see* **Note 53**). By default, the script will use the adapter sequences and read lengths described above. However, some values must be set using the option flags if differing from the default (*see* **Note 54**). The output of `adapter_trimmer.py` is two files: combined_R1.fastq and combined_R2.fastq, which have been processed to remove any Illumina adapter sequences, if present (*see* **Note 55**).

7. Feed the output of `adapter_trimmer.py` to Spats using the following command: `spats <targets.fa> RRRY` and `YYYR combined_R1.fastq combined_R2.fastq`, where `<targets.fa>` is the targets file created in **step 5** (*see* **Note 56**). The RRRY and YYYR inputs indicate that the "+" sample has the "RRRY" handle and the "–" sample has the "YYYR" handle (*see* **Note 8**). The output of Spats is a directory containing the split raw reads ($+/-$; *.fq), raw alignments (*.sam), and calculated reactivities (reactivities.out). Note that the calculated reactivities for all of the RNAs are concatenated together in the reactivities.out text file (*see* **Note 57**). Reactivities are reported as θ values for each nucleotide in a column labeled "theta".

8. Normalize the output θ_i values to ρ_i values by multiplying all of the θ_i values by one less than the original RNA length. Do not include the linker or adapter sequences in this length. These ρ reactivities are the final output SHAPE-Seq v2.0, where values between 0 and 0.5 are considered "low," 0.5–1.25 are "moderate," and >1.25 are "high" (*see* **Note 58**). These ρ_i values

can be plotted to obtain reactivity maps (Fig. 1c) or used as restraints for secondary structure prediction with RNAstructure [25] (*see* **Note 59**), using an *m*-value of 1.1 and a *b*-value of −0.3 [12] (*see* **Note 60**).

4 Notes

1. Less than 20 pmol of RNA can be used in this protocol. However, it has been optimized for 20 pmol and if less is used, more side product will be present later and will cut back on the number of usable sequencing reads. A lower concentration of RT primer can be used to partially alleviate this problem.

2. A modification of the 3′ terminal 2′-OH on the RNA of interest will prevent the RNA–DNA ligation in Subheading 3.2 from working properly. If the RNA of interest is purified directly from an in vitro transcription using T7 RNA polymerase, there are likely to be 1–3 non-templated nucleotides added to the 3′ end. The additional 3′ bases will cause an overhang mismatch during the sequence alignment step with Bowtie, which can reduce the number of usable sequencing reads. There are a few ways this problem can be dealt with: either use a ribozyme that cleaves off the 3′ end, such as the hepatitis δ ribozyme (with end healing to regenerate the 3′-OH) [12, 30], introduce a methoxy-modification near the 3′ end of the DNA template to reduce non-templated base addition [31], or add the extra non-templated bases to the targets file when performing the sequence alignment with Bowtie and assume the extra bases do not affect the RNA structure of interest.

3. Other folding buffers can be used, but should be prepared at a 3.33× concentration.

4. 1M7 is not commercially available and must be synthesized. There are two protocols currently available to do so [29, 32]. If an alternate is desired, one commercially available option is *N*-methylisatoic anhydride (NMIA; Life Technologies) [21]. However, if using NMIA, *increase* the modification time in Subheading 3.1, **step 6** from 1 to 45 min. Similarly, if benzoyl cyanide [33] is used, *reduce* the modification time from 1 min to <5 s.

5. The 1M7 solution should be prepared fresh whenever possible. However, 1M7 will retain most of its reactivity for approximately 5–6 days when stored properly in a low-moisture environment in a well-sealed tube. Degraded 1M7 will have undergone the same color change as if it was hydrolyzed as mentioned in **Note 21**.

6. Using a thermal cycler with the capability to handle 0.5 mL microcentrifuge tubes is the easiest method and will not require

tube transfers. If using thin-walled PCR tubes, you will need to transfer to a 0.5 mL microcentrifuge tube to perform EtOH precipitations and transfer back to a new PCR tube.

7. 10× T4 RNA ligase buffer and 50 % PEG 8000 solution are supplied with T4 RNA Ligase, truncated KQ when purchased from New England BioLabs.

8. The basic composition of the primer is as follows: (1) CTTTCCCTACACGACGCTCTTCCGATCT is the 3′ half of one Illumina adapter required for sequencing, the other half is added with PCR during library construction in Subheading 3.5. (Oligonucleotide sequence © 2007–2013 Illumina, Inc. All Rights Reserved.) (2) RRRY/YYYR (R for purine, Y or pyrimidine) is a degenerate pool of indexing handles used to distinguish the "+" and "−" samples during reactivity calculation. If the libraries are properly balanced during sequencing, the first four reads will also provide randomness to help calibrate the Illumina sequencing platform. (3) "xx" is a placeholder for an optional internal barcode (*see* **Note 9**). (4) TCCTTGGTGCCCGAGTG is the reverse complement to DNA adapter 1, providing an RT priming site. *See* Loughrey et al. Fig. S4 for more detailed information [12].

9. For large numbers of experiments where fewer Illumina indexes are being used (to reduce the cost of buying many expensive oligonucleotides) or a lot of barcoding options are required, an internal barcode can be included at the "xx" position. These barcodes, if used with different lengths, can also be used to shift the sequencing reading frame to improve randomness when sequencing the DNA adapter 1 sequence common to all of the experiments. For example, adding "aa" as a barcode and "c" as another, two experiments containing the same RNA sequence can be distinguished by uniquely aligning to different targets with Bowtie, one that has the "aa" present and the other that has "c" present. Note that if any barcodes are used, they need to be able to uniquely align with Bowtie. Thus, using "aa" and "a" as two different barcodes will not work, as the "a" barcode would still align to the "aa" barcode sequence. However, if "a" were replaced with any other base it would uniquely align.

10. 100 mM DTT and 5× SSIII first strand buffer are both supplied in excess with SuperScript III when purchased from Life Technologies.

11. 10× CircLigase I reaction buffer, 1 mM ATP, and 50 mM $MnCl_2$ are supplied in excess with CircLigase I when purchased from Epicentre.

12. Because of the proprietary nature of the VIC and NED fluorophores, they can only be ordered from Life Technologies.

13. If using the Applied Biosystems BioAnalyzer to perform library quality analysis instead of capillary electrophoresis with fluorescently labeled DNA, as outlined in Subheading 3.4, you will need the high sensitivity DNA chips to properly analyze the dsDNA libraries (*see* **Note 46**). Note that the resolution is lower than with the capillary electrophoresis method. Also, you will not need to acquire **items 16–21** in Subheading 2.4.

14. The Illumina TruSeq indexing system has a number of predesigned sequences as shown in Table 1. For additional indexing sequences beyond indexes 1–6, replace the "XXXXXX" with the six nucleotide indexing sequence as provided by Illumina for the TruSeq system.

15. First, the FastX toolkit and LibGTextUtils (http://hannonlab. cshl.edu/fastx_toolkit/download.html) need to be installed. The Spats pipeline also requires the alignment program Bowtie (http://sourceforge.net/projects/bowtie-bio/files/bowtie/ 0.12.8/) and the Boost software libraries (www.boost.org). The adapter_trimmer.py script mentioned in Subheading 3.6 is included with the Spats source code. Detailed installation instructions for Spats can be found at http://luckslab. github.io/spats/installation.html.

16. Use a syringe to puncture the septum of the anhydrous DMSO bottle and measure the volume of DMSO to add. It is not a problem if the DMSO/1M7 solution is briefly exposed to air afterward.

17. If using thin-walled PCR tubes and need to perform tube transfers at later steps for EtOH precipitations, etc. continue to label new tubes as "+" and "−". Always use a fresh tube when transferring.

18. If incubating at 95 °C would irreversibly denature or destroy an RNA-containing complex and/or the RNA of interest is already folded in a different buffer, skip to Subheading 3.1, **step 5**. An alternate RNA folding protocol could be inserted here instead. If so, perform the alternative folding method and then proceed to Subheading 3.1, **step 5**.

19. If the relevant temperature and folding time for analyzing the RNA of interest is not 37 °C, this step can be easily altered. However, we suggest incubating for at least a few minutes at a constant temperature to allow the temperature to come to equilibrium before modification.

20. If using a folding temperature other than 37 °C, perform the modification at the same temperature. Note that the reaction rate of 1M7 is dependent on temperature, requiring more incubation time if using a lower temperature.

21. The 1M7 reaction is self-quenching in water, and will turn from yellow to orange when the reaction is complete.

22. Pipette the PEG solution slowly and carefully, it is very viscous and it is easy to add the wrong volume by accident. However, a slight inaccuracy in the PEG volume will not likely negatively impact the ligation reaction.

23. If a different folding buffer other than the one described in Subheading 2.1 was used, EtOH precipitate the modified RNAs from Subheading 3.1, **step 6** by adding 90 µL RNase-free H_2O, 10 µL 3 M NaOAc (pH 5.5), 1 µL 20 mg/mL glycogen, and 300 µL of ice-cold absolute EtOH and store at −80 °C for 30 min. Then spin on a chilled microcentrifuge for 30 min at maximum speed and aspirate all of the EtOH, making sure that no EtOH remains. Dissolve the pellet in 10 µL of 10% DMSO in H_2O before mixing the ligation reaction in Subheading 3.2, **step 2**.

24. When aspirating large volumes of EtOH, doubling pipette tips can reduce the chance of disrupting the pellet. To do this, start with a larger volume pipette (such as 1 mL) and attach a tip. Then, plunge that tip into a low-volume tip with a fine point (such as a 10 µL tip). That way you can use the large pipette to handle the volume of EtOH present, but the fine tip to carefully withdraw EtOH from around the small pellet.

25. The glycogen should clearly distinguish the pellet, which frequently looks like a white streak at the bottom of the tube.

26. If using internal barcodes (*see* **Note 9**), add the appropriate matching barcode primer set. It is required that both the "+" and "−" samples have the same internal barcode.

27. Be careful when handling the tubes. If they are not cooled first, the pressure inside will cause them to pop open, potentially ejecting some of the sample.

28. Adding too much acid will prevent the EtOH precipitation in the next step from working properly. It is not required to fully neutralize the base.

29. The pellet after this step is frequently easy to see from some salts precipitating. However, not seeing a pellet does not necessarily mean that the reverse transcription or precipitation failed, it could simply indicate that fewer salts precipitated. The amount of cDNA product expected should not be easily visible by eye without glycogen.

30. After precipitation following the ligation step, the pellet can be seen as a rounded white dot on the bottom of the tube. Because glycogen has been added, the pellet should be clearly visible. Not seeing a pellet after this step could be an indicator that the reverse transcription did not generate much cDNA, but does not necessarily indicate complete failure. Observing a brown pellet is indicative of insufficient removal of the base following the RNA hydrolysis step, which causes the CircLigase reaction

to fail. Note, however, that extended centrifugation (much greater than 30 min) may cause a mild brown discoloration to occur in the pellet in samples that were properly ligated.

31. While the Agencourt Ampure XP beads are generally thought of as a method for purifying dsDNA, they also work very well for ssDNA. We have noticed that ssDNAs under 50 nucleotides do not bind to the beads very well, but above 50 nucleotides ssDNAs bind well. The roughly 50 nucleotide cutoff helps remove unligated adapters and unextended reverse transcription primer.

32. The bead separation will sometimes proceed slowly. If so, allow more time for the beads to completely separate. Longer incubation times are fine here, and not allowing complete separation will introduce recovery losses.

33. Allowing the beads to sit in the EtOH wash for too long can introduce recovery losses.

34. Do not overdry the beads. We have observed some recovery issues when this occurs.

35. If using the BioAnalyzer to perform quality analysis, skip this step and continue to Subheading 3.5.

36. The pellet after this step should be a clearly visible round white dot. The fluorophores present can sometimes give the pellet a pinkish hue, which is normal.

37. Other capillary electrophoresis software programs are suitable as well. We use ShapeFinder since it provides an easy-to-view window and is freely available. However, none of the specific analysis tools inherent to ShapeFinder are required. One software alternative is the freely available Peak Scanner software (Life Technologies).

38. The GeneScan 500 LIZ standard has peaks at: 35, 50, 75, 100, 139, 150, 160, 200, 250, 300, 340, 350, 400, 450, 490, and 500 nucleotides.

39. The smaller the peak at 80 nucleotides, the better the library quality. The side product is sequenced and takes away from the usable sequencing reads for alignment and reactivity calculation. While some side product is always expected, it is typically at a low enough level that data analysis is not a problem, although up to 50% side product is not unusual. However, if the library is completely dominated by side product, few reads will be usable and more material will need to be sequenced to get an adequate number of usable reads. The amount of side product visible is typically related to how well the ligation and reverse transcription steps were performed. Some RNA sequences could, however, ligate or reverse-transcribe poorly due to interference caused by secondary structures.

40. As a standard, nine cycles of PCR amplification are used to minimize potential bias introduced to the data from PCR. However, we have recently shown that up to 20 cycles can be used instead (if higher concentrations are needed) with little to no apparent bias introduced [12].

41. This cooling step is very important. If skipped, the dsDNA libraries could be partly heat-denatured and digested by ExoI when added. ExoI is not immediately heat deactivated, so skipping this cooling step will likely result in complete digestion of the dsDNA libraries.

42. This step is not explicitly required, but does help improve accuracy when measuring library concentration. Errors in quantification can affect library balancing when sequencing, especially for low concentration dsDNA libraries.

43. When eluting, be careful not to over-pipette. Frequently, traces of the surfactants present in the 5× Phusion buffer can make the final dsDNA solution appear somewhat bubbly. These bubbles will not affect the quantification or sequencing, however.

44. Libraries with less than 2 ng/μL are likely to be mostly dimer side product due to poor reverse transcription. These libraries can be sequenced, but will likely require more sequencing depth to overcome the amount of side product present. A library concentration of 10 ng/μL or higher is considered optimal for nine cycles of PCR. Be mindful that increasing the number of cycles to increase the library concentration will also increase the amount of side product and not help overcome problems with too much side product.

45. Because the raw number of reads required per "+" and "−" library pair is around 1–2 M, many pairs of libraries can be run together in a single MiSeq or HiSeq run. We recommend obtaining this many reads to overcome data losses due to sequencing the dimer side product. Many different libraries can be prepared together or separately to be sequenced all at once. However, when multiplexing many libraries together, each library pair needs to be able to uniquely align with Bowtie. Using all different TruSeq indexes (*see* **Note 14**) for each library pair will generate separate sequencing data files, thus ensuring unique alignments. If multiple library pairs share the same TruSeq index, be sure that their constituent RNA sequences are all unique, or are all barcoded to be unique (*see* **Note 9**).

46. If using the BioAnalyzer for quality analysis, run 1 μL of each of the dsDNA libraries on a high sensitivity DNA chip and use the resulting electropherograms to determine what the average fragment lengths of the "+" and "−" libraries are.

47. If the BioAnalyzer was used to determine the average lengths of the dsDNA libraries, use this formula instead: $\frac{1000 \times x}{607.4 \times L + 157.9}$.

48. The number of libraries sequenced and the sequencing platform should be chosen such that each library pair should have 1–2 M sequencing reads for downstream data analysis. This is a conservative recommendation, and fewer reads can be used, though we recommend 1–2 M when starting out with this protocol. This gives roughly 20–25 libraries for the MiSeq or 100–150 libraries per HiSeq lane.

49. To provide a certain degree of randomness for the Illumina sequencing platform, some fraction of the sequenced library should be PhiX control DNA (provided with sequencing kit). We suggest using 5 % PhiX, although higher concentrations of the PhiX control will only improve sequencing quality. Due to differences in the phasing correction between the MiSeq and HiSeq, using a higher %PhiX with the HiSeq platform may be advisable. The choice of sequencing with MiSeq or HiSeq will not alter the final data [12].

50. Because SHAPE-Seq v2.0 aligns the sequencing data to a file of known RNA targets, only a short stretch of bases are required to confidently align the sequencing reads. Longer reads would only be necessary if the RNA sequence was unknown and needed to be assembled de novo.

51. gunzip can be run on the Linux/Unix command line or Mac OS X terminal with the command: gunzip *.fastq.gz. The fastq files should be named according to the provided sample name (when samples were sequenced) and TruSeq index.

52. As an example of constructing the targets file, consider an RNA of interest that contains a polyA at the 3′ end: …AAAAAAA. To include the linker sequence, add "CACTCGGGCACC AAGGAC" to the 3′ end of the RNA of interest sequence. Without any internal barcodes the targets file should read:

    >RNA_of_interest

    …AAAAAAACACTCGGGCACCAAGGAC

    If an "aa" barcode was included in the reverse transcription primer, add the reverse complement to the 3′ end, resulting in the following for a barcoded target:

    >RNA_of_interest

    …AAAAAAACACTCGGGCACCAAGGACtt

53. Detailed documentation can be found at http://github.com/ LucksLab/spats. Run time scales with the number of reads in a given fastq file pair. Under 5 M reads, the analysis should take less than an hour. For 25 M reads, the adapter trimming could

take multiple hours, mostly due to the stepwise trimming portion of `adapter_trimmer.py` (*see* **Note 55**). The screen output of the program will indicate how long each step is taking and provide an idea of how long the entire algorithm will take to complete.

54. There are a few options that can be added to the `adapter_trimmer.py` command to specify variables important to the analysis. Use the "-h" or "--help" options to reveal all of them. Most of the options will be unnecessary for most users of this protocol. Two options may be useful. The first is "--read-len $<N>$", where N is the $2 \times N$ bp paired-end read length, to be included if something other than 2×35 is used (which is the default value). The other is "--trim-match $<N>$", where N, in this case, is the number of bases used to search for Illumina adapter sequence (*see* **Note 55**). The "trim-match" variable only needs to be increased from the default value, 6, if any of the RNAs of interest contain the beginning of an Illumina adapter sequence. It can be manually changed if this is the case or, more easily, optimally determined using the `targets_analyzer.py` script included in the Spats source code from http://github.com/LucksLab/spats.

55. `adapter_trimmer.py` works by first determining if a sequencing read pair aligns to any of the targets provided. If not, the read pair is searched to determine if it contains a portion of the Illumina adapter sequence based on the *trim-match* variable (*see* **Note 54**). If no adapter sequence is found, base-by-base sequential trimming is used to determine if only a few bases of adapter are present in the sequencing read (shorter than the *trim-match* length). By exhaustively searching all of the sequencing reads in this manner, all adapter sequences are removed that perfectly match any length of the adapter sequence.

56. Spats runs much more quickly than `adapter_trimmer.py` (*see* **Note 53**) and should take less than an hour to calculate reactivities for 25 M reads.

57. The reactivities.out file should show a range of reactivities (θ) for all nucleotides in an RNA. Typically, a fair number of values are "0", but the total number of 0s should generally not exceed 80% or so. Reads aligned to every nucleotide in both the "+" and "−" samples should be observed, although the exact number of reads will vary from nucleotide to nucleotide. Because reactivities are calculated using fragment distributions [22, 23], it is possible to see positions where the "+" sample alignments exceed the "−" sample, but the reactivity is "0". Also, aligned reads tend to accumulate at the 3′ end of the RNA due to abortive reverse transcription. Thus, the reactivities of the last four nucleotides in an RNA sequence may show unusual patterns. If no reads are aligning in either the "+" or "−" sam-

ples, the targets file should be the first place to look for issues. Common problems include miscopied RNA sequence and incorrect reverse complementarity for the linker/internal barcode sequences. Comparing the raw fastq files in Read 1 to the 3′ ends of the targets is generally the best place to look for inconsistencies between the targets file and the sequencing data. If the targets file contains all the correct sequence, extensive sequencing errors (having degenerate bases appear, for example) could cause poor alignment. If these errors occur at the 3′ end of either the Read 1 or Read 2 reads, they can be trimmed off using `fastx_trimmer` from the FastX toolkit without affecting data calculation. Lastly, poor alignment of one sample could be due to an underabundance of that sample, typically caused by addition of the wrong RT primer, pipetting errors when preparing the library mix for sequencing, or incorrect balancing calculations/average length determination.

58. A repository of chemical probing data, including SHAPE-Seq v2.0, can be found at the RNA Mapping Database (rmdb. stanford.edu/repository/) [13]. We highly recommend that users of this method deposit their data in this database after publication for easy community access. See Loughrey et al. for locations of example SHAPE-Seq v2.0 data [12].

59. Bar charts of the reactivity values, ρ, can serve as "fingerprints" for an RNA structure. Clusters of highly reactive positions are strong indicators of loop regions that are very flexible. Likewise, clusters of very low reactivity positions can indicate base-paired nucleotides. One typical pattern to observe contains clusters of low reactivity, followed by high then low again, which suggest a stem-loop. Note that tertiary interactions and noncanonical base pairs can also affect nucleotide reactivity and make data interpretation more difficult. Further, these types of interactions are usually not included in RNA folding algorithms and can lead to oversimplified views of predicted RNA structures. Thus, we typically focus on the reactivity map as the final form of SHAPE-Seq data, supplemented with a number of possible interpretations without relying on a single minimum free energy structure.

60. RNAstructure [25] has long supported SHAPE reactivity values as restraints for secondary structure prediction. RNAStructure can be accessed via web server or downloaded as a GUI or command line executable (http://rna.urmc.rochester.edu/RNAstructure.html). To include restraints, a reactivities file must first be generated. To do this, create a text file with two tab-separated columns, where the first column has numbers from 1 to the exact length of the RNA being folded and the second has the reactivity (ρ) value. Use the value "−999" for bases to ignore or if there is no data present for that base. Save this file as *.shape instead of *.txt, then

input the *.shape file and the values 1.1 for *m* and –0.3 for *b* to the SHAPE Constraints subsection of the Optional Data section of the RNAtructure webserver (http://rna.urmc.rochester.edu/RNAstructureWeb/Servers/Predict1/Predict1.html) when folding the RNA. The output will be restrained with the SHAPE-Seq reactivities. The *Fold* algorithm of RNAstructure adds an extra pseudo-free energy term of the form $\Delta G_{\text{SHAPE}} = m\ln(\rho + 1) + b$ during total free energy calculation. The values *m* and *b* were heuristically determined to be 1.1 and –0.3, respectively, for SHAPE-Seq v2.0 using a panel of well-characterized RNAs [12]. Alternatively, *ShapeKnots*, which includes pseudoknots, can be used in place of *Fold* [34].

Acknowledgements

We thank Alex Settle for assistance on experimental procedures, Peter Schweitzer and the Cornell Life Sciences Core facility for sequencing support, and David Loughrey and James Chappell for helpful comments in reviewing this manuscript. This work was supported by the National Science Foundation Graduate Research Fellowship Program (grant number DGE-1144153 to K.E.W.); the Cornell University Center for Life Sciences Enterprises, a New York State Center for Advanced Technology supported by New York State and industrial partners (grant number C110124 to J.B.L.); and a New Innovator Award through the National Institute of General Medical Sciences of the National Institutes of Health (grant number DP2GM110838 to J.B.L.). K.E.W. is a Fleming Scholar in the Robert F. Smith School of Chemical and Biomolecular Engineering at Cornell University. J.B.L. is an Alfred P. Sloan Research Fellow.

References

1. Weeks KM (2010) Advances in RNA structure analysis by chemical probing. Curr Opin Struct Biol 20:295–304
2. Butcher SE, Pyle AM (2011) The molecular interactions that stabilize RNA tertiary structure: RNA motifs, patterns, and networks. Acc Chem Res 44:1302–1311
3. Duncan CDS, Weeks KM (2008) SHAPE analysis of long-range interactions reveals extensive and thermodynamically preferred misfolding in a fragile group I intron RNA. Biochemistry 47:8504–8513
4. McGinnis JL, Weeks KM (2014) Ribosome RNA assembly intermediates visualized in living cells. Biochemistry 53:3237–3247
5. Rouskin S, Zubradt M, Washietl S et al (2014) Genome-wide probing of RNA structure reveals active unfolding of mRNA structures in vivo. Nature 505:701–705
6. Ding Y, Tang Y, Kwok CK et al (2014) In vivo genome-wide profiling of RNA secondary structure reveals novel regulatory features. Nature 505:696–700
7. Talkish J, May G, Lin Y et al (2014) Mod-seq: high-throughput sequencing for chemical probing of RNA structure. RNA 20:713–720
8. Siegfried NA, Busan S, Rice GM et al (2014) RNA motif discovery by SHAPE and mutational profiling (SHAPE-MaP). Nat Methods 11:959–965
9. Homan PJ, Tandon A, Rice GM et al (2014) RNA tertiary structure analysis by 2′-hydroxyl molecular interference. Biochemistry 53:6825–6833

10. Cheng C, Chou FC, Kladwang W et al (2015) Consistent global structures of complex RNA states through multidimensional chemical mapping. eLife 4, e07600

11. Byrne RT, Konevega AL, Rodnina MV, Antson AA (2010) The crystal structure of unmodified tRNAPhe from Escherichia coli. Nucleic Acids Res 38:4154–4162

12. Loughrey D, Watters KE, Settle AH, Lucks JB (2014) SHAPE-Seq 2.0: systematic optimization and extension of high-throughput chemical probing of RNA secondary structure with next generation sequencing. Nucleic Acids Res 42:e165

13. Cordero P, Lucks JB, Das R (2012) An RNA mapping DataBase for curating RNA structure mapping experiments. Bioinformatics 28:3006–3008

14. Peattie DA, Gilbert W (1980) Chemical probes for higher-order structure in RNA. Proc Natl Acad Sci U S A 77:4679–4682

15. McGinnis JL, Dunkle JA, Cate JHD, Weeks KM (2012) The mechanisms of RNA SHAPE chemistry. J Am Chem Soc 134:6617–6624

16. Culver GM, Noller HF (1998) Directed hydroxyl radical probing of 16S ribosomal RNA in ribosomes containing Fe(II) tethered to ribosomal protein S20. RNA 4:1471–1480

17. Brunel C, Romby P (2000) Probing RNA structure and RNA-ligand complexes with chemical probes. Methods Enzymol 318:3–21

18. Mortimer SA, Weeks KM (2007) A fast-acting reagent for accurate analysis of RNA secondary and tertiary structure by SHAPE chemistry. J Am Chem Soc 129:4144–4145

19. Spitale RC, Flynn RA, Torre EA et al (2014) RNA structural analysis by evolving SHAPE chemistry. Wiley Interdiscip Rev RNA 5:867–881

20. Wilkinson KA, Merino EJ, Weeks KM (2006) Selective 2'-hydroxyl acylation analyzed by primer extension (SHAPE): quantitative RNA structure analysis at single nucleotide resolution. Nat Protoc 1:1610–1616

21. Merino EJ, Wilkinson KA, Coughlan JL, Weeks KM (2005) RNA structure analysis at single nucleotide resolution by selective 2'-hydroxyl acylation and primer extension (SHAPE). J Am Chem Soc 127:4223–4231

22. Aviran S, Trapnell C, Lucks JB et al (2011) Modeling and automation of sequencing-based characterization of RNA structure. Proc Natl Acad Sci U S A 108:11069–11074

23. Aviran S, Lucks JB, Pachter L (2011) RNA structure characterization from chemical mapping experiments. 49th annual Allerton Conference on communication, control, and computing. pp 1743–1750. doi:10.1109/Allerton.2011.6120379

24. Steen K-A, Rice GM, Weeks KM (2012) Fingerprinting noncanonical and tertiary RNA structures by differential SHAPE reactivity. J Am Chem Soc 134:13160–13163

25. Mathews DH, Disney MD, Childs JL et al (2004) Incorporating chemical modification constraints into a dynamic programming algorithm for prediction of RNA secondary structure. Proc Natl Acad Sci U S A 101:7287–7292

26. Low JT, Weeks KM (2010) SHAPE-directed RNA secondary structure prediction. Methods 52:150–158

27. Vasa SM, Guex N, Wilkinson KA et al (2008) ShapeFinder: a software system for high-throughput quantitative analysis of nucleic acid reactivity information resolved by capillary electrophoresis. RNA 14:1979–1990

28. Lucks JB, Mortimer SA, Trapnell C et al (2011) Multiplexed RNA structure characterization with selective 2'-hydroxyl acylation analyzed by primer extension sequencing (SHAPE-Seq). Proc Natl Acad Sci U S A 108:11063–11068

29. Mortimer SA, Trapnell C, Aviran S et al (2012) SHAPE-Seq: high-throughput RNA structure analysis. Curr Protoc Chem Biol 4:275–297

30. Avis JM, Conn GL, Walker SC (2012) Cis-acting ribozymes for the production of RNA in vitro transcripts with defined 5' and 3' ends. Methods Mol Biol 941:83–98

31. Kao C, Zheng M, Rüdisser S (1999) A simple and efficient method to reduce nontemplated nucleotide addition at the 3 terminus of RNAs transcribed by T7 RNA polymerase. RNA 5:1268–1272

32. Turner R, Shefer K, Ares M (2013) Safer one-pot synthesis of the "SHAPE" reagent 1-methyl-7-nitroisatoic anhydride (1m7). RNA 19:1857–1863

33. Mortimer SA, Weeks KM (2009) Time-resolved RNA SHAPE chemistry: quantitative RNA structure analysis in one-second snapshots and at single-nucleotide resolution. Nat Protoc 4:1413–1421

34. Hajdin CE, Bellaousov S, Huggins W et al (2013) Accurate SHAPE-directed RNA secondary structure modeling, including pseudoknots. Proc Natl Acad Sci U S A 110:5498–5503

Chapter 10

Experiment-Assisted Secondary Structure Prediction with RNAstructure

Zhenjiang Zech Xu and David H. Mathews

Abstract

Experimental probing data can be used to improve the accuracy of RNA secondary structure prediction. The software package RNAstructure can take advantage of enzymatic cleavage data, FMN cleavage data, traditional chemical modification reactivity data, and SHAPE reactivity data for secondary structure modeling. This chapter provides protocols for using experimental probing data with RNAstructure to restrain or constrain RNA secondary structure prediction.

Key words Thermodynamics, RNA structure prediction, SHAPE, Chemical modification data

1 Introduction

Techniques are available for determining RNA structure, including X-ray crystallography [1], NMR [2], and cryo-electron microscopy [3]. While providing high-resolution information for RNA structure, they require a large amount of human labor and expertise. Thus, RNA structure determination lags behind fast-paced genomic and transcriptomic sequencing [4–6].

Alternatively, enzymatic and chemical probing are commonly used to experimentally map secondary and tertiary RNA structure, as they are quicker to perform and can be read using widely available sequence techniques. In a probing experiment, folded RNA molecules are exposed to the probing reagent. The reagent either cleaves the RNA or prevents read-through by reverse transcriptase. Traditionally, the positions and extent of modification were then determined by polyacrylamide gel electrophoresis (PAGE), but now capillary electrophoresis [7] or deep sequencing [8–11] can be used. The modification pattern then is compared to that of the untreated RNA as a control. Because the reactivities of nucleotides to the reagent depend on the context of the local structure, the changes in the extent of modification can help detect nucleotides

Douglas H. Turner and David H. Mathews (eds.), *RNA Structure Determination: Methods and Protocols*, Methods in Molecular Biology, vol. 1490, DOI 10.1007/978-1-4939-6433-8_10, © Springer Science+Business Media New York 2016

that participate in RNA secondary and tertiary structure interactions, as well as RNA–protein contacts. Excellent reviews on RNA structure probing are available in the literature [12–17].

Chemical reagents have been available for over 30 years [15, 18]. Dimethylsulfate (DMS) is one of the most widely used chemicals for RNA structure probing. One reason for this is that it can readily penetrate cells without prior membrane permeabilization and modify RNA under in vivo conditions at N1 of adenosine and N3 of cytosine [10, 19–21]. Other popular probing reagents include, but are not limited to, 1-cyclohexyl-(2-morpholinoethyl) carbodiimide metho-*p*-toluene sulfonate (CMCT, which primarily modifies U at N3 and G at N1), diethyl pyrocarbonate (DEPC, which primarily modifies A at N7), and kethoxal (which primarily modifies G at N1 and N2). They all covalently modify the accessible nucleotides in a structure-dependent way, which can be detected by blockage of reverse transcriptase during primer extension.

Other reagents, including as RNases [14, 22] and flavin mononucleotide (FMN) [23], are able to cleave RNA molecules at specific sites. RNases selectively cleave at unpaired or base paired nucleotides. FMN specifically photocleaves RNA at uridines in G-U base pairs. Additionally, hydroxyl radicals generated by Fe(II)-EDTA can break the sugar–phosphate backbone independent of secondary structure and is used to probe structured nucleotides buried in tertiary configurations or protected by protein interactions [24–26].

New tools, such as in-line probing [27] and selective 2′-hydroxyl acylation analyzed by primer extension (SHAPE) [7, 28], have been introduced more recently to facilitate RNA structure determination. They both act independently of base identity and react at the 2′-hydroxyl group in each ribose ring. In-line probing measures local nucleotide flexibility by quantifying the rates of spontaneous cleavage. It is often used to quantify RNA structure changes due to ligand binding. SHAPE also reports local nucleotide dynamics at all positions in RNA by attacking the ribose 2′ hydroxyl with an electrophile. The reactivity of the 2′-hydroxyl is sensitive to the local nucleotide conformation, and unpaired nucleotides tend to react to a greater extent than base paired nucleotides. The adducts can be detected by primer extension and sequencing. SHAPE allows rapid determination of RNA structures comprehensively at single nucleotide resolution and is used in time-resolved structure dynamics analysis [29].

Computational prediction is often indispensable to build models of RNA structure. This is true even when experimental probing data are available because experiments are often noisy and do not in themselves determine the detailed structure. For example, some nucleotides are not chemically or enzymatically reactive because they are inaccessible due to crowding in vivo, protein binding, or experimental limitations. RNAstructure is an RNA structure prediction package that includes facilities for experimental-assisted structure determination. Algorithms have been implemented to employ data from (1) SHAPE, (2) chemical modification, (3) enzymatic and FMN cleavage, and (4) other general experiments or human insight.

The SHAPE reactivity of a nucleotide is inversely correlated with the probability that the nucleotide is base paired and thus can be converted to a pseudo-free energy change term for each base pair stack. The pseudo-free energy change is then used in dynamic programming algorithms in RNAstructure in addition to the thermodynamic nearest neighbor parameters [28]. This algorithm predicted greater than 90% of the known base pairs for the *E. coli* 16S rRNA and other smaller RNAs that are poorly predicted by computational methods alone. It was also successfully applied to modeling the structure of the whole HIV genome [30].

Chemical reagents like CMCT, DMS, and kethoxal modify nucleotides that are unpaired, in A-U or G-C pairs at helix ends, in G-U pairs, or adjacent to G-U pairs. The modifications can be ranked according to strength. Strong and moderate modifications can be used as hard constraints in folding and the recursions of the structure prediction algorithm prevent conformations that conflict with the constraints. Weak modifications are ignored because they can occur in nucleotides buried in helices. FMN photocleaves RNA specifically at uridine in G-U pairs, and that information can be used to constrain structure prediction. For enzymatic cleavage, a nucleotide is constrained to be paired or unpaired (depending of the specificity of the nuclease) only if it is cut on both its immediate 5' and 3' sides. These constraints are also applied into the structure prediction algorithm to prevent any predictions that conflict with the constraints. Additionally, one or more nucleotides can be required to be paired or unpaired in structure prediction if information from other sources suggests so. All of the above algorithms are rigorously implemented in RNAstructure to predict lowest free energy structure or base pair probabilities [21, 31]. One caveat of applying chemical modification or enzymatic constraints is that they are hard constraints and thus incorrect constraints might direct algorithms to the wrong prediction.

This chapter focuses on how to use the RNAstructure package to model RNA secondary structure with experimental data included as part of a structure prediction calculation. The high accuracies of the methods explained here [21, 28, 31] were demonstrated by comparing the predicted structures to reference secondary structures derived from comparative sequence analysis [32] as measured with sensitivity and positive predictive value (PPV) [33]. Sensitivity is the percentage of true base pairs that are predicted and PPV is the percentage of predicted base pairs that are in the reference structure. The download and installation of the RNAstructure package and the input and output file formats are described in detail in chapter 2. An online help page is available at http://rna.urmc.rochester.edu/RNAstructureHelp.html.

2 Protocols

2.1 RNAstructure Graphical User Interface for Experimental Data

Several modules in the RNAstructure graphical user interface are capable of utilizing experimental data for RNA secondary structure prediction. These modules include single sequence free energy minimization and partition function calculation (*see* Chapter 2 of this volume). Although the following two sections only describe the protocols and examples for the free energy minimization module, they are similar for the partition function calculation. And the results from a partition function calculation with integrated experimental data can then be used for structure prediction with MaxExpect [34] or ProbKnot [35].

2.2 Incorporating Traditional Chemical and Enzymatic Constraints into Secondary Structure Prediction

RNAstructure is capable of incorporating chemical and enzymatic experimental data into dynamic programming algorithms for RNA secondary structure prediction. After choosing a module under the "RNA" menu for secondary structure prediction, a "Force" menu option will be available to set experimental constraints. For example, clicking "RNA" → "Fold RNA Single Strand" will make the "Force" menu item available. Users can then input the "Sequence File" and "CT File" (as described in Chapter 2) and specify chemical constraints, enzymatic constraints, FMN cleavages and SHAPE reactivities with the "Force" menu as shown in Fig. 1. After inputing constraints, the constraint information is temporarily stored in the program and only associated with the current prediction. The constraints need to be input again when starting another

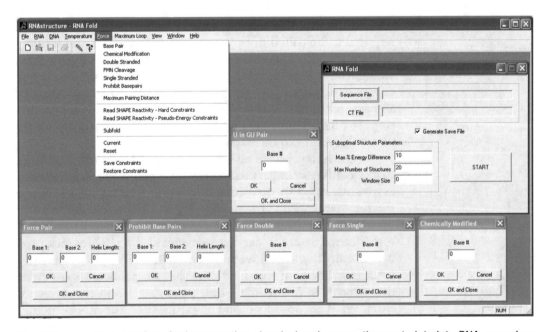

Fig. 1 The graphical interface for incorporating chemical and enzymatic constraints into RNA secondary structure prediction

prediction. One convenient way to do this is to save the inputted constraints to disk using "Force" → "Save Constraints". These can then be subsequently restored from the saved file by clicking "Force" → "Restore Constraints". It is also recommended that the constraints are saved, not only to save clicking and typing later, but also to provide a record of what was entered. The format of the saved constraint file, a plain text, is described below.

To provide constraints, the following steps are used:

1. Chemical modification. A small dialog window titled "Chemically Modified" is opened by clicking "Force" → "Chemical Modification". Input the position of a modified nucleotide (where 1 is the 5′-most nucleotide) and click the button labeled "OK" to input another modified nucleotide until there is no more to add. Then click the "OK and Close" button to close the window. In the structure prediction, each specified nucleotide will be unpaired, at a helix end, or in or adjacent to a G-U pair. Prior modification studies demonstrate that the nucleotides at these positions are accessible to probing chemicals CMCT, DMS, and kethoxal. Users are advised to use only strong and moderate modifications and ignore weak ones because they can occur in nucleotides buried in helices.

2. FMN cleavage. Users can specify FMN cleavage sites by clicking "Force" → "FMN Cleavage". A window titled "U in GU Pair" pops up as FMN specifically cleaves at uridine in G-U pairs. Users can input the position of the cleaved uridine, which then will be forced to pair with a guanosine in the prediction. Again, click the button "OK" to input another cleaved uridine. After inputting all the FMN cleavage sites, click "OK and Close".

3. Enzymatice cleavage. For enzymatic cleavages, it is recommended that a nucleotide is constrained to be paired or unpaired (depending of the specificity of the nuclease) only if it is cut on both on its immediate 5′ and 3′ sides. Users can choose the menu item "Force" → "Single Stranded" or "Force" → "Double Stranded" to input the nucleotides cleaved by nucleases. This opens a "Force Single" or "Force Double" window. The input manner is the same as that explained above for chemical modification or FMN cleavage.

4. Force base pairs and prohibit base pairs. Specific base pairs can be forced to occur or prohibited from occurring by choosing the menu items "Force" → "Base Pair" or "Force" → "Prohibit Basepairs", respectively. Users first input the positions of the two bases that pair at the start of the forced or prohibited helix and then the length of the helix. Press "OK" to input for another helix and press "OK and Close" to finish the input. While there are no specific experiments that can provide these data, this information can be gleaned from sequence alignment or intuition.

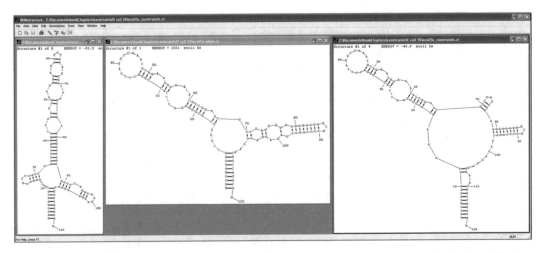

Fig. 2 The secondary structures prediction of *E. coli* 5S rRNA by RNAstructure with chemical modification constraints. *Left*: the lowest free energy structure predicted without modification constraints; *middle*: the reference secondary structure from comparative sequence analysis; *right*: the lowest free energy structure predicted with modification constraints [21]. The percentage of known base pairs in the predicted structure increased from 26.3 to 86.8 %. The sequence file and constraint file used for this figure come as examples with the RNAstructure package

After inputting all the experimental data, users can confirm that the input is correct by clicking "Force" → "Current" to show the currently specified constraints. If there is anything wrong or users want a prediction without experimental data, clicking "Force" → "Reset" will erase all the constraints.

RNAstructure is restrictive with the input constraints and will prohibit prediction of any secondary structures conflicting with the constraints outlined above. Thus users should be cautious not to provide erroneous constraints to force RNAstructure to predict possibly wrong structures. Usually the accuracies of predictions assisted with experimental data are higher than for those without experimental data, especially for the sequences poorly predicted by computation alone [21]. Figure 2 shows an example of *E. coli* 5S rRNA. The percentage of known base pairs in the predicted structure increased from 26.3 to 86.8 % by using modification constraints [21].

2.3 Incorporating SHAPE Data into Secondary Structure Prediction

SHAPE is a widely used approach to quantitatively probe RNA structure. It measures nucleophilic reactivity of the ribose 2′-hydroxyl at nucleotide resolution. The reactivities are strongly correlated with the local nucleotide flexibility. Thus SHAPE reactivity of each nucleotide can be converted to a pseudo-free energy change term because there is an inverse correlation to the probability of the nucleotide forming a base pair. For nucleotide *i*, the pseudo-free energy can be described as the following equation:

$$"G_{\text{SHAPE}} = m \ln(k_i + 1) + b$$

where ki is the SHAPE reactivity of the nucleotide, and m and b are the slope and the intercept parameters. The ΔG_{SHAPE} is applied for each nucleotide in each base pair stack. This SHAPE pseudo-free energy change term, in conjunction with nearest neighbor thermodynamic parameters, is incorporated into dynamic programming algorithms in RNAstructure for RNA secondary structure prediction.

This SHAPE-assisted structure prediction is also available under the "Force" menu item as shown in Fig. 1. Taking the free energy minimization method for a single sequence as an example, after choosing "Fold RNA Single Strand" under the "RNA" menu item and specifying the SEQ and CT file names (described in "Fold" module in Chapter 2 of this volume), users can choose the "Force" → "Read SHAPE Reactivities—Pseudo-Energy Constraints" menu option. This will open the window as shown in Fig. 3. Click "SHAPE Datafile" to input the data file containing

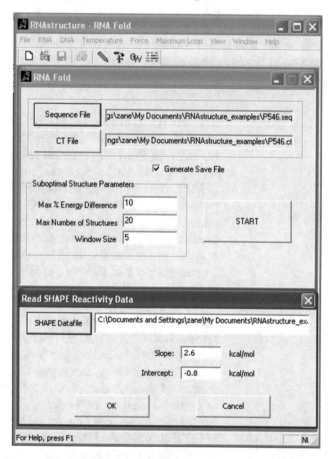

Fig. 3 The graphical user interface for SHAPE-directed RNA secondary structure prediction

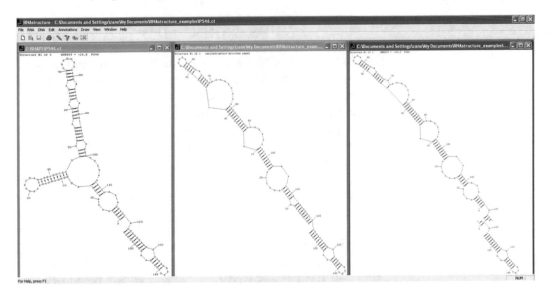

Fig. 4 The secondary structure prediction of the P546 domain of the bl3 group I intron by RNAstructure with SHAPE data. *Left*: the lowest free energy structure predicted without SHAPE data; *middle*: the reference secondary structure from comparative sequence analysis [57]; *right*: the lowest free energy structure predicted with SHAPE data modeled as pseudo-free energy changes [28]. The sensitivity and PPV of prediction with SHAPE data are improved from 42.9 % and 44.4 % to 96.4 % and 98.2 %, respectively. The sequence file and SHAPE data file for this figure come as examples with the RNAstructure package

SHAPE reactivities (the file format is explained in the following section). The "Slope" and "Intercept" parameters are m and b, respectively, from the equation above. The default values were previously found to balance the nearest neighbor parameters and SHAPE data and were parameterized against a database of structures [36]. Then click the "OK" button to finish the input and close the window. Finally, click the "START" button to start the prediction and a calculation progress bar will appear. Figure 4 is an example prediction for the P546 domain of the bI3 group I intron. The sensitivity and PPV of SHAPE assisted prediction is improved to 96.4 % and 98.2 %, respectively.

Alternatively, SHAPE data can be used as hard constraints in the recursions of dynamic programming algorithm. In this approach, nucleotides with SHAPE reactivity equal or above a specified threshold are forced single stranded. Additionally, nucleotides below that reactivity, but equal or above a second threshold, are treated as though they were accessible to chemical modification, i.e., not allowed to be buried in a helix. This is implemented in RNAstructure and can be accessed by choosing the "Force" → "Read SHAPE Reactivity—Hard Constraints" menu option. This option is available for testing and may be useful in specialized applications, but this has not been well tested.

Another way to employ SHAPE information is to color anno-tate an RNA secondary structure diagram according to the SHAPE reactivities of its nucleotides. After a structure is drawn, the "Annotations" → "Add SHAPE Annotation" menu item can be chosen to color-annotate a secondary structure. This is useful because it can show any inconsistencies between SHAPE reactivities and the predicted structure.

2.4 File Formats

Folding constraints are saved in plain text, and with a .CON file extension by default. These can be hand edited. There are different types of constraints—"DS", "SS", "Mod", "FMN", "Pairs", "Forbids", which stand for "Double Stranded", "Single Stranded", "Chemical Modification", "FMN Cleavage", "Base Pairs", and "Prohibit Basepairs" on the "Force" menu option. A sample of this file format is shown in Fig. 5. There can be multiple entries of each type of constraint with each entry listed on a separate line. When there is no constraint of a type, there are no lines required. After specifying entries for a type of constraint, it should be ended by a line of "–1" or "–1 –1". For "Base Pairs" and "Prohibit Basepairs", the first argument should be the lower nucleotide index (the more 5′ nucleotide) in the pair.

SHAPE reactivities need to be normalized before being input to RNAstructure. Specifically, the nucleotides with reactivities larger than 1.5 times the inter-quartile range are identified as outli-ers. All the nucleotide reactivities are then divided by the average intensity of the 10 % most highly reactive nucleotides without outliers [28]. The file format for SHAPE reactivity comprises two columns separated by any white space. The first column is the nucleotide position, and the second is the reactivity. Nucleotides for which there is no SHAPE data can either be left out of the file, or the reactivity can be entered as less than –500. A sample of the SHAPE reactivity file format is shown in Fig. 5. By default, RNAstructure looks for SHAPE data files to have the file extension ".SHAPE", but any plain text file can be read.

2.5 Alternative Protocols: Text User Interface

All the protocols described above have command-line interfaces for Windows, GNU/Linux, and Mac OS-X operating systems. Their command-line versions also have the same sets parameters as the graphical user interface. Some other modules, such as Dynalign [37] and Multilign [38], are able to take experimental data in the text interface but are not able to use experimental data with the graphical user interface. They require a configuration file in the command line, in which users can optionally specify the folding constraints file and the SHAPE data file in addition to input sequences, output CT and other parameters. The formats for those configuration files can be found in the online help page: http://rna.urmc.rochester.edu/Text/index.html.

Constraint File Sample	SHAPE Reactivity File Sample	
DS:	19	-999
15	20	-999
25	21	0.67157407
-1	22	0.55462963
SS:	23	0.51401852
17	24	0.53527778
35	25	0.3362963
-1	26	0.43446296
Mod:	27	0.1537037
2	28	0.16041296
15	29	-999
-1	30	0
Pairs:	31	-999
16 26	32	-999
-1 -1	33	0.042816
FMN:	34	0.15027
-1	35	0
Forbids:	36	0
15 27	37	0.16201
-1 -1	38	-999

Fig. 5 Constraint and SHAPE data file formats for RNAstructure. **Constraint file sample**: Nucleotides 15 and 25 will be predicted double-stranded. Nucleotide 17 and 35 will be single-stranded. Nucleotides 2 and 15 are accessible to chemical modification and will be predicted to be unpaired, in A-U or G-C pairs at helix end, in G-U pairs anywhere, or adjacent to G-U pairs. No nucleotide is accessible to FMN cleavage. Nucleotide 16 will be forced to pair with nucleotide 26. Nucleotide 15 will not be paired with nucleotide 27. **SHAPE file sample**: Nucleotides 1 through 20, 29, 31, 32 and 38 have no reactivity information. There are reactivities for all other nucleotides shown. Note that some nucleotides (30, 35, and 36) have normalized SHAPE reactivities of 0, which does not mean there is no data for those nucleotides

3   Notes

Prediction of structures conserved in multiple sequences (described in Chapter 3 of this volume) and prediction assisted with experimental data are two effective ways to improve RNA secondary structure prediction. RNA structure analysis by chemical probing is usually reliable and accurate, but requires human labor and expertise. It is often time consuming to apply to large-scale structure determination. Recently, parallel analysis of RNA structures (PARS) [9] and fragmentation sequencing (FragSeq) [8], which combine the classic RNA structure probing techniques with high-throughput sequencing, have been reported to profile RNA structures genome-wide. SHAPE also enables high-throughput RNA structure characterization when coupled with deep sequencing technology [11, 39].

Besides RNAstructure, an algorithm is also reported to reconcile experimental data, including SHAPE, DMS, and PARS as restraints with the thermodynamic model to improve RNA structure prediction [40]. In addition, a "Sample and select" approach is proposed to sample a large number of structures from predicted Boltzmann ensemble and select a structure with the minimum distance to experimental data [41]. This uncoupling between structure prediction and selection is more robust to experimental noise and constraint errors. BayesFold is another program that uses Bayes Theorem to predict the probabilities of RNA secondary structure given the experimental data [42].

Accuracies of structure prediction, constrained or restrained with experimental data, are improved as compared to prediction without data, especially for those RNA sequences poorly predicted by computational methods alone. Additionally, probing experiments have other uses. Combined with probing experiments done in different conditions, predictions can reveal conformation dynamics that may be induced by binding of proteins or ligands or other perturbations [43, 44]. Secondly, constraints are useful to identify pseudoknots because constraints generally reduce the number of suboptimal structures, making possible human inspection of suboptimal structures to spot pseudoknot candidates [45–47]. Thirdly, experimental data may contain structural information of high-order or long-range interactions, providing valuable insight in interpreting the predicted structures [48]. Last but not least, the time-resolved chemistry can be used to obtain RNA structure snapshots for kinetic studies such as RNA folding pathways [29, 49].

There are other types of experiments that can be utilized for RNA structure determination. NMR spectroscopy is widely used to obtain information about the structure and dynamics of nucleic acid molecules. NAPSS is a program that integrates NMR data into RNA secondary structure prediction and improves prediction accuracy [50, 51] (*see* Chapter 11 of this volume). Nucleotide analog interference mapping (NAIM) allows mapping of important functional groups [52, 53]. Microarrays are also able to improve RNA secondary structure prediction by RNAstructure [54]. The mutate-and-map method that combines systematic mutagenesis and chemical mapping is also able to probe RNA secondary structure [55, 56].

Acknowledgement

This protocol was developed with the support of National Institutes of Health Grant R01GM076485 to D.H.M.

References

1. Holbrook SR, Kim SH (1997) RNA crystallography. Biopolymers 44(1):3–21. doi:10.1002/(SICI)1097-0282(1997)44:1<3::AID-BIP2>3.0.CO;2-Z

2. Furtig B, Richter C, Wohnert J, Schwalbe H (2003) NMR spectroscopy of RNA. Chembiochem 4(10):936–962. doi:10.1002/cbic.200300700

3. Bai XC, McMullan G, Scheres SH (2015) How cryo-EM is revolutionizing structural biology. Trends Biochem Sci 40(1):49–57. doi:10.1016/j.tibs.2014.10.005

4. Tang F, Barbacioru C, Wang Y, Nordman E, Lee C, Xu N, Wang X, Bodeau J, Tuch BB, Siddiqui A, Lao K, Surani MA (2009) mRNA-Seq whole-transcriptome analysis of a single cell. Nat Methods 6(5):377–382. doi:10.1038/nmeth.1315

5. Martin JA, Wang Z (2011) Next-generation transcriptome assembly. Nat Rev Genet 12(10):671–682. doi:10.1038/nrg3068

6. Grabherr MG, Haas BJ, Yassour M, Levin JZ, Thompson DA, Amit I, Adiconis X, Fan L, Raychowdhury R, Zeng Q, Chen Z, Mauceli E, Hacohen N, Gnirke A, Rhind N, di Palma F, Birren BW, Nusbaum C, Lindblad-Toh K, Friedman N, Regev A (2011) Full-length transcriptome assembly from RNA-Seq data without a reference genome. Nat Biotechnol 29(7):644–652. doi:10.1038/nbt.1883

7. Merino EJ, Wilkinson KA, Coughlan JL, Weeks KM (2005) RNA structure analysis at single nucleotide resolution by selective 2′-hydroxyl acylation and primer extension (SHAPE). J Am Chem Soc 127(12):4223–4231

8. Underwood JG, Uzilov AV, Katzman S, Onodera CS, Mainzer JE, Mathews DH, Lowe TM, Salama SR, Haussler D (2010) FragSeq: transcriptome-wide RNA structure probing using high-throughput sequencing. Nat Methods 7(12):995–1001. doi:10.1038/nmeth.1529

9. Kertesz M, Wan Y, Mazor E, Rinn JL, Nutter RC, Chang HY, Segal E (2010) Genome-wide measurement of RNA secondary structure in yeast. Nature 467(7311):103–107. doi:10.1038/nature09322

10. Ding Y, Tang Y, Kwok CK, Zhang Y, Bevilacqua PC, Assmann SM (2014) In vivo genome-wide profiling of RNA secondary structure reveals novel regulatory features. Nature 505(7485):696–700. doi:10.1038/nature12756

11. Lucks JB, Mortimer SA, Trapnell C, Luo S, Aviran S, Schroth GP, Pachter L, Doudna JA, Arkin AP (2011) Multiplexed RNA structure characterization with selective 2′-hydroxyl acylation analyzed by primer extension sequencing (SHAPE-Seq). Proc Natl Acad Sci U S A 108(27):11063–11068. doi:10.1073/pnas.1106501108

12. Ziehler WA, Engelke DR (2001) Probing RNA structure with chemical reagents and enzymes. Curr Protoc Nucleic Acid Chem Chapter 6: Unit 6 1. doi:10.1002/0471142700.nc0601s00

13. Low JT, Weeks KM (2010) SHAPE-directed RNA secondary structure prediction. Methods 52(2):150–158. doi:10.1016/j.ymeth.2010.06.007

14. Knapp G (1989) Enzymatic approaches to probing RNA secondary and tertiary structure. Methods Enzymol 180:192–212

15. Ehresmann C, Baudin F, Mougel M, Romby P, Ebel J, Ehresmann B (1987) Probing the structure of RNAs in solution. Nucleic Acids Res 15:9109–9128

16. Ding Y, Kwok CK, Tang Y, Bevilacqua PC, Assmann SM (2015) Genome-wide profiling of in vivo RNA structure at single-nucleotide resolution using structure-seq. Nat Protoc 10(7):1050–1066. doi:10.1038/nprot.2015.064

17. Sloma MF, Mathews DH (2015) Improving RNA secondary structure prediction with structure mapping data. Methods Enzymol 553:91–114. doi:10.1016/bs.mie.2014.10.053

18. Peattie DA, Gilbert W (1980) Chemical probes for higher-order structure in RNA. Proc Natl Acad Sci U S A 77(8):4679–4682

19. Tijerina P, Mohr S, Russell R (2007) DMS footprinting of structured RNAs and RNA-protein complexes. Nat Protoc 2(10):2608–2623. doi:10.1038/nprot.2007.380

20. Zaug AJ, Cech TR (1995) Analysis of the structure of Tetrahymena nuclear RNAs in vivo: telomerase RNA, the self-splicing rRNA Intron, and U2 snRNA. RNA 1:363–374

21. Mathews DH, Disney MD, Childs JL, Schroeder SJ, Zuker M, Turner DH (2004) Incorporating chemical modification constraints into a dynamic programming algorithm for prediction of RNA secondary structure. Proc Natl Acad Sci U S A 101:7287–7292

22. Daou-Chabo R, Condon C (2009) RNase J1 endonuclease activity as a probe of RNA secondary structure. RNA 15(7):1417–1425. doi:10.1261/rna.1574309

23. Burgstaller P, Famulok M (1997) Flavin-dependent photocleavage of RNA at G.U base pairs. J Am Chem Soc 119:1137–1138

24. Tullius TD, Dombroski BA (1986) Hydroxyl radical "footprinting": high-resolution information about DNA-protein contacts and application to lambda repressor and Cro protein. Proc Natl Acad Sci U S A 83(15):5469–5473

25. Culver GM, Noller HF (2000) Directed hydroxyl radical probing of RNA from iron(II) tethered to proteins in ribonucleoprotein complexes. Methods Enzymol 318:461–475

26. Shcherbakova I, Mitra S, Beer RH, Brenowitz M (2006) Fast Fenton footprinting: a laboratory-based method for the time-resolved analysis of DNA, RNA and proteins. Nucleic

Acids Res 34(6):e48. doi:10.1093/nar/gkl055

27. Regulski EE, Breaker RR (2008) In-line probing analysis of riboswitches. Methods Mol Biol 419:53–67. doi:10.1007/978-1-59745-033-1_4

28. Deigan KE, Li TW, Mathews DH, Weeks KM (2009) Accurate SHAPE-directed RNA structure determination. Proc Natl Acad Sci U S A 106(1):97–102. doi:10.1073/pnas.0806929106

29. Mortimer SA, Weeks KM (2008) Time-resolved RNA SHAPE chemistry. J Am Chem Soc 130(48):16178–16180. doi:10.1021/ja8061216

30. Watts JM, Dang KK, Gorelick RJ, Leonard CW, Bess JW Jr, Swanstrom R, Burch CL, Weeks KM (2009) Architecture and secondary structure of an entire HIV-1 RNA genome. Nature 460(7256):711–716. doi:10.1038/nature08237

31. Mathews DH, Sabina J, Zuker M, Turner DH (1999) Expanded sequence dependence of thermodynamic parameters provides improved prediction of RNA secondary structure. J Mol Biol 288:911–940

32. Pace NR, Thomas BC, Woese CR (1999) Probing RNA structure, function, and history by comparative analysis. In: Gesteland RF, Cech TR, Atkins JF (eds) The RNA world, 2nd edn. Cold Spring Harbor, Cold Spring Harbor Laboratory Press, pp 113–141

33. Mathews DH (2004) Using an RNA secondary structure partition function to determine confidence in base pairs predicted by free energy minimization. RNA 10:1178–1190

34. Lu ZJ, Gloor JW, Mathews DH (2009) Improved RNA secondary structure prediction by maximizing expected pair accuracy. RNA 15:1805–1813

35. Bellaousov S, Mathews DH (2010) ProbKnot: fast prediction of RNA secondary structure including pseudoknots. RNA 16:1870–1880. doi:10.1261/rna.2125310

36. Hajdin CE, Bellaousov S, Huggins W, Leonard CW, Mathews DH, Weeks KM (2013) Accurate SHAPE-directed RNA secondary structure modeling, including pseudoknots. Proc Natl Acad Sci U S A 110(14):5498–5503. doi:10.1073/pnas.1219988110

37. Mathews DH, Turner DH (2002) Dynalign: an algorithm for finding the secondary structure common to two RNA sequences. J Mol Biol 317:191–203

38. Xu Z, Mathews DH (2011) Multilign: an algorithm to predict secondary structures conserved in multiple RNA sequences. Bioinformatics 27(5):626–632. doi:10.1093/bioinformatics/btq726

39. Aviran S, Trapnell C, Lucks JB, Mortimer SA, Luo S, Schroth GP, Doudna JA, Arkin AP, Pachter L (2011) Modeling and automation of sequencing-based characterization of RNA structure. Proc Natl Acad Sci U S A 108(27):11069–11074. doi:10.1073/pnas.1106541108

40. Wu Y, Shi B, Ding X, Liu T, Hu X, Yip KY, Yang ZR, Mathews DH, Lu ZJ (2015) Improved prediction of RNA secondary structure by integrating the free energy model with restraints derived from experimental probing data. Nucleic Acids Res 43(15):7247–7259. doi:10.1093/nar/gkv706

41. Quarrier S, Martin JS, Davis-Neulander L, Beauregard A, Laederach A (2010) Evaluation of the information content of RNA structure mapping data for secondary structure prediction. RNA 16(6):1108–1117. doi:10.1261/rna.1988510

42. Knight R, Birmingham A, Yarus M (2004) BayesFold: Rational 2° folds that combine thermodynamic, covariation, and chemical data for aligned RNA sequences. RNA 10(9):1323–1336

43. Moazed D, Stern S, Noller HF (1986) Rapid chemical probing of conformation in 16S ribosomal RNA and 30S ribosomal subunits using primer extension. J Mol Biol 187:399–416

44. Matsuura M, Noah JW, Lambowitz AM (2001) Mechanism of maturase-promoted group II intron splicing. EMBO J 20:7259–7270

45. Mathews DH (2005) Predicting a set of minimal free energy RNA secondary structures common to two sequences. Bioinformatics 21:2246–2253

46. Wuchty S, Fontana W, Hofacker IL, Schuster P (1999) Complete suboptimal folding of RNA and the stability of secondary structures. Biopolymers 49:145–165

47. Zuker M (1989) On finding all suboptimal foldings of an RNA molecule. Science 244:48–52

48. Brunel C, Romby P, Westhof E, Ehresmann C, Ehresmann B (1991) Three-dimensional model of Escherichia coli ribosomal 5 S RNA as deduced from structure probing in solution and computer modeling. J Mol Biol 221:293–308

49. Mathews DH, Turner DH (2002) Use of chemical modification to elucidate RNA folding pathways. In: Beaucage SL, Bergstrum DE, Glick GD, Jones RA (eds) Current protocols in nucleic acid chemistry. Wiley, New York, pp 11.19.11–11.19.14

50. Chen JL, Bellaousov S, Tubbs JD, Kennedy SD, Lopez MJ, Mathews DH, Turner DH (2015) Nuclear magnetic resonance-assisted prediction of secondary structure for RNA: incorporation of direction-dependent chemical shift constraints. Biochemistry 54(45):6769–6782. doi:10.1021/acs.biochem.5b00833

51. Hart JM, Kennedy SD, Mathews DH, Turner DH (2008) NMR-assisted prediction of RNA secondary structure: identification of a probable pseudoknot in the coding region of an R2 retrotransposon. J Am Chem Soc 130(31):10233–10239. doi:10.1021/ja8026696

52. Ryder SP, Ortoleva-Donnelly L, Kosek AB, Strobel SA (2000) Chemical probing of RNA by nucleotide analog interference mapping. Methods Enzymol 317:92–109

53. Waldsich C (2008) Dissecting RNA folding by nucleotide analog interference mapping (NAIM). Nat Protoc 3(5):811–823. doi:10.1038/nprot.2008.45

54. Kierzek E, Kierzek R, Turner DH, Catrina IE (2006) Facilitating RNA structure prediction with microarrays. Biochemistry 45(2): 581–593

55. Kladwang W, VanLang CC, Cordero P, Das R (2011) A two-dimensional mutate-and-map strategy for non-coding RNA structure. Nat Chem 3(12):954–962. doi:10.1038/nchem.1176

56. Kladwang W, Cordero P, Das R (2011) A mutate-and-map strategy accurately infers the base pairs of a 35-nucleotide model RNA. RNA 17(3):522–534. doi:10.1261/rna.2516311

57. Michel F, Westhof E (1990) Modeling of the three-dimensional architecture of group I catalytic introns based on comparative sequence analysis. J Mol Biol 216:585–610

Chapter 11

RNA Secondary Structure Determination by NMR

Jonathan L. Chen, Stanislav Bellaousov, and Douglas H. Turner

Abstract

Dynamic programming methods for predicting RNA secondary structure often use thermodynamics and experimental restraints and/or constraints to limit folding space. Chemical mapping results typically restrain certain nucleotides not to be in AU or GC pairs. Two-dimensional nuclear magnetic resonance (NMR) spectra can reveal the order of AU, GC, and GU pairs in double helixes. This chapter describes a program, NMR-assisted prediction of secondary structure and chemical shifts (NAPSS-CS), that constrains possible secondary structures on the basis of the NMR determined order and 5′–3′ direction of AU, GC, and GU pairs in helixes. NAPSS-CS minimally requires input of the order of base pairs as determined from nuclear Overhauser effect spectroscopy (NOESY) of imino protons. The program deduces the 5′–3′ direction of the base pairs if certain chemical shifts are also input. Secondary structures predicted by the program provide assignments of input chemical shifts to particular nucleotides in the sequence, thus facilitating an important step for determination of the three dimensional structure by NMR. The method is particularly useful for revealing pseudoknots and an example is provided. The method may also allow determination of secondary structures when a sequence folds into two structures that exchange slowly.

Key words NAPSS, NMR, RNA secondary structure, Chemical shifts

1 Introduction

RNA typically folds in a hierarchical manner, from sequence to secondary structure, then tertiary structure [1, 2]. For a long time, secondary structure has been predicted from sequence with computational algorithms that utilize various thermodynamic models [3–8]. Currently, folding of single sequences is usually accomplished by coupling the INN-HB model [9] with a dynamic programming algorithm to identify structures by free energy minimization [10–12]. To model secondary structures of RNAs, constraints from NMR [13] and/or constraints or restraints from chemical and/or enzymatic mapping [11, 14, 15] can be coupled with thermodynamic models.

Helical regions of RNA may be identified with imino proton connectivities within the imino region of 2D NOESY spectra [13, 16]. Cromsigt et al. [17] observed a dependence of the AH2

Douglas H. Turner and David H. Mathews (eds.), *RNA Structure Determination: Methods and Protocols*, Methods in Molecular Biology, vol. 1490, DOI 10.1007/978-1-4939-6433-8_11, © Springer Science+Business Media New York 2016

chemical shift in an AU pair on the identity of the 5′ and 3′ neighboring nucleotides in a triplet of canonical base pairs, i.e., the orientation of the flanking base pairs. They hypothesized that the AH2 chemical shift is influenced by ring currents from neighboring base pairs. Analysis of GH1 chemical shifts of GC and GU pairs revealed a similar dependence [18]. A greater dependence of NMR chemical shifts on the orientation of AU and GU pairs within a triplet of base pairs was observed when their UH3 and UH5 chemical shifts were also considered [18]. From this information, the orientation of a canonical base pair in the middle of a triplet in A-form helixes may be deduced. Each neighboring base pair is classified according to the base that is adjacent to the A or G of the middle base pair, i.e., as a purine (R=A or G) or a pyrimidine (Y=C or U). For example, a triplet with a middle AU pair, 5′CAA3′/3′GUU5′, and one with a middle GU pair, 5′AGC3′/3′UUG5′ are classified as 5′YAR3′ and 5′RGY3′, respectively.

This chapter describes a protocol for using the program NAPSS-CS, which incorporates NMR constraints into a dynamic programming algorithm to predict RNA secondary structure from sequence. A separate program supplied with NAPSS-CS converts chemical shift(s) to direction-dependent base pair triplets according to chemical shift patterns and uses them as constraints [18]. Chemical and/or enzymatic mapping restraints may also be applied to limit the folding space of a sequence [11, 14, 15]. These programs may be compiled locally on a computer running a Unix-based operating system, such as Unix, Linux, or Mac OS X.

1.1 NAPSS-CS Calculation

NAPSS-CS accepts constraints consisting of imino proton walks and optional chemical shifts of AH2, UH3, and UH5 of AU pairs; GH1, UH3, and UH5 of GU pairs; and GH1 of GC pairs for base pairs in helical walks. The program applies NMR constraints to a dynamic programming algorithm to identify matching helixes. If available, chemical mapping, including SHAPE restraints [14, 15] are applied alongside NMR constraints. NAPSS-CS does not accept chemical shift constraints for bases at the end of an imino proton helical walk since these resonances may be from terminal base pairs of a helix and therefore not in the middle of a base pair triplet. Chemical exchange with water may prevent detection of imino protons of terminal base pairs and/or NOEs to those protons from adjacent base pairs from being observed and included in imino walk constraints [16]. Therefore, the algorithm extends helixes to adjacent canonical base pairs after matching constrained helixes. NAPSS-CS then folds the RNA and calculates free energies with the INN-HB model [9, 19] for non-pseudoknotted structures and with the ShapeKnots energy and INN-HB models for pseudoknotted structures [15]. From these structures, the program identifies the lowest free energy structure and also suboptimal structures.

2 Materials

Local compilation of NAPSS-CS from source code requires a Unix-based operating system and C++ compiler, such as GNU GCC. The program may be compiled with a Makefile provided with RNAstructure (http://rna.urmc.rochester.edu/RNAstructure.html) or as a separate component. The program for converting chemical shifts to triplet constraints must be compiled separately.

3 Methods

3.1 Protocol for Compiling Program

NAPSS-CS can be downloaded as part of the RNAstructure package from the Mathews Lab website at http://rna.urmc.rochester.edu. Create a directory named RNAstructure and extract the program to the directory with the command "unzip RNAstructure.zip-d/RNAstructure". An environmental variable needs to be set to the location of the tables of thermodynamic parameters and chemical shift constraints, which are in the directory /RNAstructure/data_tables. This is accomplished by adding the following line to the .bashrc file in BASH:

```
export DATAPATH = [directory where RNAstructure
resides]/RNAstructure
/data_tables
```

Enter the RNAstructure directory and type "make all" to build all components of RNAstructure. If other components have already been compiled, enter the napss directory and type "make napss" to only compile NAPSS-CS. The import_linux program to convert chemical shift constraints to triplet constraints is compiled separately by executing "make import_linux" in the napss directory.

3.2 Creating Sequence and Constraint Files

NAPSS-CS requires input files with an RNA sequence and helical walk constraints (*see* **Note 1**). Figures 1, 2, 3, and 4 provide an example. The sequence file should use the .seq format, where the first line must be a comment line denoted by a ";" (Fig. 1). Any number of comment lines is permitted. A title must be given on one line after the comment lines. After the title line, the sequence is written from 5′ to 3′. Bases should be written in uppercase letters; lowercase bases will be constrained as unpaired. The sequence must end with a 1. All input files must have UNIX line endings; files may be converted from Windows to Unix line endings with the dos2unix tool.

```
;
B. mori R2 fragment
GGCCCGAUGGACGGA
CCGCGAGGACCGUCA
AGCCUAGCAGGUACC
UUCGGGUGGGCCCUU
GCGAUACCUGCGGG1
```

Fig. 1 Input sequence file format for NAPSS-CS for a 74-nt fragment of the
B. mori R2 retrotransposon (Fig. 2) [13]

a	b
66(12.93 0 0)6(13.29 0 0)6(13.50 0 0)6	6666(-YGR)6
65(7.547 14.39 0)6(12.75 0 0)6(12.34 0 0)6	65666
66	66
66(12.43 0 0)5(6.927 13.27 0)6(12.80 0	665(-RAY)66556
0)6(13.07 0 0)5(7.558 13.33 0)5(6.874	
14.25 0)6	

Fig. 2 (a) Input NMR constraints file format for NAPSS-CS with helical walk and chemical shift constraints for
a 74-nt fragment of the *B. mori* R2 retrotransposon [13]. Imino walks are displayed in an NMR spectrum in
Fig. 4. *Colors* of helical walk constraints correspond to *colors* of base pairs in Fig. 3 and *lines* in Fig. 4. These
constraints consist of four imino proton walks and chemical shifts for base pairs flanked by other base pairs
within each walk. **(b)** NMR constraints file format for the same RNA after chemical shift constraints are converted to triplet constraints

The helical walk constraints file should be written with a
sequence of numbers to represent base pairs, where "5", "6", and
"7" are AU, GC, and GU pairs, respectively (Figs. 2, 3, and 4).
(see **Note 1**). As shown in Figs. 2–4, chemical shift data for each
base pair not at the end of an imino proton walk may be supplied
after the base pair according to the following format for each base
pair (without square brackets):

AU pair	([AH2 shift] [UH3 shift] [UH5 shift])
GC pair	([GH1 shift] 0 0)
GU pair	([GH1 shift] [UH3 shift] [UH5 shift])

Each set of chemical shift(s) should have three values. Any
unknown chemical shifts within the parentheses should be indicated by a "0". For GC pairs, the user must type the second and
third "0" in the parentheses because chemical shift constraints are
only available for GH1. Chemical shift constraints for any base pair
may be omitted if not desired. Helical walk constraints can be
entered in any sequential order, but any chemical shift constraints
must immediately follow their corresponding base pair.

Chemical shift constraints may be converted to triplet constraints by running import_linux (without square brackets or
parentheses):

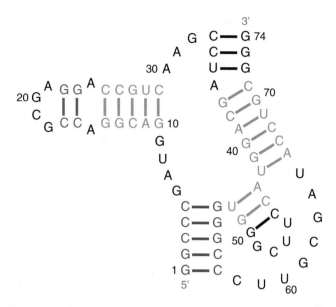

Fig. 3 Secondary structure of a 74-nt fragment of the *B. mori* R2 retrotransposon [13]. *Colored* base pairs correspond to imino proton walks with the same *line patterns* in Fig. 4. Helixes consisting of base pairs G37:C71 to U42:A66 and A43:U52 to C44:G51 are coaxially stacked and observed in a single imino proton walk

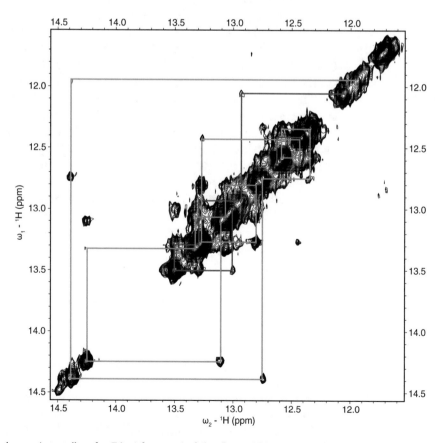

Fig. 4 Imino proton walks of a 74-nt fragment of the *B. mori* R2 retrotransposon [13]. *Lines* correspond to regions with the same *colors* in Fig. 3. Spectrum was acquired at 15 °C with 200 ms mixing time and an S-pulse [26] to suppress the water signal

```
./import_linux [name of input NMR constraints
file] [name of output NMR constraints file] [AU
constraints (1: yes; 0: no)] [GC constraints
(1: yes; 0: no)] [GU constraints (1: yes; 0:
no)]
```

The user must type "1" or "0" (indicating yes or no) to include or exclude, respectively, chemical shift constraints for AU, GC, or GU base pairs. If in the constraint file generated by import_linux, a triplet is preceded by a "+", then NAPSS-CS requires a matching helix in the dot plot. If a triplet is preceded by a "−", then NAPSS-CS requires a matching helix does not have that triplet. The resulting file with triplets can be used as the NMR constraints file by NAPSS-CS in the RNAstructure/exe directory. Chemical reactivity restraints must be typed in a separate plain text file that follows the reactivity data file format that RNAstructure uses for SHAPE data.

3.3 Running NAPSS-CS

NAPSS-CS can be run with the minimum command (no square brackets):

./NAPSS [sequence file] [NMR constraints file] [output ct file]

Structures are outputted in the .ct file format by default. The name of the sequence, NMR constraints, and output CT files must be typed in the order defined in the minimum command, but additional options may be specified anywhere in the command (*see* **Note 2**). A full list of options is in Table 1. Many of these options are the same as in RNAstructure [11, 20]. Structures in the output CT file and optional positions paired file are sorted by increasing free energy. NAPSS-CS may be specified not to generate pseudoknots, although this feature is off by default. Pseudoknots may be visualized with a program that accepts positions paired formatted files, such as PseudoViewer [21]. The program might take a long time to run if it finds a large number of matches. Table 2 has example calculation times and memory requirements on a quad-core 2.33 GHz Intel Xeon E5410 with 8 GB RAM and Ubuntu Linux (*see* **Note 3**). Consistent with NMR structures reported in the literature, NAPSS-CS permits walks across bulges [22, 23] and coaxially stacked helixes [13] (*see* **Note 4**).

4   Notes

1. Helical walk constraints must be at least two base pairs long. At least three base pairs must be present in a helical walk to apply any chemical shift constraints. The set of chemical shift constraints may be modified in the chemshiftranges.dat file in the data_tables directory as needed or if new constraints are identified. NOEs between both G and U of a GU pair and each neighboring base pair may be present in an NMR spectrum, but

Table 1
Option flags for running NAPSS-CS. Some commands are the same as in RNAstructure

Flag(s)	Definition
-c/-C/--constraint	Specify a chemical and/or enzymatic mapping constraints file to be applied. Default is no constraints.
-d/-D/--DotPercent	Specify maximum percent energy difference from MFE structures without pseudoknots that selected base pairs on the dot plot that match constraints will have. Default is 5 %.
-m/-M/--Maximum	Specify a maximum number of structures to be generated per matched constraints set. Default is 100 structures.
-p/-P/--percent	Specify maximum percent energy difference in free energy above MFE structure for generating suboptimal structures. Default is 0 to generate all output structures.
-p1/-P1/--Penalty1	Specify P1 for calculating entropic free energy penalty of pseudoknot formation. Default is 0.35 kcal/mol [15].
-p2/-P2/--Penalty2	Specify P2 for calculating entropic free energy penalty of pseudoknot formation. Default is 0.65 kcal/mol [15].
-pp/-PP/--posPaired	Specify the name of an output file in the positions paired format. Default is no file output.
-sh/-SH/-SHAPE	Specify a SHAPE constraints file. Default is no SHAPE constraints.
-si/-SI/--SHAPEintercept	Specify an intercept for SHAPE constraints. Default is –0.8 kcal/mol [15].
-sm/-SM/--SHAPEslope	Specify a slope for SHAPE constraints. Default is 2.6 kcal/mol [15].
-w/-W/--window	Specify a window size. Default is 0 nucleotides.
-h/-H/--help	Display help file.
-pf/-PF/-pseudoknotFree	Specify no pseudoknot prediction. Default is to predict pseudoknots.
-v/-V/--version	Display version and copyright information for the program.

each GU pair should only be entered once (as a single "7") in a helical walk constraint.

2. Typically, -*d* (Table 1) should be increased until structures start to be generated. It has the most effect on the number of matches generated. Pseudoknotted structures with a lower minimum free energy than non-pseudoknotted structures generated with Fold can be generated when -*d* is increased because helixes involved in pseudoknots can be added to the dot plot and the pseudoknotted energies calculated. For a given set of helixes that match constraints, the number of suboptimal structures after the structures are refolded may be controlled with the -*m*,

Table 2
Example calculation time and memory requirements for NAPSS-CS

Structure	Length (nt)	Time (s)	Memory (MB)	Reference
B. mori R2 retrotransposon PK (74-nt)	74	6.20	12.2	[13]
B. mori R2 retrotransposon PK (75-nt)	75	6.67	12.2	[18]
Bovine tRNA^{Trp}	75	0.12	12.0	[27]
Human HAR1 MBL	124	1.42	12.8	[18]
Human HDV ribozyme PK	63	14.95	12.1	[28]
Influenza A segment 7 MBL	61	0.16	11.8	[23]
Moloney MLV core encapsidation signal MBL	101	0.70	12.4	[22]
S. pneumoniae preQ$_1$-II riboswitch PK	59	0.23	11.8	[29]

-*p*, and -*w* flags (Table 1). Increasing -*p* may generate more suboptimal structures, but setting it to zero (which is not expressed as a percent) generates all possible suboptimal structures. The -*w* flag (Table 1) determines how different suboptimal structures must be from each other [20]. A value of zero for this term allows all possible suboptimal structures.

3. NAPSS-CS was tested on 18 structures, including nine pseudoknots. The average sensitivity and PPV were 96% and 92%, respectively, for all 18 structures and 95% and 88%, respectively, for base pairs creating the pseudoknots [18].

4. There will be cases where NAPSS-CS will not return a secondary structure or perhaps an incorrect structure. For example, NAPSS-CS does not identify matches with helical walks across single base pairs or across coaxially stacked helixes that generate a pseudoknot. However, little evidence of walks across these types of helixes exists in the literature aside from two cases [24, 25] where no structures were returned when tested with the program. The program may not predict helixes or loops accurately that form from tertiary interactions facilitated by modified nucleotides, such as in tRNAs, but these bases can be constrained as single-stranded in the sequence file. The current version of NAPSS-CS cannot predict structures that form from more than one sequence.

References

1. Tinoco I, Bustamante C (1999) How RNA folds. J Mol Biol 293(2):271–281. doi:10.1006/jmbi.1999.3001

2. Turner DH, Sugimoto N, Freier SM (1988) RNA structure prediction. Annu Rev Biophys Biophys Biochem 17:167–192. doi:10.1146/annurev.bb.17.060188.001123

3. Tinoco I Jr, Uhlenbeck OC, Levine MD (1971) Estimation of secondary structure in ribonucleic acids. Nature 230(5293):362–367. doi:10.1038/230362a0

4. Borer PN, Dengler B, Tinoco I, Uhlenbeck OC (1974) Stability of ribonucleic acid

double-stranded helices. J Mol Biol 86(4):843–853. doi:10.1016/0022-2836(74)90357-X

5. Pipas JM, McMahon JE (1975) Method for predicting RNA secondary structure. Proc Natl Acad Sci U S A 72(6):2017–2021. doi:10.1073/pnas.72.6.2017

6. Nussinov R, Jacobson AB (1980) Fast algorithm for predicting the secondary structure of single-stranded RNA. Proc Natl Acad Sci U S A 77(11):6309–6313. doi:10.1073/pnas.77.11.6309

7. Zuker M, Stiegler P (1981) Optimal computer folding of large RNA sequences using thermodynamics and auxiliary information. Nucleic Acids Res 9(1):133–148. doi:10.1093/nar/9.1.133

8. Zuker M (1989) On finding all suboptimal foldings of an RNA molecule. Science 244(4900):48–52. doi:10.1126/science.2468181

9. Xia TB, SantaLucia J, Burkard ME, Kierzek R, Schroeder SJ, Jiao XQ, Cox C, Turner DH (1998) Thermodynamic parameters for an expanded nearest-neighbor model for formation of RNA duplexes with Watson-Crick base pairs. Biochemistry 37(42):14719–14735. doi:10.1021/bi9809425

10. Mathews DH, Sabina J, Zuker M, Turner DH (1999) Expanded sequence dependence of thermodynamic parameters improves prediction of RNA secondary structure. J Mol Biol 288(5):911–940. doi:10.1006/jmbi.1999.2700

11. Mathews DH, Disney MD, Childs JL, Schroeder SJ, Zuker M, Turner DH (2004) Incorporating chemical modification constraints into a dynamic programming algorithm for prediction of RNA secondary structure. Proc Natl Acad Sci U S A 101(19):7287–7292. doi:10.1073/pnas.0401799101

12. Lorenz R, Bernhart SH, Höner zu Siederdissen C, Tafer H, Flamm C, Stadler PF, Hofacker IL (2011) ViennaRNA Package 2.0. Algorithm Mol Biol 6:26–26. doi:10.1186/1748-7188-6-26

13. Hart JM, Kennedy SD, Mathews DH, Turner DH (2008) NMR-assisted prediction of RNA secondary structure: identification of a probable pseudoknot in the coding region of an R2 retrotransposon. J Am Chem Soc 130(31):10233–10239. doi:10.1021/ja8026696

14. Deigan KE, Li TW, Mathews DH, Weeks KM (2009) Accurate SHAPE-directed RNA structure determination. Proc Natl Acad Sci U S A 106(1):97–102. doi:10.1073/pnas.0806929106

15. Hajdin CE, Bellaousov S, Huggins W, Leonard CW, Mathews DH, Weeks KM (2013) Accurate SHAPE-directed RNA secondary structure modeling, including pseudoknots. Proc Natl Acad Sci U S A 110(14):5498–5503. doi:10.1073/pnas.1219988110

16. Fürtig B, Richter C, Wohnert J, Schwalbe H (2003) NMR spectroscopy of RNA. ChemBioChem 4(10):936–962. doi:10.1002/cbic.200300700

17. Cromsigt JAMTC, Hilbers CW, Wijmenga SS (2001) Prediction of proton chemical shifts in RNA—their use in structure refinement and validation. J Biomol NMR 21(1):11–29. doi:10.1023/A:1011914132531

18. Chen JL, Bellaousov S, Tubbs JD, Kennedy SD, Lopez MJ, Mathews DH, Turner DH (2015) Nuclear magnetic resonance-assisted prediction of secondary structure for RNA: incorporation of direction-dependent chemical shift constraints. Biochemistry 54(45):6769–6782. doi:10.1021/acs.biochem.5b00833

19. Turner DH, Mathews DH (2010) NNDB: the nearest neighbor parameter database for predicting stability of nucleic acid secondary structure. Nucleic Acids Res 38:D280–D282. doi:10.1093/nar/gkp892

20. Reuter JS, Mathews DH (2010) RNAstructure: software for RNA secondary structure prediction and analysis. BMC Bioinformatics 11:129. doi:10.1186/1471-2105-11-129

21. Han K, Lee Y, Kim W (2002) PseudoViewer: automatic visualization of RNA pseudoknots. Bioinformatics 18(Suppl 1):S321–S328. doi:10.1093/bioinformatics/18.suppl_1.S321

22. D'Souza V, Dey A, Habib D, Summers MF (2004) NMR structure of the 101-nucleotide core encapsidation signal of the Moloney murine leukemia virus. J Mol Biol 337(2):427–442. doi:10.1015/j.jmb.2004.01.037

23. Jiang T, Kennedy SD, Moss WN, Kierzek E, Turner DH (2014) Secondary structure of a conserved domain in an intron of influenza A M1 mRNA. Biochemistry 53(32):5236–5248. doi:10.1021/bi500611j

24. Houck-Loomis B, Durney MA, Salguero C, Shankar N, Nagle JM, Goff SP, D'Souza VM (2011) An equilibrium-dependent retroviral mRNA switch regulates translational recoding. Nature 480(7378):561–564. doi:10.1038/nature10657

25. Cash DD, Cohen-Zontag O, Kim N-K, Shefer K, Brown Y, Ulyanov NB, Tzfati Y, Feigon J (2013) Pyrimidine motif triple helix in the *Kluyveromyces lactis* telomerase RNA pseudoknot is essential for function *in vivo*. Proc Natl Acad Sci U S A 110(27):10970–10975. doi:10.1073/pnas.1309590110

26. Smallcombe SH (1993) Solvent suppression with symmetrically-shifted pulses. J Am Chem Soc 115(11):4776–4785. doi:10.1021/ja00064a043

27. Gong Q, Guo Q, Tong K-L, Zhu G, Wong JT-F, Xue H (2002) NMR analysis of bovine tRNA^{Trp}. J Biol Chem 277(23):20694–20701. doi:10.1074/jbc.M202299200

28. Tanaka Y, Hori T, Tagaya M, Sakamoto T, Kurihara Y, Katahira M, Uesugi S (2002) Imino proton NMR analysis of HDV ribozymes: nested double pseudoknot structure and Mg^{2+} ion-binding site close to the catalytic core in solution. Nucleic Acids Res 30(3):766–774. doi:10.1093/nar/30.3.766

29. Kang M, Eichhorn CD, Feigon J (2014) Structural determinants for ligand capture by a class II preQ$_1$ riboswitch. Proc Natl Acad Sci U S A 111(6):E663–E671. doi:10.1073/pnas.1400126111

Chapter 12

Modeling Small Noncanonical RNA Motifs with the Rosetta FARFAR Server

Joseph D. Yesselman and Rhiju Das

Abstract

Noncanonical RNA motifs help define the vast complexity of RNA structure and function, and in many cases, these loops and junctions are on the order of only ten nucleotides in size. Unfortunately, despite their small size, there is no reliable method to determine the ensemble of lowest energy structures of junctions and loops at atomic accuracy. This chapter outlines straightforward protocols using a webserver for Rosetta Fragment Assembly of RNA with Full Atom Refinement (FARFAR) (http://rosie.rosettacommons.org/rna_denovo/submit) to model the 3D structure of small noncanonical RNA motifs for use in visualizing motifs and for further refinement or filtering with experimental data such as NMR chemical shifts.

Key words RNA 3D structure prediction, RNA Motifs

1 Introduction

RNA plays critical roles in all living systems through its ability to adopt complex 3D structures and perform chemical catalysis [1]. RNA structure appears modular in nature, defined through base pairing interactions. Nucleotides can either form structured helices composed of canonical Watson–Crick base pairs or small unpaired or noncanonical base paired regions in the form of junctions and loops (motifs) [2–4]. Helices are, for the most part, structurally similar to each other, leaving noncanonical motifs to define the vast complexity of RNA structure and function. These noncanonical elements define the topology of the 3D structure of RNA by orienting the helices to which they connect and by forming long-range tertiary contacts that can lock specific global RNA conformations in place. In addition to defining the overall 3D structure of RNA [5, 6], noncanonical motifs are the sites of small molecule binding and chemical catalysis [7–10]. Many noncanonical motifs are on the order of only ten nucleotides in size. Unfortunately, despite their small size, there is no reliable method to determine the ensemble of lowest energy structures of junctions

Douglas H. Turner and David H. Mathews (eds.), RNA Structure Determination: *Methods and Protocols*, Methods in Molecular Biology, vol. 1490, DOI 10.1007/978-1-4939-6433-8_12, © Springer Science+Business Media New York 2016

and loops at near atomic accuracy. Nevertheless, to model RNA at high resolution, it is critical to achieve accurate solutions for these small motifs.

When their structures are solved experimentally, most motifs turn out to form complex arrangements of non Watson–Crick hydrogen bonds and a wide range of backbone conformations. Due to the large number of interactions possible and each nucleotide's many degrees of internal freedom, it remains difficult to determine the lowest energy conformation [11]. Fragment assembly of RNA with full atom refinement (FARFAR) was an early attempt to help address this problem. FARFAR adapted the well-developed Rosetta framework for protein structure modeling to predict and design RNA noncanonical motifs [12]. Out of a 32-target test set, 14 cases gave at least one out of five models that were better than 2.0 Å all-heavy-atom RMSD to the experimentally observed structure. While not perfect, this level of accuracy can be combined with even sparse experimental data, such as ^{1}H chemical shifts, to obtain high confidence structural models, as was demonstrated recently in blind predictions with the CS-ROSETTA-RNA method [13]. The motif models can also form building blocks for modeling more complex RNAs and has been tested in the RNA-Puzzles trials [14]. Application of FARFAR method for large RNAs with complex folds has been reviewed recently [15]. The current bottleneck for some of these motifs and for larger RNAs is the difficulty of complete conformational sampling [11]. On-going work with stepwise assembly (SWA) attempts to resolve this issue [16], but this more advanced procedure requires greater computational expense and a complex workflow that is not yet straightforward to implement on a public server, except in the special case of one-nucleotide-at-a-time crystallographic refinement [17]. Stepwise assembly is available in the main Rosetta codebase, but is not further discussed here.

This chapter outlines straightforward protocols that are enabling expert scientists and citizen scientists in the Eterna platform [18] to access FARFAR 3D RNA modeling through a simple web server. FARFAR (RNA De Novo) is part of the Rosetta Online Server that Includes Everyone (ROSIE) software, a push to give wide access to the algorithms found in the Rosetta 3.x framework [19]. The web server requires no initial setup for the user; all that is needed is to supply a sequence and an optional secondary structure to obtain all-atom models for an RNA motif of interest.

1.1 FARFAR Calculation

The FARFAR structure-modeling algorithm is based on two discrete steps. First, the RNA is assembled using 1–3 nucleotide fragments from existing RNA crystal structures whose sequences match subsequences of the target RNA. Fragment Assembly of RNA (FARNA) uses a Monte Carlo process guided by a low-resolution knowledge-based energy function [20]. Afterwards, these models can be further refined in an all-atom potential to yield structures with hydrogen bonds with realistic geometries and fewer clashes; the resulting energies are also better at discriminating native-like conformations from non-native conformations [12]. The two-stage protocol is called fragment assembly of RNA with full atom refinement (FARFAR).

2   Materials

FARFAR (RNA De Novo) is a webserver implementation of the Rosetta RNA fragment assembly algorithm server using the ROSIE framework. ROSIE is a web front-end for Rosetta 3 software suite, which provides experimentally tested and rapidly evolving tools for the high-resolution 3D modeling of nucleic acids, proteins, and other biopolymers. FARFAR (RNA De Novo) can be reached using any of the standard web browsers such as Apple Safari, Microsoft Internet Explorer, Mozilla Firefox, and Google Chrome here: http://rosie.rosettacommons.org/rna_denovo/submit.

3   Methods

This protocol outlines the steps to use the FARFAR (RNA De Novo) webserver located on the ROSIE website. Although it is possible to submit jobs without creating an account, having an account yields numerous benefits, such as email alerts when jobs are finished, as well as the ability to create private jobs that are not visible to other users. It is highly recommended to create an account when first visiting ROSIE. In addition to the FARFAR webserver, ROSIE also hosts many other Rosetta based applications with a continuous stream of novel applications in development.

3.1   Main Page Form

This demonstration of FARFAR (RNA De Novo) uses the GCAA tetraloop; the whole structure was determined through NMR spectroscopy by Jucker et al. (PDB 1ZIH) [21]. This tetraloop has a sequence of gggcgcaagccu and secondary structure of (((((....))))) in dot parentheses notation (Fig. 1). Figure 2 shows the main submission form for the RNA De Novo server. The only required input is the sequence, from 5′ to 3′. This is typically in lowercase letters, but uppercase letters are acceptable and will be converted. Use a space, *, or + between strands (see below for a test case with multiple strands). Note that this sequence is treated as RNA so that any T's that appear in the sequence are automatically converted to U's for the calculation. Next, enter the secondary structure, in dot-parentheses notation. This is optional for single-stranded motifs, but required for multi-strand motifs. Note that even if a location is "unpaired" in the input secondary structure (given by a dot, "."), it is not forced to remain unpaired. Although this is optional for single stranded motifs, the results improve with the addition of the correct secondary structure. If uncertain about the

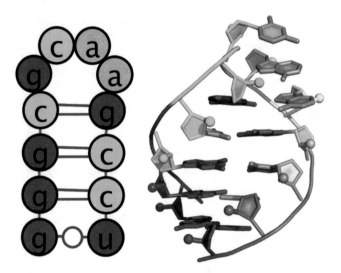

Fig. 1 (*Left*) secondary structure of GCAA tetraloop. (*Right*) 3D structure of GCAA tetraloop (PDB: 1ZIH)

secondary structure, consider utilizing the Vienna RNAfold web-server [22] (http://rna.tbi.univie.ac.at/cgi-bin/RNAfold.cgi) or other utilities described in this book. Alternatively, use chemical mapping techniques to estimate the secondary structure these methods have been recently tested in blind trials for their accuracy [23, 24]. In addition, note that there is currently a size submission limit of 32 nucleotides for FARFAR (RNA De Novo), as the amount of computation greatly increases as a function of number of residues.

There are two more optional arguments. First is a file containing the ¹H chemical shifts determined by NMR spectroscopy. The format of this file follows the STAR v2.1 format used by the Biological Magnetic Resonance Data Bank (BMRB) [25]. An example of the format is displayed in Fig. 3 with an explanation of each column. In addition, it is possible to supply a native structure for RMSD calculations. This file must be in PDB format, and for this case it is possible to download the structure from http://pdb.org/pdb/explore/explore.do?structureId=1zih. To supply a native structure, click the "Choose file" button next to native PDB-formatted file and select the appropriate file from your local hard drive.

There are two ways of running a FARFAR (RNA De Novo) job. The first is a trial run, which generates only one structure with a limited number of fragment assembly steps. This is for testing purposes only, and allows confirmation that the job is set up properly. The second is a full run that takes more computational time to complete and produces thousands of models. It is advised when setting up a job for a new sequence and secondary structure to always first run the job as a trial. Then, using www.pymol.org or your favorite viewer, open the PDB file; we use the PyMOL

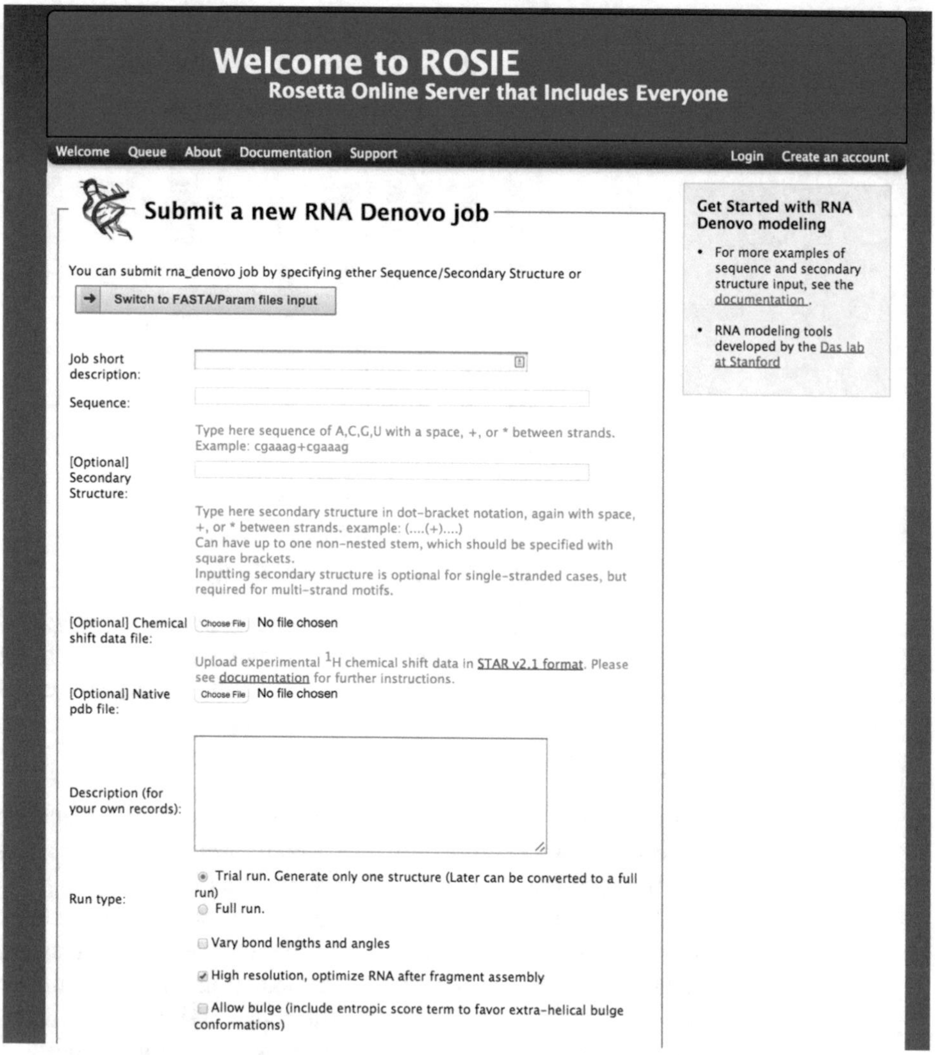

Fig. 2 Main page of the FARFAR (RNA De Novo) webserver. Here the user can enter a sequence and secondary to submit a job to generation an all atom model of their construct

visualization script rr() available as part of the RiboVis package (https://ribokit.github.io/RiboVis/). This is particularly important if you have a multi-stranded motif—check that the strands are separated, and that any specified Watson–Crick pairs are reasonably paired. Once this is set up, go to the bottom of the page and click "Submit FARFAR (RNA De Novo) job". Upon submission, a temporary status page will load (Fig. 4).

3.2 Advanced Options

In addition to the options discussed above, there are a few additional options that may be used occasionally. First is "Vary bond lengths and angles"; typically each residue has a set of bond lengths and angles between atoms that are based on idealized parameters. Checking this option will allow these parameters to vary slightly based on the Rosetta force field energy. This can increase

1	2	2 G	H1'	H	5.62	.	.
2	2	2 G	H2'	H	3.74	.	.
3	2	2 G	H3'	H	4.75	.	.
4	2	2 G	H4'	H	4.37	.	.
5	2	2 G	H5'	H	4.57	.	.
6	2	2 G	H5''	H	4.14	.	.
7	2	2 G	H8	H	7.55	.	.
8	3	3 G	H1'	H	5.89	.	.
9	3	3 G	H2'	H	4.93	.	.
10	3	3 G	H3'	H	4.85	.	.
11	3	3 G	H4'	H	4.52	.	.
12	3	3 G	H5'	H	4.50	.	.
13	3	3 G	H5''	H	4.18	.	.
14	3	3 G	H8	H	8.02	.	.

Fig. 3 Example chemical shift data. Column description is as follows. (1) Atom entry number. (2) Residue author sequence code. (3) Residue sequence code. (4) Residue label. (5) Atom name. (6) Atom type. (7) Chemical shift value. (8) Chemical shift value error. (9) Chemical shift ambiguity code

conformational search space if you are interested in a specific interaction between residues and was used in previous benchmark studies, but requires more computational time [12].

When checked, "High resolution, optimize RNA after fragment assembly" will perform the all-atom refinement after fragment assembly; it is not recommended to uncheck this unless you are interested in quickly seeing the initial results or would like to perform your own high-resolution optimization. "Allow bulge (include entropic score term to favor extra-helical bulge conformations)", will include conformations with residues bulged out and not interacting with other residues. If a residue is known to be extruded from the helix, this might be a good option to try to reduce the conformational space searched. When "Allow bulge (include entropic score term to favor extra-helical bulge conformations)" is checked, please note that residues that are bulged out will not be present in the final pdb model. "Number of structures to generate", will change the number of final models, which will also greatly increase the time each run takes. "Number of Monte Carlo cycles", controls the quality of each model; if models generated for a specific run have wildly different structures, then FARFAR has poor confidence in the accuracy (*see* next section). Increasing the number of Monte Carlo cycles can increase convergence, at the expense of greater computation.

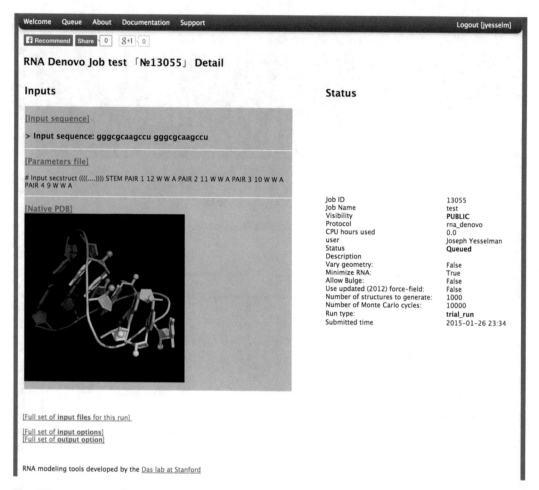

Fig. 4 The status page for a submitted FARFAR (RNA De Novo) job

3.3 Server Results

The server returns pictures of the best-scoring models from the five best-scoring clusters from the run in rank order by energy (Fig. 5). The clustering radius is 2.0 Å by default. Click on the [Model-N] link to download the PDB file. The server returns cluster centers (without pictures) for the next 95 clusters as, as well as the top 20 lowest-energy structures. These may be valuable if you are filtering models based on experimental data. The server also returns a "scatter plot" of the energies of all the models created. The x-axis is a distance measure from the native/reference model in RMSD (root mean-squared deviation) over all heavy atoms; if a reference model is not provided, then the RMSD is computed relative to the lowest energy model discovered by FARFAR. The y-axis is the score (energy) of the structure. In runs where a native structure is not supplied, the x-axis is a distance measure from the best scoring model found. As with nearly every Rosetta application, a hallmark of a successful run is convergence, visible as an energetic

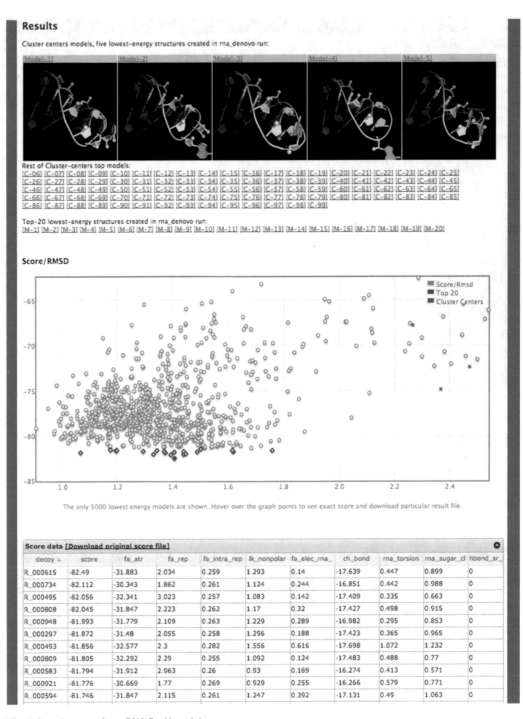

Fig. 5 Results page for a RNA De Novo job

"funnel" of low-energy structures clustered around a single position. That is, near the lowest energy model there are additional models within ~2 Å RMSD. In such runs, the lowest energy cluster centers have a reasonable chance of covering native-like structures for the motif, based on our benchmarks. A hallmark of an unsuccessful

Table 1
Score terms reported on RNA De Novo results page

Term	Definition
Score	Final total score
fa_atr	Lennard-Jones attractive between atoms in different residues
fa_rep	Lennard-Jones repulsive between atoms in different residues
fa_intra_rep	Lennard-Jones repulsive between atoms in the same residue
lk_nonpolar	Lazaridis–Karplus solvation energy, over nonpolar atoms
fa_elec_rna_phos_phos	Simple electrostatic repulsion term between phosphates
ch_bond	Carbon hydrogen bonds
rna_torsion	RNA torsional potential
rna_sugar_close	Term that ensures that ribose rings stay closed during refinement
hbond_sr_bb_sc	Backbone-sidechain hbonds close in primary sequence
hbond_lr_bb_sc	Backbone-sidechain hbonds distant in primary sequence
hbond_sc	Sidechain-sidechain hydrogen bond energy
geom_sol	Geometric solvation energy for polar atoms
linear_chainbreak	For "temporary" chainbreaks, penalty term that keeps chainbreaks closed
N_WC	Number of Watson–Crick base pairs
N_NWC	Number of non-Watson–Crick base pairs
N_BS	Number of base stacks
Following are provided if the user gives a native structure	
rms	All-heavy-atom RMSD to the native structure
rms_stem	All-heavy-atom RMSD to helical segments in the native structure
f_natWC	Fraction of native Watson–Crick base pairs recovered
f_natNWC	Fraction of native non-Watson–Crick base pairs recovered
f_natBP	Fraction of native base pairs recovered

run is a lack of convergence—few structures within 2 Å RMSD of the lowest energy model. Below the scatter plot, there is a detailed table of all the score terms used to calculate the final score as well as the RMSD to the native structure (if supplied). A description of the meaning of each term can be found in Table 1.

Visual representation of convergence of the models generated by FARFAR (RNA De Novo) can be found in Fig. 6. As the figure demonstrates, there is high convergence in the top models found throughout the run. In addition, if one has ^{1}H chemical shift data, those measurements can also be supplied, as described above; this can increase the convergence and accuracy of an FARFAR prediction run. Fig. 6 illustrates these improvements through a simple GA

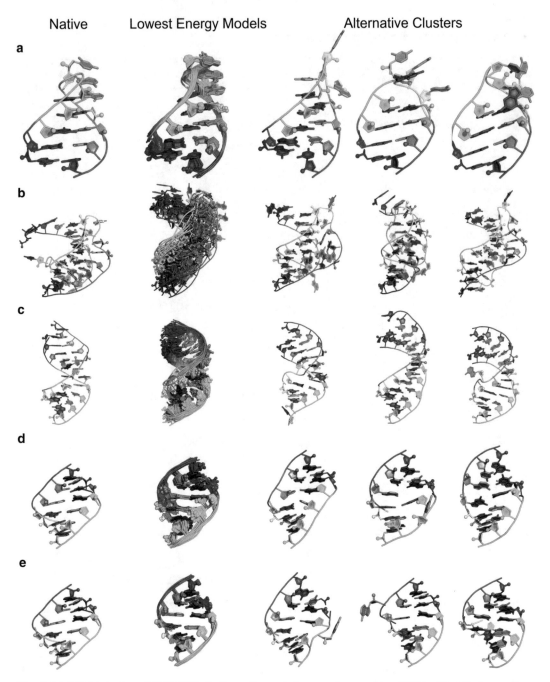

Fig. 6 (**a**) GCAA tetraloop (1ZIH): RNA De Novo (through fragment assembly of RNA with full atom refinement, FARFAR) gives lowest energy models displaying structural convergence. (**b**) Pseudoknot (1L2X) [27], less converged then tetraloop–but also a larger RNA–gives models that are still within 3 Å heavy-atom RMSD for top model. (**c**) 4 × 4 internal loop solved by NMR at PDB ID 2L8F [28], converges despite presenting four noncanonical base pairs. (**d**) Tandem GA (1MIS) [26] without application of ^{1}H chemical shifts. (**e**) Tandem GA with ^{1}H chemical shifts, demonstrates the improved convergence with the addition of ^{1}H chemical shift

tandem motif; first generating models without ^{1}H chemical shift data (Fig. 6d) yields the correct overall fold of the structure while incorrectly predicting the GA base pairs to be sheared instead of forming hydrogen bonds through their Watson-Crick edge [26]. The ^{1}H chemical shift data adds sufficient restraints to resolve the base pairing discrepancy, with all top 20 models having the correct base pairing as the NMR solved structure. Both the native PDB and the chemical shift file can be downloaded from http://rosie.rosettacommons.org/documentation/rna_denovo.

Acknowledgments

We thank Sergey Lyskov for thoughtful discussions and expert assistance with the ROSIE platform development. We thank G. Kapral as well as elNando888 and Eterna players for testing and comments. Writing of this work was supported by a Burroughs-Wellcome Foundation Career Award and National Institutes of Health Grant R01GM100953.

References

1. Cech TR, Steitz JA (2014) The noncoding RNA revolution—trashing old rules to forge new ones. Cell 157(1):77–94

2. Leontis NB, Westhof E (2003) Analysis of RNA motifs. Curr Opin Struct Biol 13(3):300–308

3. Hendrix DK, Brenner SE, Holbrook SR (2006) RNA structural motifs: building blocks of a modular biomolecule. Q Rev Biophys 38(03):221

4. Leontis NB, Lescoute A, Westhof E (2006) The building blocks and motifs of RNA architecture. Curr Opin Struct Biol 16(3):279–287

5. Moore PB (1999) Structural motifs in RNA. Annu Rev Biochem 68(1):287–300

6. Brion P, Westhof E (1997) Hierarchy and dynamics of RNA folding. Annu Rev Biophys Biomol Struct 26(1):113–137

7. Lauhon CT, Szostak JW (1995) RNA aptamers that bind flavin and nicotinamide redox cofactors. J Am Chem Soc 117(4):1246–1257

8. Paige JS, Wu KY, Jaffrey SR (2011) RNA mimics of green fluorescent protein. Science 333(6042):642–646

9. Doudna JA, Lorsch JR (2005) Ribozyme catalysis: not different, just worse. Nat Struct Mol Biol 12(5):395–402

10. Lilley DM (2005) Structure, folding and mechanisms of ribozymes. Curr Opin Struct Biol 15(3):313–323

11. Sripakdeevong P, Beauchamp K, Das R (2012) Why Can't We Predict RNA structure at atomic resolution? Nucleic Acids and Molecular Biology. Springer, Berlin, Heidelberg, pp 43–65

12. Das R, Karanicolas J, Baker D (2010) Atomic accuracy in predicting and designing noncanonical RNA structure. Nat Methods 7(4):291–294

13. Sripakdeevong P, Cevec M, Chang AT, Erat MC, Ziegeler M, Zhao Q et al (2014) Structure determination of noncanonical RNA motifs guided by 1H NMR chemical shifts. Nat Methods 11(4):413–416

14. Cruz JA, Blanchet MF, Boniecki M, Bujnicki JM, Chen SJ, Cao S et al (2012) RNA-Puzzles: A CASP-like evaluation of RNA three-dimensional structure prediction. RNA 18(4):610–625

15. Cheng CY, Chou FC, Das R (2015) Modeling complex RNA tertiary folds with Rosetta. Methods Enzymol 553:35–64

16. Sripakdeevong P, Kladwang W, Das R (2011) An enumerative stepwise ansatz enables atomic-accuracy RNA loop modeling. Proc Natl Acad Sci U S A 108(51):20573–20578

17. Chou F-C, Sripakdeevong P, Dibrov SM, Hermann T, Das R (2013) Correcting pervasive errors in RNA crystallography through enumerative structure prediction. Nat Methods 10(1):74–76

18. Lee J, Kladwang W, Lee M, Cantu D, Azizyan M, Kim H, Limpaecher A, Yoon S, Treuille A, Das R, EteRNA Participants (2014) RNA design rules from a massive open laboratory. Proc Natl Acad Sci U S A 111(6): 2122–2127

19. Lyskov S, Chou F-C, Conchúir SÓ, Der BS, Drew K, Kuroda D et al (2013) Serverification of molecular modeling applications: the Rosetta Online Server That Includes Everyone (ROSIE). PLoS One 22;8(5)

20. Das R, Baker D (2007) Automated de novo prediction of native-like RNA tertiary structures. Proc Natl Acad Sci U S A 104(37): 14664–14669

21. Jucker FM, Heus HA, Yip PF, Moors EH, Pardi A (1996) A network of heterogeneous hydrogen bonds in GNRA tetraloops. J Mol Biol 264(5):968–980

22. Gruber AR, Lorenz R, Bernhart SH, Neuböck R, Hofacker IL (2008) The Vienna RNA websuite. Nucleic Acids Res 36(Web Server issue):W70–W74

23. Kladwang W, Cordero P, Das R (2011) A mutate-and-map strategy accurately infers the base pairs of a 35-nucleotide model RNA. RNA 17(3):522–534

24. Miao Z, Adamiak RW, Blanchet M-F, Boniecki M, Bujnicki JM, Chen S-J et al (2015) RNA-Puzzles Round II: assessment of RNA structure prediction programs applied to three large RNA structures. RNA 21:1066–1084

25. Ulrich EL, Akutsu H, Doreleijers JF, Harano Y, Ioannidis YE, Lin J et al (2008) BioMagResBank. Nucleic Acids Res 36(Database issue):D402–D408

26. Wu M, Turner DH (1996) Solution structure of (rGCGGACGC)2 by two-dimensional NMR and the iterative relaxation matrix approach. Biochemistry 35(30):9677–9689

27. Egli M, Minasov G, Su L, Rich A (2002) Metal ions and flexibility in a viral RNA pseudoknot at atomic resolution. Proc Natl Acad Sci U S A 99(7):4302–4307

28. Lerman YV, Kennedy SD, Shankar N, Parisien M, Major F, Turner DH (2011) NMR structure of a 4×4 nucleotide RNA internal loop from an R2 retrotransposon: identification of a three purine-purine sheared pair motif and comparison to MC-SYM predictions. RNA 17(9):1664–1677

Chapter 13

Automated RNA 3D Structure Prediction with RNAComposer

Marcin Biesiada*, Katarzyna J. Purzycka*, Marta Szachniuk, Jacek Blazewicz, and Ryszard W. Adamiak

Abstract

RNAs adopt specific structures to perform their activities and these are critical to virtually all RNA-mediated processes. Because of difficulties in experimentally assessing structures of large RNAs using NMR, X-ray crystallography, or cryo-microscopy, there is currently great demand for new high-resolution 3D structure prediction methods. Recently we reported on RNAComposer, a knowledge-based method for the fully automated RNA 3D structure prediction from a user-defined secondary structure. RNAComposer method is especially suited for structural biology users. Since our initial report in 2012, both servers, freely available at http://rnacomposer.ibch.poznan.pl and http://rnacomposer.cs.put.poznan.pl have been often visited. Therefore this chapter provides guidance for using RNAComposer and discusses points that should be considered when predicting 3D RNA structure. An application example presents current scope and limitations of RNAComposer.

Key words RNA tertiary structure, RNA three-dimensional structure, RNA modeling

1 Introduction

RNAs adopt specific structures to perform their activities, beginning with transcription and ending with turnover. RNA structure is critical to virtually all RNA-mediated processes ranging from splicing to viral replication in eukaryotes. Studying RNA structure helps understanding how it guides RNA function. The ability of RNA strands to fold back on themselves and to form stable tertiary architectures is fundamental to RNA function. In many cases, the RNA tertiary structure is crucial for recognition by cellular factors. RNA structure is influenced by primary sequence, cellular environment, trans-acting factors, or ion homeostasis. These factors

*These authors contributed equally to this work.

Dedication: This work is dedicated to Professor David Shugar, one of the pioneers in the field of molecular biophysics, on the occasion of his 100th birthday anniversary.

Douglas H. Turner and David H. Mathews (eds.), *RNA Structure Determination: Methods and Protocols*, Methods in Molecular Biology, vol. 1490, DOI 10.1007/978-1-4939-6433-8_13, © Springer Science+Business Media New York 2016

contribute to the difficulty of obtaining RNA 3D structures using X-ray crystallography or NMR.

Recent advancements in RNA secondary structure probing, including new reagents or structure mapping integrated with systematic mutagenesis, allowed to determine secondary structures of large RNAs with reasonable accuracy [1, 2]. The bottleneck is an RNA 3D structure determination. One possibility to overcome this limitation is RNA 3D structure prediction. Computational methods for RNA tertiary structure prediction are based on simulation of RNA folding (DMD [3], NAST [4]), comparative modeling (ModeRNA [5]) or fragment assembly (FARNA [6], MC-Fold/MC-Sym [7]). Most of them are time-consuming and require high level of expertise to accomplish prediction of 3D model. Few methods are automated (Vfold [8], iFoldRNA [9], 3dRNA [10]) and among them is our method called RNAComposer [11]. All available approaches have substantial limitations, but the field of computational methods for RNA tertiary structure prediction is currently coming into bloom.

1.1 RNA 3D Structure Prediction with RNAComposer

The RCSB PDB [12] database contains over 2500 spatial structures of RNA, and this number still increases. Every spatial structure has corresponding secondary structure. Every RNA secondary structure contains single and double stranded regions, and these can be classified as loops, stems, etc. If we divide RNA secondary structures into specific elements, like stems or loops, many of these elements will be identical or similar. The idea of RNAComposer [11] is based on the observation that many of these elements repeat. Therefore unknown 3D structures can be predicted and built based on the known elements derived from the solved 3D structures. RNAComposer predicts 3D structures of RNA molecules based on their sequence and secondary structure topology. It uses a dedicated database (a dictionary of structure elements) that contains 3D RNA fragments derived from RNA FRABASE [13, 14]. The dictionary relates RNA secondary and tertiary structure elements. In the first step, secondary structure provided by the user is divided into fragments according to its graph representation [15]. Next, RNAComposer algorithm searches through the dictionary of elements to find best matching 3D structure fragments with the RNA secondary structure of interest. Initial 3D model is built by assembling selected 3D structural elements. Next, it is refined to the final 3D structure by minimization in torsion angle space and in Cartesian atom coordinate space using CHARMM force field (both steps use incorporated X-Plor suite [16]).

RNAComposer is based on the concept of machine translation. It is a knowledge-based method that employs fully automated fragment assembly based on the user-specified secondary RNA structure. Structure prediction is very fast and accomplished using web-servers: http://rnacomposer.ibch.poznan.pl and mirror http://rnacomposer.cs.put.poznan.pl.

Two procedures are implemented in RNAComposer web-server to obtain RNA 3D structures. The interactive mode, for fast inspection of RNA molecule of interest is dedicated to all visitors, while the batch mode allows modeling larger RNA structures in large-scale. Batch mode is available after registration.

2 Materials

RNAComposer should be run via an Internet web browser. It has been implemented in the client–server model and requires from the user (i.e., the client side) to have an Internet access and a web browser installed locally. The system works with most of the available browsers. Windows users can execute it in Microsoft Internet Explorer (from version 8.0), Mozilla Firefox (from version 3.6), Opera (from version 10.53), or Google Chrome (from version 5.0), whereas for those working under Linux or Mac OS, Mozilla Firefox (from version 3.6) and Opera (from version 10.53) are suggested. In every case, the latest versions of web browsers are strongly recommended. In the interactive mode, RNAComposer provides a possibility to display the output 3D model. The visualization is performed by the incorporated Jmol [17] applet that runs on a web browser's Java Virtual Machine. Therefore, an installation of Java (www.java.com), preferably its latest version, is required to execute this option.

3 Methods

3.1 RNAComposer Website at a Glance

When opening the RNAComposer website, one can see Homepage with interactive mode activated, vertical menu panel displayed on the left side, and bottom bar with quick links (Fig. 1).

Menu panel contains Main Menu, login area, visitor counter, and links to supporting institutions. Main menu allows to navigate between the system pages: "Home", "Tools", "Help", "About", "References", "Links", and "Contact us". "Home" is the starting page. Its main content, in both modes, is the task entry box, where the input sequence and secondary structure topology should be typed in. Three examples are available at hand for quick upload and processing. Clicking on "Compose" button runs the process of 3D structure modeling. "Tools" page provides support for users having their secondary structures encoded in CT or BPSEQ format. Two converters from these notations to dot–bracket are available there. "Help" gives a detailed description of the system, including usage scenarios, input and output data formats with examples, and user account. RNAComposer authors, developers, supporting team, and funders are acknowledged on the "About" page. "References" enumerate RNAComposer-related publications for

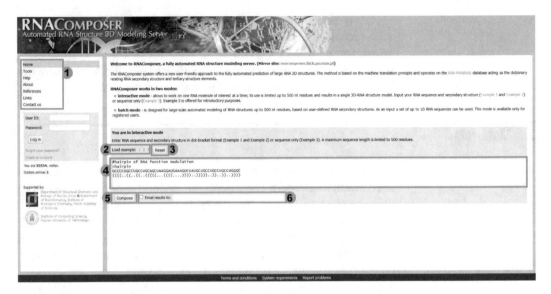

Fig. 1 RNAComposer interactive mode homepage (http://rnacomposer.cs.put.poznan.pl). (1) Main menu. (2) Examples. (3) Reset button. (4) Entry box with input example. (5) Compose button. (6) E-mail address box

citation. On the "Links" page we have collected links to selected tools for RNA structure storage, analysis and processing. Finally, "Contact us" provides the message form to be used in case of questions, problems, or suggestions concerning RNAComposer. Messages typed here are e-mailed to the RNAComposer team members.

Login area differs between modes. In the interactive mode it allows to register within the system ("Create an account" option), reset forgotten password ("Forgot your password?" option), and enter the batch mode by logging into the system. In the batch mode it provides links to access user workspace and account settings page.

Quick links located on the bottom bar direct the user to "Terms and conditions", "System requirements", and "Report problems" pages. The first page collects information about policy of using RNAComposer system. Software requirements that should be met to make the use of RNAComposer possible are reported on "System requirements" page. Finally, the "Report problems" link directs to the contact page, similarly as "Contact us" option in the Main Menu.

3.2 Getting Started: How to Prepare the Input Data

RNAComposer requires sequence and defined secondary structure topology as an input. RNA length is limited to 500 nucleotides. Input consists of three clearly defined lines. The first line serves to identify the molecule while following two lines are critical for the three-dimensional structural model building. The first line begins with the right angle bracket ">" and identifies the RNA strand of interest. After ">" only basic letters "A–Z", "a–z", numbers 0–9, underscore "_" and colon ":" signs are accepted. The next line contains RNA sequence annotated in four-letter ribonucleotide code: "A, C, G, U". Modified bases cannot be marked. The third line represents RNA secondary structure topology encoded in dot–bracket notation. This notation represents secondary structure of RNA in a simple way, but few principles must be followed to prepare correct input. In this notation, dots are assigned to unpaired nucleotides or noncanonical pairing. Parentheses are assigned to canonical-paired nucleotides so that left "(" represents first nucleotide from the base-pair (closer to the RNA 5′-end) and the right ")" is attributed to the nucleotide closing this pair (Fig. 2a). If the secondary structure is more complicated, e.g., contains structural elements of higher order, it is necessary to use other brackets for the structure representation. The square brackets "[]", braces "{}", or angle brackets "<>" are allowed. For example first order pseudoknot within RNA structure should be annotated using square brackets.

Lines 2 and 3 must have equal number of characters and each dot or bracket sign from the third line should correspond with the letter identifying the base and located above this sign. Only canonical A-U, C-G and a wobble G-U base pairs are permitted in the input data. Any additional comments can be added in any new line starting with hash "#" sign. An example of the correct input data (structure of RNA function modulator, PDB id: 4K27 [18]) is shown on Fig. 2a. Its secondary structure is visualized on panel b.

Three examples are available in the web-server interactive mode to display correct input data. First example is a model hairpin, the second shows RNA structure with the pseudoknot and the third one exemplifies the use of the secondary structure prediction program (described in detail in Subheading 3.3). Button "Reset" above the entry box allows to clear the entry box contents.

In the batch mode the user can provide a batch of up to ten RNA sequences with 1–10 secondary structure topologies for

a

```
#hairpin of RNA function modulation
>hairpin
GCCCCUGCCUGCCUGCAGCUAAGGAUGAAAGUCUAUGCUGCCUGCCUGCCUGGGC
(((((..((..((..(((((...(((((....)))))..)))))..))..))..)))))
```

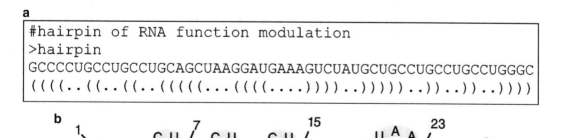

Fig. 2 Example of correct input data. (**a**) Secondary structure of functional modulator hairpin in dot–bracket notation and (**b**) its PseudoViewer visualization

every sequence. Secondary structure topology is represented in dot–bracket notation. Each sequence must be introduced with a new line containing sequence identifier following the angle bracket. Every additional dot–bracket notation of the secondary structure must be written in separated line directly under the sequence line.

To present correct input data in the batch mode, three examples are provided on the RNAComposer website. The first example is a 274 nts RNA containing pseudoknot, based on the crystal structure of tetrahymena ribozyme (PDB id 1X8W). The second example is a 120 nts RNA, based on 5S rRNA *E. coli* mutant (12C>12A; PDB id 2AWB). For this RNA, three different secondary structures are predefined. Example 3 is oriented towards high-throughput approach available in RNAComposer and exemplifies input of multiple sequences of pre-miRNA with several defined secondary structures for each sequence.

If the above described rules are not obeyed, the computation is stopped and the error messages are displayed under the entry box. Non-critical errors (displayed in yellow) like presence of non-canonical base pairs in secondary structure topology or lowercase letter in the sequence can be automatically corrected or ignored. If ignored, the RNAComposer treats noncanonical base pair as the canonical one and the lowercase letter is changed to the capital. Critical errors (written in red) obstruct launching of the computation and this type of error must be repaired.

3.3 Structure Modeling in the Interactive Mode

Interactive mode (Fig. 1), available without registration is dedicated mostly to the inexperienced users who are interested in the fast inspection of simple structures or want to test RNAComposer performance. Interactive mode is useful for smaller and not complex RNAs that are readily predicted in silico (*see* **Notes 1** and **2**).

Before launching structure modeling, correct input data are required (*see* Subheading 3.2). Secondary structure topology of RNA can be entered by the user in dot–bracket notation. However, in this mode, the secondary structure can be also predicted making use of one of three programs: RNAstructure [19], CONTRAfold [20], or RNAfold [21] that have been incorporated into RNAComposer system. For this purpose the name of selected program should be provided in the third line instead of dot–bracket representation (example 3 in the RNAComposer interactive mode).

Pushing "Compose" button results in opening the "Task progress information" page (Fig. 3). In this page, the user obtains output information containing: task identifier and input data, information about the task processing phases released in real-time with partial and completed computing times, and two links. First link allows to download "pdb" file with coordinates of the predicted 3D model (Fig. 4). The second link allows for instant 3D visualization of the model using Jmol [17] applet. Additionally, upon user request, the pdb and log files may be sent to the supplied e-mail

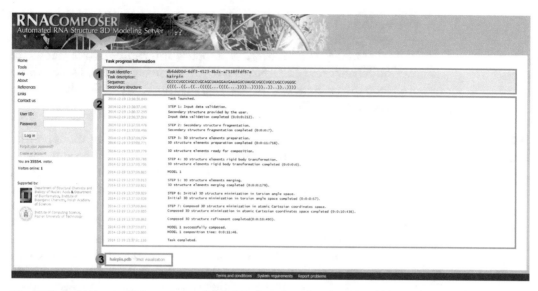

Fig. 3 The task progress information page (http://rnacomposer.cs.put.poznan.pl). (1) Task identifier and input data. (2) Information about task processing phases. (3) Links to output data: pdb file and Jmol visualization

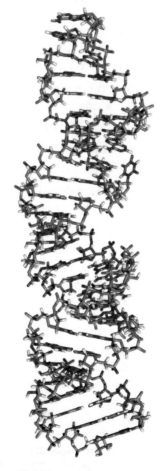

Fig. 4 3D representation of hairpin model

address. This is possible when the appropriate option is set in the user workspace.

One query in RNAComposer's interactive mode allows to build only one 3D RNA model. It is usually accomplished within seconds to minutes, depending on the RNA molecule size and complexity [11].

3.4 Creating User Account

For the purpose of using the RNAComposer batch mode, a user should register in the system by creating a personal account. Upon selecting "Create an account" option, located in the menu panel login area (Fig. 1), an account creation page is launched. The user is required to provide an e-mail address, unique username (user ID), and password (all of them are case sensitive). After quick data validation, an e-mail with activation link is sent to the user. Clicking onto the link ends the registration. Immediately after that, the new account is available and ready to use. Logged user can change the account settings, like e-mail address, password, and notification about completed batches. Three options are defined for e-mail notifications: no notifications, notifications with or without prediction results attached.

3.5 Structure Modeling in the Batch Mode

Batch mode (Fig. 5) is designed for RNA 3D structure prediction in large scale and allows to use additional RNAComposer functionality:

– Single input with multiple sequences defined and multiple secondary structures for each sequence

– Prediction of multiple models for one secondary structure

– Addition of distance restraints

– User workspace for short term storage of obtained data

– Detailed information about prediction steps and results provided in the log file (*see* **Note 3**)

Process of RNA structure prediction in the batch mode is similar to the interactive mode. However, in this mode the user can provide a batch of up to ten sequences with 1–10 secondary structure topologies for every sequence. No limit has been defined for a number of batches that can be run by the user. All batches are queued in the system and served according to the queuing protocol. Similarly to the interactive mode, the secondary structure topology is presented in dot–bracket notation (*see* **Notes 1** and **2**). In the single batch prediction, the user can launch as many as 100 tasks (one task consists of one sequence and secondary structure) that would have to be introduced separately in the interactive mode. Additionally, for each of these tasks RNAComposer can compute up to ten structural models, resulting in 1000 RNA 3D structural models that can be generated at a time, upon a single batch. The user can choose the required number of

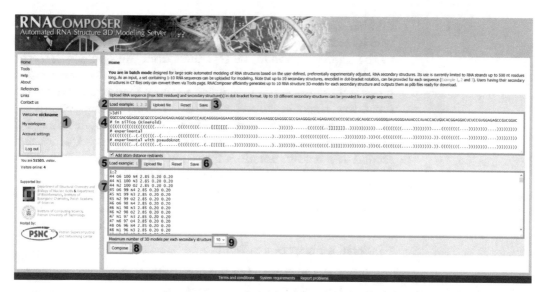

Fig. 5 RNAComposer batch mode homepage (http://rnacomposer.ibch.poznan.pl). (1) Batch mode's login area. (2) Examples. (3, 5, 6) Action buttons. (4) Entry box with input example of lysine riboswitch. (7) Example of correct atom distance restraints. (8) Compose button. (9) Drop-down list of maximum number of 3D models

structures by selecting option "maximum number of 3D models per each secondary structure" (Fig. 5). The predicted models are ranked based on the following criteria:

– Secondary structure topology compliance

– Similarity of the input and output sequences

– Purine–pyrimidine compatibility

– Source structure resolution

– Energy

The first output model is the one with best values of all the above criteria. In case of other models, the resolution and energy criteria are omitted.

3.5.1 Atom Distance Restraints

In addition to the sequence and secondary structure input, atom distance restraints can be optionally provided in the batch mode. Information about interatomic distances in RNA can be obtained experimentally or from analysis of particular databases, e.g., RNA FRABASE [13, 14]. Long range contacts or information about base-pairs can be revealed using UV or chemically induced crosslinking [22], nuclear magnetic resonance (NMR) [23], fluorescence resonance energy transfer (FRET) [24], or electron paramagnetic resonance (EPR) [25] studies. Such information can greatly improve 3D structure prediction. Atom distance restraints can be entered into additional entry box (Fig. 5). Format of atom distance restraints for RNAComposer is strictly defined and divided into two parts. The first part is a headline that defines the sequence number and the number of the secondary structure topology for which restraints will be applied. Numbers (from 1 to 10) referring to the sequences should be separated from those referring to the topologies by semicolons (example 3 in the RNAComposer batch mode). If the restraints are applied to more than one sequence (or secondary structure topology), then the sequences (topologies) should be separated by commas. As shown in Fig. 5, headline: 1;2 indicates that restraints will be applied to the first sequence and second dot–bracket notation. Every new description of interatomic distances must be specified under new headline.

In the second part, the user provides restraints as rigid atom distances. One line corresponds to the single restraint and consists of seven fields separated by spaces. The following fields represent:

- Serial number of first residue
- Name of the atom from the first residue
- Serial number of second residue
- Name of the atom from the second residue
- Interatomic distance value [Å]
- Allowable lower deviation from distance value [Å]
- Allowable upper deviation from distance value [Å]

Number of nucleotide residue and name of the atom can be described by at most four characters. Numbers of nucleotide residues correspond to nucleotides in chain from 5′ to 3′ end. Names of the atoms consist of the atom symbol and its number ascribed in accordance with IUPAC rules. Values defining distances must be described in %5.2f format, which means that the total number of digits is five, and number of decimal points is 2. No limit is set to the number of distance restraints that can be defined for single headline. Input data in specified format can be introduced into the entry boxes by pasting, writing or uploading text file. Additionally, "Save" button allows writing input data on hard disk (Fig. 5).

3.5.2 RNA 3D Structure Prediction Results

When the computation of query finishes, the user can download the results. Results are provided in pdb and log files. Pdb file contains atom coordinates of RNA 3D structural model(s). Log is a text file with data and parameters describing obtained model(s) and all steps of the 3D structure prediction. It contains:

- Input data
- Processing phases with partial and completed computing times
- Secondary structure elements resulting from the fragmentation of the input secondary structure
- 3D structure elements selected for the model building with their PDB IDs and similarity (%) to the structure provided by the user (*see* **Notes 4** and **5**)

Table 1
Approximate energy values of the final 3D structure expected for different RNA strand lengths

RNA length (nt)	Energy (kcal/mol)
30–100	−300 to −2000
100–200	−2000 to −4000
200–300	−4000 to −6000
300–400	−6000 to −8000
400–500	−8000 to −10,000

- 3D structure energy after every 100 steps of minimization in the Cartesian coordinates space
- Final energy of the 3D structure

Included information allows evaluation of model accuracy. The log file should be thoroughly analyzed by the user and several points should be taken under consideration. A good indicator of the 3D structural model quality is the final structure energy. Expected energy values were estimated in the original report [11] and are summarized in Table 1.

Log file contains also information about structural elements that due to the absence in the RNAComposer dictionary (although containing nearly half million of 3D structure elements) were generated de novo by the system. It should be noted that 3D structures containing such elements are usually of lower accuracy. Additional experimental data should be provided in such cases to help refine the structure and make the prediction more reliable (*see* **Note 6**). RNAComposer does not require homologs of RNA in question to predict the 3D structure. However, structure prediction accuracy tends to be better if the homology of the fragments used for the structure assembly is higher. Especially more complex elements, such as multi-helical junctions, should be inspected for the level of similarity. This information is provided as a percentage for every fragment in the log file.

3.6 Application Example

Usage of the RNAComposer batch mode is presented on the example of the lysine riboswitch. This RNA regulates biosynthesis and transport of amino acids, mainly lysine [26, 27]. Active domain of *Thermotoga maritima* lysine riboswitch RNA contains 174 nts and its secondary and three-dimensional structures have been solved [28] (PDB id 3DIL). The core of this RNA consists of a five-way junction leading to four hairpins and helix formed by pairing of the 5′ and 3′ ends. This RNA is also stabilized by the

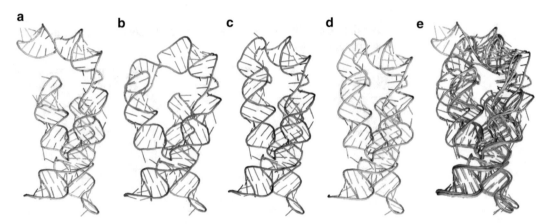

Fig. 6 3D structure representation of lysine riboswitch models obtained from (**a**) experimental data without pseudoknot, (**b**) experimental data with pseudoknot determined as atom distance restraints, (**c**) experimental data with pseudoknot determined as brackets. (**d**) Reference crystal structure of lysine riboswitch (PDB id. 3DIL). (**e**) Superposition of obtained models and crystal structure

pseudoknot between two hairpin apical loops. (Fig. 6). This RNA is an interesting example of complex structure and was therefore chosen to present scope and limitations of RNAComposer. To simulate a situation in which 3D structure of unknown RNA is predicted we removed all structural elements derived from 3DIL from the RNAComposer dictionary.

Correct secondary structure information is critical for the prediction of 3D structure. To present RNAComposer dependence on the input secondary structure we have undertaken two approaches: (1) secondary structure of lysine riboswitch RNA was predicted in silico or (2) was based on the experimental data from probing experiments [27, 29].

Different web-accessible tools were used for the in silico experiment. Secondary structure predicted using KineFold [30] was most similar to that observed in the crystal structure with the Matthews correlation coefficient (MCC) [31] of 0.877. This structure was used for further analyses (Fig. 5 entry box).

Secondary structure probing experiments provide valuable information that help to develop RNA secondary structure models. Recent advancement in probing methods, including new reagents [32] and experiments prepared in high-throughput fashion, made it possible to obtain good quality secondary structure models of large RNAs [33–35]. However, these methods still have limitations. In most cases complex elements, like pseudoknots, require additional analysis to confirm their existence [36]. In the case of lysine riboswitch RNA loop–loop interaction was postulated [27] and further confirmed [29]. To reflect this situation in our tests, experimentally supported structure was used in two options: without and with pseudoknot (Fig. 5 entry box). RNAComposer allows to annotate pseudoknots using square brackets (Fig. 5) or by providing appropriate distance restraints (Fig. 5). In summary, the following input options for 3D structure prediction of lysine riboswitch were used:

Case 1. The *in silico* predicted secondary structure.

Case 2. Experimentally supported secondary structure without pseudoknot.

Case 3. Experimentally supported secondary structure with the pseudoknot annotated using distance restraints.

Case 4. Experimentally supported secondary structure with the pseudoknot annotated using square brackets notation.

For each RNA secondary structure 10 three-dimensional structural models were predicted. Entire prediction took 26 min, thus single 3D structure was predicted in about 40 s. For clarity, we analyze here in detail only model no. 1 generated for each case.

According to the previously reported estimation [11] total energy calculated by RNAComposer for the 174 nts RNA should not exceed −3474 kcal/mol. Examination of the log file showed that all of the models meet this criterion suggesting that they can be further analyzed.

Case 1.

During the modeling of 3D structure using in silico predicted RNA secondary structure input, one 3D element ought to be generated by the RNAComposer engine. The 3D element representing required secondary structure topology of the five-way junction predicted in silico was not present in the RNAComposer dictionary. The predicted 3D model showed departure from the RNA crystal structure, as demonstrated by RMSD of 24.82 Å (Table 2). This could be anticipated since an input secondary structure was inaccurate. In such case total energy criterion might not be informative. Moreover, this case confirms that the quality of the predicted 3D models is strongly dependent on the RNAComposer dictionary content.

Case 2.

When the correct secondary structure was used as input but the pseudoknot was omitted, calculated RMSD of 6.91 Å (Table 2)

Table 2

Energy and global RMSD of models obtained for lysine riboswitch compared with crystal structure of 3DIL

RNA secondary structure model	RMSD (Å)	Energy (kcal/mol)
In silico predicted	24.82	−3642.483
Experimental without pseudoknot	6.91	−4494.975
Experimental with atom distance restraints	5.82	−4245.223
Experimental with square brackets	1.72	−4628.297

showed that predicted 3D model closely resembled RNA crystal structure (Fig. 6a, e). Local departure from the correct structure was observed within the region corresponding to the apical loops forming pseudoknot in lysine riboswitch RNA, underlying the importance of the fully correct input secondary structure. It is important to note that five-way junction was well predicted and therefore correct orientation of all helices was observed.

Case 3.

To correct prediction in Case 2 model, distances between residues involved in pseudoknot formation were fixed (Fig. 5). For this purpose RNA helix with the sequence identical to the loop–loop interaction was extracted from RNA FRABASE [13, 14] and distances between atoms characteristic for this helix were used to restrain the prediction. Use of this additional RNAComposer functionality allowed to obtain model with slightly better global RMSD (5.82 Å) (Table 2). However, kink introduced by the restraints within one of the hairpins affected conformation of adjoining structural elements (Fig. 6b, e). Sequence similarity between input structure and element used by RNAComposer for loop 1 (nts 41–54) was 42.86 %, while for the loop 2 (nts 93–101) it was 66.67 %. Still, predicted and crystal structure showed good overall agreement.

Case 4.

When correct input secondary structure was used and loop–loop interaction was annotated with square brackets predicted structure showed global RMSD of 1.72 Å (Table 2, Fig. 6c, e) demonstrating predictive power of RNAComposer.

3.7 User Workspace

Registered users have the opportunity to view their latest batches in the personal workspace. It is accessible after login and selecting "My workspace" option in the login area of menu panel. Also after running a new batch, the user is immediately taken to the workspace. There, the list of all uploaded batches that are unfinished or were finished less than 2 weeks ago, is displayed. For every batch in the list, the user can see the time of its uploading to the system (i.e., the time of pressing "Compose" button), its launching (i.e., actual time in which it left the queue and started to be processed), and its completion. The details concerning batch input data can be recalled after clicking on its identifier which takes the user to batch details page. Batch processing results (pdb and log files) can be saved to a local disk upon selecting the "Download" option. Every completed batch, together with its results, can be removed from the system after selecting it from the list and pressing the "Delete selected" button. Otherwise, it is stored in the system for 2 weeks and next removed after notifying the user with a warning e-mail.

4 Notes

RNAComposer fidelity was validated on 40 RNA 3D structures of different complexity and ranging in length from 33 to 161 nts [11]. The method is fully applicable to the prediction of 3D structures of large RNA, up to 500 nucleotides [36], including folding intermediates [37]. RNAComposer is being instantly developed and its dictionary volume increases, thus predictions are more accurate. However several points should be considered.

Note 1. As demonstrated in the application example, correct secondary structure is critical to obtain accurate 3D structure.

Note 2. The in silico RNA structure prediction of larger RNA should be reinforced by incorporation of the restraints obtained in RNA structure probing experiments.

Note 3. Log file should be thoroughly examined by the user. Total energy value is an important indicator of prediction quality. High total energy value disqualifies the model.

Note 4. Models containing 3D elements generated by RNAComposer usually show lower accuracy.

Note 5. In general, RNAComposer prediction does not depend on fragments homology. However if low homology fragments are used by RNAComposer for critical structural elements like multihelical junctions, quality of the predicted structure might be lower.

Note 6. Users might want to test predicted models experimentally. Possibilities include hydroxyl radical probing or introduction of mutations that would compromise predicted long-range contacts in RNA 3D models [36]. In addition, RNAComposer can be used to derive models based on NMR experimental data [38].

Acknowledgments

This work was supported by the National Science Center Poland [MAESTRO 2012/06/A/ST6/00384 (to R.W.A)] and Ministry of Science and Higher Education [0492/IP1/2013/72 (to K.J.P.)].

References

1. Spitale RC, Flynn RA, Torre EA, Kool ET, Chang HY (2014) RNA structural analysis by evolving SHAPE chemistry. Wiley Interdiscip Rev RNA 5(6):867–881. doi:10.1002/wrna.1253

2. Tian S, Cordero P, Kladwang W, Das R (2014) High-throughput mutate-map-rescue evaluates

SHAPE-directed RNA structure and uncovers excited states. RNA 20(11):1815–1826. doi:10.1261/rna.044321.114

3. Ding F, Sharma S, Chalasani P, Demidov VV, Broude NE, Dokholyan NV (2008) Ab initio RNA folding by discrete molecular dynamics: from structure prediction to folding mechanisms.

RNA   14(6):1164–1173.   doi:10.1261/rna.894608

4. Jonikas MA, Radmer RJ, Laederach A, Das R, Pearlman S, Herschlag D, Altman RB (2009) Coarse-grained modeling of large RNA molecules with knowledge-based potentials and structural filters. RNA 15(2):189–199. doi:10.1261/rna.1270809

5. Rother M, Rother K, Puton T, Bujnicki JM (2011) ModeRNA: a tool for comparative modeling of RNA 3D structure. Nucleic Acids Res 39(10):4007–4022. doi:10.1093/nar/gkq1320

6. Das R, Baker D (2007) Automated de novo prediction of native-like RNA tertiary structures. Proc Natl Acad Sci U S A 104(37):14664–14669. doi:10.1073/pnas.0703836104

7. Parisien M, Major F (2008) The MC-Fold and MC-Sym pipeline infers RNA structure from sequence data. Nature 452(7183):51–55. doi:10.1038/nature06684

8. Cao S, Chen SJ (2011) Physics-based de novo prediction of RNA 3D structures. J Phys Chem B 115(14):4216–4226. doi:10.1021/jp112059y

9. Sharma S, Ding F, Dokholyan NV (2008) iFoldRNA: three-dimensional RNA structure prediction and folding. Bioinformatics 24(17):1951–1952. doi:10.1093/bioinformatics/btn328

10. Zhao Y, Huang Y, Gong Z, Wang Y, Man J, Xiao Y (2012) Automated and fast building of three-dimensional RNA structures. Sci Rep 2:734. doi:10.1038/srep00734

11. Popenda M, Szachniuk M, Antczak M, Purzycka KJ, Lukasiak P, Bartol N, Blazewicz J, Adamiak RW (2012) Automated 3D structure composition for large RNAs. Nucleic Acids Res 40(14):e112. doi:10.1093/nar/gks339

12. Berman HM, Westbrook J, Feng Z, Gilliland G, Bhat TN, Weissig H, Shindyalov IN, Bourne PE (2000) The protein data bank. Nucleic Acids Res 28(1):235–242

13. Popenda M, Blazewicz M, Szachniuk M, Adamiak RW (2008) RNA FRABASE version 1.0: an engine with a database to search for the three-dimensional fragments within RNA structures. Nucleic Acids Res 36(Database issue):D386–D391. doi:10.1093/nar/gkm786

14. Popenda M, Szachniuk M, Blazewicz M, Wasik S, Burke EK, Blazewicz J, Adamiak RW (2010) RNA FRABASE 2.0: an advanced web-accessible database with the capacity to search the three-dimensional fragments within RNA structures. BMC Bioinformatics 11:231. doi:10.1186/1471-2105-11-231

15. Gan HH, Pasquali S, Schlick T (2003) Exploring the repertoire of RNA secondary motifs using graph theory; implications for RNA design. Nucleic Acids Res 31(11):2926–2943

16. Schwieters CD, Kuszewski JJ, Tjandra N, Clore GM (2003) The Xplor-NIH molecular structure determination package. J Magn Reson 160(1):65–73

17. Herraez A (2006) Biomolecules in the computer: Jmol to the rescue. Biochem Mol Biol Educ 34(4):255–261. doi:10.1002/bmb.2006.494034042644

18. Childs-Disney JL, Yildirim I, Park H, Lohman JR, Guan L, Tran T, Sarkar P, Schatz GC, Disney MD (2014) Structure of the myotonic dystrophy type 2 RNA and designed small molecules that reduce toxicity. ACS Chem Biol 9(2):538–550. doi:10.1021/cb4007387

19. Mathews DH (2014) RNA secondary structure analysis using RNAstructure. Curr Protoc Bioinformatics 46:12.16.11–12.16.25. doi:10.1002/0471250953.bi1206s46

20. Do CB, Woods DA, Batzoglou S (2006) CONTRAfold: RNA secondary structure prediction without physics-based models. Bioinformatics 22(14):e90–e98. doi:10.1093/bioinformatics/btl246

21. Hofacker IL, Fontana W, Stadler PF, Bonhoeffer LS, Tacker M, Schuster P (1994) Fast folding and comparison of RNA secondary structures. Monatshefte Fur Chem 125(2):167–188. doi:10.1007/Bf00818163

22. Sergiev PV, Dontsova OA, Bogdanov AA (2001) Chemical methods for the structural study of the ribosome: judgment day. Mol Biol 35(4):472–495. doi:10.1023/A:1010506522897

23. Furtig B, Richter C, Wohnert J, Schwalbe H (2003) NMR spectroscopy of RNA. Chembiochem 4(10):936–962. doi:10.1002/cbic.200300700

24. Wozniak AK, Nottrott S, Kuhn-Holsken E, Schroder GF, Grubmuller H, Luhrmann R, Seidel CA, Oesterhelt F (2005) Detecting protein-induced folding of the U4 snRNA kink-turn by single-molecule multiparameter FRET measurements. RNA 11(10):1545–1554. doi:10.1261/rna.2950605

25. Frolow O, Endeward B, Schiemann O, Prisner TF, Engels JW (2008) Nitroxide spin labeled RNA for long range distance measurements by EPR-PELDOR. Nucleic Acids Symp Ser (Oxf) 52:153–154. doi:10.1093/nass/nrn078

26. Huang LL, Serganov A, Patel DJ (2010) Structural insights into ligand recognition by a

sensing domain of the cooperative glycine ribo-switch. Mol Cell 40(5):774–786. doi:10.1016/j.molcel.2010.11.026

27. Grundy FJ, Lehman SC, Henkin TM (2003) The L box regulon: lysine sensing by leader RNAs of bacterial lysine biosynthesis genes. Proc Natl Acad Sci U S A 100(21):12057–12062. doi:10.1073/pnas.2133705100

28. Serganov A, Huang L, Patel DJ (2008) Structural insights into amino acid binding and gene control by a lysine riboswitch. Nature 455(7217):1263–1267. doi:10.1038/nature07326

29. Blouin S, Lafontaine DA (2007) A loop-loop interaction and a K-turn motif located in the lysine aptamer domain are important for the riboswitch gene regulation control. RNA 13(8):1256–1267. doi:10.1261/Rna.560307

30. Xayaphoummine A, Bucher T, Isambert H (2005) Kinefold web server for RNA/DNA folding path and structure prediction including pseudoknots and knots. Nucleic Acids Res 33(Web Server issue):W605–W610. doi:10.1093/nar/gki447

31. Matthews BW (1975) Comparison of the predicted and observed secondary structure of T4 phage lysozyme. Biochim Biophys Acta 405(2):442–451

32. Spitale RC, Crisalli P, Flynn RA, Torre EA, Kool ET, Chang HY (2013) RNA SHAPE analysis in living cells. Nat Chem Biol 9(1):18–20. doi:10.1038/nchembio.1131

33. Purzycka KJ, Pachulska-Wieczorek K, Adamiak RW (2011) The in vitro loose dimer structure and rearrangements of the HIV-2 leader RNA. Nucleic Acids Res 39(16):7234–7248. doi:10.1093/nar/gkr385

34. Legiewicz M, Zolotukhin AS, Pilkington GR, Purzycka KJ, Mitchell M, Uranishi H, Bear J, Pavlakis GN, Le Grice SF, Felber BK (2010) The RNA transport element of the murine musD retrotransposon requires long-range intramolecular interactions for function. J Biol Chem 285(53):42097–42104. doi:10.1074/jbc.M110.182840

35. Purzycka KJ, Legiewicz M, Matsuda E, Eizentstat LD, Lusvarghi S, Saha A, Le Grice SF, Garfinkel DJ (2013) Exploring Ty1 retrotransposon RNA structure within virus-like particles. Nucleic Acids Res 41(1):463–473. doi:10.1093/nar/gks983

36. Huang Q, Purzycka KJ, Lusvarghi S, Li D, Legrice SF, Boeke JD (2013) Retrotransposon Ty1 RNA contains a 5′-terminal long-range pseudoknot required for efficient reverse transcription. RNA 19(3):320–332. doi:10.1261/rna.035535.112

37. Lusvarghi S, Sztuba-Solinska J, Purzycka KJ, Pauly GT, Rausch JW, Grice SF (2013) The HIV-2 Rev-response element: determining secondary structure and defining folding intermediates. Nucleic Acids Res 41(13):6637–6649. doi:10.1093/nar/gkt353

38. Krahenbuhl B, Lukavsky P, Wider G (2014) Strategy for automated NMR resonance assignment of RNA: application to 48-nucleotide K10. J Biomol NMR 59(4):231–240. doi:10.1007/s10858-014-9841-3

Chapter 14

RNA 3D Structure Modeling by Combination of Template-Based Method ModeRNA, Template-Free Folding with SimRNA, and Refinement with QRNAS

Pawel Piatkowski, Joanna M. Kasprzak, Deepak Kumar, Marcin Magnus, Grzegorz Chojnowski, and Janusz M. Bujnicki

Abstract

RNA encompasses an essential part of all known forms of life. The functions of many RNA molecules are dependent on their ability to form complex three-dimensional (3D) structures. However, experimental determination of RNA 3D structures is laborious and challenging, and therefore, the majority of known RNAs remain structurally uncharacterized. To address this problem, computational structure prediction methods were developed that either utilize information derived from known structures of other RNA molecules (by way of template-based modeling) or attempt to simulate the physical process of RNA structure formation (by way of template-free modeling). All computational methods suffer from various limitations that make theoretical models less reliable than high-resolution experimentally determined structures. This chapter provides a protocol for computational modeling of RNA 3D structure that overcomes major limitations by combining two complementary approaches: template-based modeling that is capable of predicting global architectures based on similarity to other molecules but often fails to predict local unique features, and template-free modeling that can predict the local folding, but is limited to modeling the structure of relatively small molecules. Here, we combine the use of a template-based method ModeRNA with a template-free method SimRNA. ModeRNA requires a sequence alignment of the target RNA sequence to be modeled with a template of the known structure; it generates a model that predicts the structure of a conserved core and provides a starting point for modeling of variable regions. SimRNA can be used to fold small RNAs (<80 nt) without any additional structural information, and to refold parts of models for larger RNAs that have a correctly modeled core. ModeRNA can be either downloaded, compiled and run locally or run through a web interface at http://genesilico.pl/modernaserver/. SimRNA is currently available to download for local use as a precompiled software package at http://genesilico.pl/software/stand-alone/simrna and as a web server at http://genesilico.pl/SimRNAweb. For model optimization we use QRNAS, available at http://genesilico.pl/qrnas.

Key words RNA structure, Comparative modeling, Homology modeling, Free modeling, De novo modeling, Monte Carlo simulation, Statistical potential

---

The authors wish it to be known that the three first authors (P.P., J.M.K., and D.K.) should be regarded as joint first authors.

Douglas H. Turner and David H. Mathews (eds.), *RNA Structure Determination: Methods and Protocols*, Methods in Molecular Biology, vol. 1490, DOI 10.1007/978-1-4939-6433-8_14, © Springer Science+Business Media New York 2016

1   Introduction

Advances in high-throughput nucleic acid sequencing resulted in a rapid growth of RNA sequence information. Unfortunately, this growth of sequence information has not been paralleled by structure determination, and for the large majority of known RNA sequences, the 3D structures remain unknown. The experimental determination of RNA structures is difficult and expensive; currently it is significantly more challenging than protein structure determination [1]. This situation resembles a similar problem concerning protein sequences and structures, and both these problems have been approached by the development of computational methods for predicting 3D structures from the sequence information [2].

There exist a wide variety of methods for macromolecular 3D structure prediction that are applicable to RNA and they can be classified in various ways. One classification divides structure modeling methods into those that use information about potential similarity to known structures of other RNA molecules (the "Babylonian science" approach), and those that do not (the "Greek science" approach) [3]. All methods developed have various strengths and limitations, as observed in the recently initiated RNA Puzzles experiment.

The "Babylonian science" approach that exploits databases for macromolecular structure prediction has a long tradition and has been implemented in many different ways. Most commonly it utilizes the results of observations that evolutionarily related (homologous) molecules usually retain the same three-dimensional structure despite the accumulation of divergent mutations. This type of modeling has been developed initially for protein 3D structures and later adapted to model RNAs and is often referred to as "comparative modeling," "homology modeling," or "template-based modeling" [2]. There, a model is built for an RNA molecule with an unknown structure based on an experimentally determined structure of another RNA molecule, expected to be evolutionarily related, with the assumption that both molecules exhibit a similar structure. For this type of modeling, the sequence of a "target" RNA molecule to be modeled must be aligned to the sequence of a "template" RNA molecule with a known 3D structure (to define the correspondence between target and template residues), and then the sequence of the template is replaced with the sequence of the target in the context of the target structure. Thus, the major limitation of that method is that it can accurately predict RNA structures only if a similar structure is provided as a template, along with a sequence alignment between the target and the template molecules. However, as mentioned earlier, experimentally determined RNA 3D structures are sparse; hence, template-based modeling is currently possible for only a small fraction of RNA sequences.

We developed a template-based method ModeRNA that builds models of RNA 3D structure using information from structures of homologous RNAs used as templates [4, 5]. A highlight of ModeRNA is that it can model not only RNAs composed of the four canonical residues, but can also handle post-transcriptional modifications.

The "Greek science" approach that employs the fundamental laws of physics without information from databases is based on first principles and is often referred to (not fully correctly) as "ab initio." This type of modeling is accurate, at least for small molecules, but computationally very expensive, and hence very slow. One way to reduce the computational cost is to reduce the number of adjustable parameters that characterize a model. A drastic improvement in speed of calculations can be achieved by coarse-graining, where groups of atoms may be treated as single interaction centers or "pseudoatoms," so that a smaller number of elements and interactions need to be considered [6]. It must be emphasized that simplifications of the model representation and the energy function enhances the modeling speed usually at the cost of accuracy of the structures obtained. Thus, it is not practical to expect that a folding simulation with a coarse-grained representation will always faithfully predict a native-like RNA structure with a precisely estimated energy. On the other hand, these methods offer keen insights into the main features of the folding process over long time scales at a comparatively modest cost in computational resources, data storage and time. The use of simplified methods may be the most practical way to computationally fold a structure that is too complex for typical methods utilizing a full-atom representation and a physical potential that is more expensive to calculate.

We developed a coarse-grained method for RNA folding simulations and 3D structure prediction dubbed SimRNA, which has been inspired by the success of coarse-grained methods of protein structure prediction, in particular CABS [7] and REFINER [8]. SimRNA allows for RNA 3D structure prediction from sequence alone, and can use additional structural information, if available, in the form of restraints on the local arrangement of certain atoms, secondary structure, and other types of contacts.

The protocol for the combination of template-based and template-free modeling was initially developed for protein 3D structure prediction [9] and is now implemented for RNA 3D structure modeling.

In this tutorial we describe a case study of predicting the tertiary structure of a phage Twort group I intron RNA. We used a crystal structure of an Azoarcus group I intron (PDB ID: 1ZZN) as a template for the initial modeling with ModeRNA, followed by refolding of poorly modeled regions with SimRNA. For model optimization, we use QRNAS. Comparison of the model to the known crystal structure (PDB ID: 1Y0Q) serves to highlight strengths and limitations of template-based and template-free modeling approaches.

2 Materials

ModeRNA is written in Python and can be run either via a web server or locally from a Python script. The installable package of ModeRNA is available from http://genesilico.pl/moderna/ and its use is free for all users. For local use, the package can be run on Linux, Windows (XP, 7, 8), or Mac OS X operating systems as long as they have Python 2.6 or higher installed. The web server can be found under the link: http://genesilico.pl/modernaserver/. The use of a standard web browser, such as Apple Safari, Microsoft Internet Explorer, or Mozilla Firefox is required.

SimRNA is written in C++ and currently is only available for the Linux and Mac OS X operating systems. The compiled Linux binaries for Intel and AMD (32-bit and 64-bit) are available from http://genesilico.pl/software/stand-alone/simrna/. The use of SimRNA is free for noncommercial use by academic users. Nonacademic users and those interested in commercial use must contact J.M.B. to obtain a commercial license. The multiprocessor version of SimRNA code requires OpenMP. The Mac OS X binaries are compiled with OS X.6/7 support and are compatible with system versions 10.6 and above. Users interested in obtaining compiled SimRNA binaries for other distributions must contact the authors. While this article was processed for publication, a web server version of SimRNA (SimRNAweb) was published, which allows structure prediction and model clustering to be performed online. The tutorial outlined here can be accomplished using SimRNAweb instead of SimRNA (see http://iimcb.genesilico.pl/SimRNAweb/doc for details) [10].

QRNAS is written in C++. It is available from http://genesilico.pl/qrnas/ and its use is free for all users. For compilation of QRNAS, a C++ compiler, such as GNU g++ is required. A bash shell script is provided for compilation of the package.

Files
All files used in the tutorial can be downloaded from ftp://genesilico.pl/iamb/tutorial/groupI_intron_modeling.

3 Methods

3.1 Template Search

The first step in template-based modeling of RNA is to identify an appropriate template, i.e., a related RNA molecule with known structure, which is expected to be similar to the (unknown) structure to be modeled. Sequence similarity between the target and the template is an important factor influencing the accuracy of the model. In general, molecules with a higher sequence similarity tend to exhibit structures that are more similar to each other. Besides, for highly similar sequences it is generally easier to generate a correct alignment (to find homologous residues between the target and the template). Therefore, the use of templates with high sequence similarity is recommended. The simplest and probably most commonly used method to find RNA sequences with high similarity to the target is to apply simple sequence database searching tools such as nucleotide BLAST [11] on sequences of RNA molecules with known structures. However, high sequence similarity is not an absolute prerequisite for template-based modeling. In fact, RNA molecules can exhibit very similar structures even if their sequence identity is almost nil; hence it is possible to create accurate template-based models even for target RNA molecules with very low sequence similarity to the template(s).

Ideally, both the target and the template should be evolutionarily related (e.g., belong to the same RNA family) and exhibit similar structure: there should be an experimentally determined template structure that roughly fits the target to be predicted. A recommended advanced way to identify potential template RNAs that combine evolutionary relationship and structural similarity is to compare the target sequence with the Rfam database of RNA sequence families [12] (http://rfam. xfam.org/). For each family of sequences potentially related to the target, representatives with a known 3D structure can be aligned to the target sequence; e.g., using Infernal [13], with the aid of a covariance model corresponding to the family of the template candidate. The covariance models represents correlated base exchanges over the entire family and can be derived; for example, from sequence alignments in the Rfam database.

For various RNA families, specialized databases exist that combine sequences and structures and often include additional information, such as evolutionary relationships, which may guide template selection. In the case study presented in this tutorial, we used the Group I intron Sequence and Structure Database (GISSD) [14] (http://www.rna.whu.edu.cn/gissd/).

In practice:
The aim of the exercise presented in this chapter is to predict the tertiary structure of a phage Twort group I intron RNA using the crystal structure of an Azoarcus group I intron RNA (PDB ID: 1ZZN) as a template. The structure of the Twort intron has been determined experimentally (PDB ID: 1Y0Q), and is available to validate the accuracy of the modeling done here. Download the files containing coordinates of both structures in PDB format from the RCSB Protein Data Bank (http://www.rcsb.org/) and save them locally as 1ZZN.pdb and 1Y0Q.pdb.

The group I intron sequence is the following:

```
AAAUAAUUGAGCCUUUAUACAGUAAUGUAUAUCGAAAAA
UCCUCUAAUUCAGGGAACACCUAAACAAACUAAGAUGUAGGC
AAUCCUGAGCUAAGCUCUUAGUAAUAAGAGAAAGUGCAA
CGACUAUUCCGAUAGGAAGUAGGGUCAAGUGACUCG
AAAUGGGGAUUACCCUUCUAGGGUAGUGAUAUAGUCUGA
ACAUAUAUGGAAACAUAUAGAAGGAUAGGAGU
AACGAACCUAUUCGUAACAUAAUUG
```

3.2 Preparation of the Template Structure for Modeling

Files downloaded from the PDB database usually contain more than just one copy of the RNA molecule of interest and often include some small molecules, water or metal ions. All the data that is not essential for modeling of the target structure may impair the modeling process. Thus, a recommended practice for typical modeling tasks involving single RNA molecules is to "clean" the template structure of the additional small molecules until all that remains is the one chain that is supposed to be used as a modeling template. It is also important to remember that sequences of molecules in the PDB database often contain various modifications (e.g., extended or truncated termini, and various mutations) introduced to improve crystallization, and some elements of the target sequence may be "invisible" in the structure due to intrinsic disorder (thus, some residues may be missing). Hence, the sequence of the template is not necessarily identical to the sequence of the RNA under consideration that exists in nature.

In practice:
Open the `1ZZN.pdb` file in a macromolecule structural viewer, e.g., PyMOL. The structure consists of four chains: A: protein, B: intron RNA, C: 3′ exon RNA, and D: 5′ exon RNA. Chain A contains nonstandard residues: a GTP (residue 1) and an A23 (adenosine-5′-phosphate-2′,3′-cyclic phosphate; residue 190) and ions. In addition, an inserted fragment containing residues numbered 1001–1014 ("CCAUUGCACUCCGG") is placed after the sequence of the intron, rather in the position where the insertion actually takes place. Hence, for the purpose of modeling, a series of modifications must be introduced to standardize the order, numbering, and nomenclature of all residues. Apply the following procedures to prepare the template:

1. Change modified residue names (GTP into G and A23 into A).

2. Move the 1001–1014 sequence fragment to the relevant position in the structure (between residues 107 and 112).

3. Merge the 3′ exon from chain C.

4. Make two "gaps" (change the numbering of the template) for the fragments that will be inserted into the model.

5. Save the template as `1ZZN_cleaned.pdb` (chain A).

To perform these operations with ModeRNA, follow the Python interface below:

```
$ python
>>> from moderna import *
>>> t = load_template("1ZZN.pdb", "B")
>>> t.get_modified_residues()
{'1': <Residue 1 GTP>, '190': <Residue 190 23pA>}
>>> remove_modification(t["1"])
>>> remove_modification(t["190"])
```

```
>>> clean_structure(t)
Chain OK
>>> m = create_model()
>>> # Add the first residue of chain B
>>> m.add_residue(t["1"])
>>> # Add the first fragment of chain B (residues 5-107)
>>> for i in range(5, 108): m.add_residue(t[str(i)])
...

>>> # Add and renumber the second fragment (residues
    1001-1014)
>>> for i in range(1, 15): m.add_residue(t[str(i +
    1000)], str(107 + i))
...

>>> # Add and renumber the last fragment (residues
    112-190)
>>> for i in range(112, 191): m.add_residue(t[str(i)],
    str(i + 10))
...

>>> # Merge 3' exon (chain C)
>>> t_ex = load_template("1ZZN.pdb", "C")
>>> for i in range(191, 207): m.add_residue(t_ex[str(i)],
    str(i + 10))
...

>>> # Insert gap between residues 145 and 146 for
    future insertion
>>> for i in range(146, 217): m.renumber_residue(str(i),
    str(i + 100))
...

>>> # Insert gap between 307 and 308
>>> for i in range(308, 317): m.renumber_residue(str(i),
    str(i + 100))
...
>>> m.write_pdb_file("1ZZN_cleaned.pdb")
>>> m.get_sequence()
GGCCGUGUGCCUUGCGCCGGGAAACCACGCAAGGGAUGGU
GUCAAAUUCGGCGAAACCUAAGCGCCCGCCCGGGCGUAUGGCAA
CGCCGAGCCAAGCUUCGCAGCCAUUGCACUCCGGCUGCGAUGAAGG
UGUAGAGACUAGACGGCACCCACCUAAGGCAAACGCUAUGGUGAAGG
CAUAGUCCAGGGAGUGGCGA_AAGCCACACAAACCAG
```

Alternatively, the ModeRNA server can be used in the "Analyse Structure" mode (http://genesilico.pl/modernaserver/submit/analyse/) with the option "clean structure". If need be, the "Convert Format" mode can be used (http://genesilico.pl/modernaserver/submit/convert/) to adjust the formatting of the PDB files: in particular, to switch between "old" and "new" formats that involve different nomenclatures of ribose atoms and phosphate groups.

3.3 Target-Template Alignment

In order to build a model of a given target sequence, ModeRNA requires (as an input) the atomic 3D coordinates of a template RNA molecule, and a user-specified sequence alignment between the target and the template. The accuracy of the alignment will ultimately determine the quality of the resulting model. The alignment can be generated automatically with "*Find Template*" and "*Prepare Alignment*" procedures in ModeRNA server. The first approach uses Infernal [13] with covariance models taken from the Rfam database, and the second approach uses R-Coffee [15]. However, for remotely related sequences, alignments generated automatically usually contain various errors. The recommended practice is to verify whether the alignment correctly reproduces the correspondence between functionally important sequence motifs, secondary structure elements, and local structural motifs. If possible, alignments from curated databases should be used, where such verification has already been carried out by experts.

In practice:
The sequence alignment between the target (Twort intron) and the template (Azoarcus intron) has to be prepared in the FASTA format, in which the target sequence is positioned first in the file, followed by the template sequence. In the exercise described here, we use the full sequence of a phage Twort group I intron RNA obtained from the GISSD database (the modeling target), and the sequence extracted from the PDB 1ZZN file as the template. To obtain the target sequence from GISSD, click the "*Search*" tab and enter *Staphylococcus phage* Twort as organism. In ModeRNA server's main window, click "*Prepare alignment*" and enter both sequences.

Bear in mind that an automatically generated alignment might contain errors such as gaps in secondary structure elements or misaligned structural motifs. For this reason it is recommended to edit the alignment manually and improve its quality.

One possibility is to obtain the target-template alignment from an external source, such as the Rfam database. Search the Rfam database with the Twort group I intron RNA sequence as a target, using the Infernal (http://rfam.xfam.org/, "sequence search" option). This should lead to the identification of the Intron_gpI (RF00028) family, which includes all known group I introns, including the target sequence and several experimentally determined structures. At the time of the writing of this study, the Azoarcus group I intron structure (PDB ID: 1ZZN) is not listed in the web page of the RF00028 family, in the current version of the Rfam database. The sequence of that RNA is currently included only in the full alignment that can be obtained from the Rfam database curators. Alternatively, the alignment of the target sequence to the Intron_gpI (RF00028) family can be used as a guide to improve the pairwise target-template alignment.

Experiment with the alignment file using any sequence editor (or even a plain text editor). After editing, the alignment between

```
Target    AAAUAAUUGAGCCUUUAUA-CAGUAAUGUAUAUCGAAAAAUCCUCUAAUUCAGGGAACACCUAAACAAAC
Template  --GGCCGUGUGCCUUGCGCCGGGAAACCACGCAAGGGAUGGUGUCAAAUUCGGCGAAA-CCUAAGCGCCC

Target    U--AAGAUGU-AGGCAAUCCUGAGCUAAGCUCUUAGUA-------------AUAAGAGAAAGUGCAACG
Template  GCCCGGGCGUAUGGCAACGCCGAGCCAAGCUUCGCAGCCAUUGCACUCCGGCUGCGAUGAAGGUGUAGAG

Target    ACUAUUCCGAUAGGAAGUAGGGUCAAGUGACUCGAAAUGGGGAUUACCCUUC--------UAGGGUAGUG
Template  ACUAG----------------------------ACGGCACCCACCUAAGGCAAACGCUAUGGUGAAG

Target    AUAUAGUCUGAACAUAUAUGGAAACAUAUAGAAGGAUAGGAGUAACGAACCUAUUCGUAACAUAA-UUG
Template  GCAUAGUCC-AGGGAGUGGCGAAAGCCAC--------------------------ACA-AACCAG
```

Fig. 1 Graphical illustration of the sequence alignment between the target to be modeled (Twort intron) and the template with known structure (Azoarcus intron) used as an input for comparative modeling. Residues in a given column are considered homologous and a given residue of the target sequence is going to be modeled based on coordinates of the template residue in the same column below. Gaps (indels) are indicated by *dashes* (-). Regions in the target with a "deletion" counterpart in the template will be modeled by insertion of fragments taken from a database of known RNA structures

the Twort group I intron RNA sequence and the Azoarcus group I intron sequence (corresponding to the sequence in the 1ZZN structure) may look as shown in Fig. 1. Save the alignment in the FASTA format as `alignment.fasta`.

3.4 Building a Model with ModeRNA

As an input, ModeRNA takes a PDB-formatted RNA structure file and a FASTA alignment. The alignment is decomposed into elementary operations such as copying parts from the template structure that are identical in the target, and substituting bases by adding small fragments for individual nucleotides. In this context it is noteworthy that ModeRNA is capable of modeling not only the four standard residues (A, G, C, U), but also >100 posttranscriptionally modified residues. Insertions and deletions in the alignment are modeled by inserting fragments of the appropriate length from a library of more than 100,000 fragments extracted from known RNA structures. Fragments are selected based on spatial compatibility with the rest of the molecule; i.e., geometrical match between the termini of the inserted fragment and the anchor points in the framework, and the absence of steric clashes, but no physical energy function is used to assess the resulting structure. As a result, the models may exhibit local steric problems such as a distorted backbone. In short, further refinement is often necessary.

In practice:
There are three ways to build a model with ModeRNA: using the ModeRNA server, from a command line or with the Python interpreter. The two first approaches are simpler and faster, but do not allow the user to carry out more advanced operations, such as structure editing.

In the case described in this tutorial, the use of the command-line version of ModeRNA requires only the following command:

```
python moderna.py -t 1ZZN_cleaned.pdb -c A -a
alignment.fasta -o Twort-moderna.pdb
```

Another way is to use the ModeRNA server. Open the "*Build model*" bookmark and fill in the form with the input data: choose the downloaded template file (1ZZN_cleaned.pdb), chain ID (here: A) and a previously prepared alignment file in FASTA format "alignment.fasta". Enter the title of the computing job and optionally your e-mail address if you want to be informed when the model is ready to download. Submit your job using the "*Build model*" option and wait for the result (approximately 5–6 min). When the modeling process is finished, ModeRNA visualizes the model in a Jmol viewer, provides PDB coordinates for download, and returns a report about the model's problems with geometry and stereochemistry, such as unusual bond lengths and dihedral angles. It will, however, not indicate which parts of the model are likely to be correct and which parts are almost certainly wrong. In the simplest scenario, not only residues with bad geometry and those in steric clashes, but also residues in the model that were added as insertions or whose conformation is significantly different from their counterparts in the template, should be considered potential targets for further refinement.

To create a model using ModeRNA's commands from the Python interpreter, type:

```
$ python
>>> from moderna import *
>>> t = load_template("1ZZN_cleaned.pdb", "A")
>>> a = load_alignment("alignment.fasta")
>>> m = create_model(t, a)
>>> m.renumber_chain("1")
>>> m.write_pdb_file("Twort-moderna.pdb")
```

The steps mentioned above are to generate an Intron model of the target (Twort).

3.5 Template-Free Refolding of Sequence Fragments with SimRNA

As an input, SimRNA uses a starting structure (PDB-formatted) or a sequence (ASCII-formatted) file, a configuration file that contains the basic parameters of the simulation to be performed (e.g., length of the simulation, temperature range, modifications of the parameters, etc.), and an optional file with restraints. SimRNA represents RNA using a reduced representation with only five explicit atoms per residue that generate a nearly one-to-one transformation between the reduced and the all-atom representations. It allows for simulations of a part of the system to be performed, with the conformation of the remaining part frozen or restrained. Secondary structure restraints can be specified using the multiline dots-and-brackets format, which allows for defining RNA pseudoknots. The dots-and-brackets input is parsed and internally converted into a dedicated list of restraints. If no starting structure is provided (i.e., in the template-free mode), SimRNA generates a circular conformation of the input sequence with the 5′ and 3′ ends next to each other. In the exercise described in this chapter, the modeling is initiated from a structure generated by template-based modeling with ModeRNA.

Three types of user-specified restraints are currently implemented in SimRNA: on atomic positions (immobilization or flexible pinning), on interatomic distances (flexible tethering) and on the secondary structure (base-pairing). The role of the secondary structure restraints is to specify the desired canonical Watson–Crick (*cis*), and wobble base pairs; this type of restraints may include pseudoknots of any type. By default, SimRNA does not penalize the formation of base-pairs that are not specified in the given secondary structure file of constraints.

The output of a simulation is recorded as a trajectory file (or set of files) comprising the lowest-energy conformations selected from a consecutive series of simulation steps. SimRNA is accompanied by a software package for the processing of the trajectory files. The content of the trajectory files (in the form of individual frames or a series of such frames) can be visualized, converted to PDB files, searched for structures with desired properties (lowest global energy, lowest RMSD to a reference structure), or subjected to clustering. The trajectory can be converted to a series of files in PDB format containing models in either the reduced SimRNA representation or models rebuilt to an all-atom representation. For the selection of the final model, SimRNA employs a clustering protocol. Based on our experience, we recommend to use a clustering threshold equal to 0.1 Å times the sequence length, i.e., 5 Å for a sequence of 50 residues, and we consider medoids of the three largest clusters of decoys as well as the decoy with the lowest energy. However, other protocols of clustering and data retrieval can be used depending on the purpose of the modeling (e.g., for conformational sampling, other thresholds can be used and a larger or smaller number of cluster representatives can be obtained).

In practice:

Prepare an input file for SimRNA that indicates the following regions for optimization: 1–10, 43–47, 58–81, 119–122, 125–157, 158–162, 168–180, 188–189, 192–194, 196–200, 213–216, 217–250, 252–267, so that SimRNA treats the remaining residues as "frozen." An example file is included (together with all files at ftp://ftp.genesilico.pl/iamb/tutorial/groupI_intron_modeling/) as simrna_input.pdb. The file Twort-moderna.pdb generated in Subheading 3.4 and file simrna_input.pdb are the same. The only difference is in the "occupancy" field of the PDB files. In the file simrna_input.pdb, all the residues to be optimized are set with occupancy "1.00", which is the requirement to set the residues free during SimRNA optimization, while residues with occupancy "0.00" are restricted.

- Atoms with occupancy equal to 0.000 are treated as frozen, their position is not changed during the simulation.

- Atoms with occupancy between 0.001 and 0.999 are allowed to move within a restricted radius from their starting position, with the radius defined in the B-factor column.

- Atoms with occupancy 1.000 are allowed to move without additional restrictions, unless additional restraints are applied.

Prepare an input file with the secondary structure to be used as restraints. An example file with the secondary structure of the target (Twort intron) taken from the PDB file is included as ss-constraint-file.txt.

Prior to the SimRNA simulation run, follow the steps described in *Installation of SimRNA* at the end of this chapter.

Run SimRNA with the following parameters: algorithm: Replica Exchange, number of replicas: 10, number of runs: 16, number of iterations: 16 000 000, initial temperature: 1.35, final temp: 0.9. The command-line version of SimRNA to perform optimization of the thawed residues with above parameters is:

```
SimRNA -c config.dat -P simrna_input.pdb -S ss-
constraint-file.txt -E 10 -o simrna_results &>
simrna_results.out
```

where,

- config.dat contains specific control parameters desired in a particular simulation

- '-E 10' specifies the desired number of replicas to be run in the Monte Carlo simulation.

- simrna_results is the output file generated with information about the trajectories sampled (.trafl), bonds (.bonds), and secondary structures (.ss_detected).

- simrna_results.out preserves a record of the output messages to the terminal that are generated during a simulation (helpful for checking configuration, etc.).

The above command can be used to run SimRNA optimization on local machines.

For fast and efficient optimization of the system it is recommended to run the simulations in a computer cluster environment (SGE or PBS). By default, with the command line above, SimRNA runs parallel optimizations on ten cores in a cluster node, which on the system in the authors' laboratory takes about 26 h (real time). The command to submit a SimRNA simulation run in the SGE environment is:

```
qsub -cwd -pe mpi 10 -l mem_free=450 M,h_
vmem=300 M -e simrna_results.out -b y SimRNA
-c config.dat -P simrna_input.pdb -S ss-con-
straint-file.txt -E 10 -o simrna_results
```

Similarly, simulations can be run in a PBS cluster environment too.

Once, the trajectories (.trafl) from all simulations are obtained, concatenate the files:

```
cat *.trafl > Twort-simrna.trafl
```

(the file can be obtained from the ftp repository, ftp://gene-silico.pl/iamb/tutorial/groupI_intron_modeling)

The next step is to perform "clustering" method mentioned in Subheading 3.5.

Run clustering with the following parameters:

```
clustering Twort-simrna.trafl 0.01 14.3
```

where,

- '0.01' is the fraction of lowest-energy frames taken for clustering,
- '14.3' is the RMSD threshold (0.1 Å times the sequence length as a rule of thumb).

After the clustering step is completed, the trajectory file Twort-simrna_thrs14.30A_clust01.trafl is generated.

Next, the SimRNA_trafl2pdbs is run from a command-line interface to obtain the PDB file (Twort-simrna_thrs14.30A_clust01-000001_AA.pdb) from the trafl file. The pdb file is the medoid of the cluster of the decoys.

```
SimRNA_trafl2pdbs    simrna_input.pdb    Twort-
simrna_thrs14.30A_clust01.trafl 1 AA
```

where "1" means the first frame of the cluster and the "AA" parameter generates the all-atom representation of the extracted frame.

To extract the lowest energy frame from the cluster, the following command line should be executed,

```
python trafl_extract_lowestE_frame.py Twort-
simrna_thrs14.30A_clust01.trafl
```

After this command, a file Twort-simrna_thrs14.30A_clust01_minE.trafl is generated. Next, SimRNA_trafl2pdbs program is run to obtain the PDB file (Twort-simrna_thrs14.30A_clust01_minE-000001_AA.pdb) from the trafl file.

```
SimRNA_trafl2pdbs    simrna_input.pdb    Twort-
simrna_thrs14.30A_clust01_minE.trafl 1 AA
```

Now, we have the medoid and the lowest energy frame of the cluster of the decoys. These PDB files can be taken for further structural analysis.

3.6 RNA 3D Structure Refinement

Models of RNA 3D structures obtained by modeling methods often suffer from local inaccuracies such as clashes or physically improbable bond lengths, backbone conformations, or sugar puckers. To ensure high quality of models, a procedure of refinement should be applied as a final step in the modeling pipeline. The software tool QRNAS was developed in our laboratory to perform local refinement of nucleic acid structures based on an extended version of the AMBER force field. The extensions consist of energy terms associated with introduction of explicit hydrogen bonds, idealization of base pair planarity and regularization of backbone conformation.

In practice:
The use of QRNAS is straightforward. Run the program (see *Installation of QRNAS*), using the following command

```
Twort-simrnaTwort-simrna/path/to/QRNAS/QRNA  -i
    Twort-simrna_thrs14.30A_clust01-000001_
    AA.pdb.pdb -o Twort-simrna-qrnas.pdb
```

where `Twort-simrna_thrs14.30A_clust01-000001_AA.pdb` is the file to be optimized, and `Twort-simrna-qrnas.pdb` is the optimized structure.

For more advanced usage of QRNAS, users should consult the README.txt file in the QRNAS package.

3.7 RNA 3D Structure Quality Evaluation

The evaluation of the utility of a structural model is a complex issue. In general, it depends on the precision of the question asked. Contemporary modeling methods are unable to generate very accurate models that would be suitable to answer very precise questions (e.g., the fine details of active sites). However, a general architectural level of detail or a lower-level biochemical understanding can be usefully addressed by present-day modeling tools. To evaluate the predictive success of the proposed models, two general criteria were established [16]: first, the model must be geometrically and topologically as close as possible to the experimentally determined structure used as the reference, and second, the model must be stereochemically correct (bond distances, angles and intermolecular contacts should be close to the values typically observed in experimentally determined structures). The geometrical and topological similarity of the model to the "true" structure can be assessed only if a suitable reference is known. In the absence of the reference structure, only statistical properties of the model may be assessed. In addition, the validity of the model may be tested by its assessment against independently obtained data, e.g., from biochemical experiments.

Here, the availability of the reference structure for the Azoarcus group I intron allows us to calculate both the statistical parameters as well as to assess the relative similarity of the model to the reference. Figure 2. illustrates subsequent modeling steps, from the original

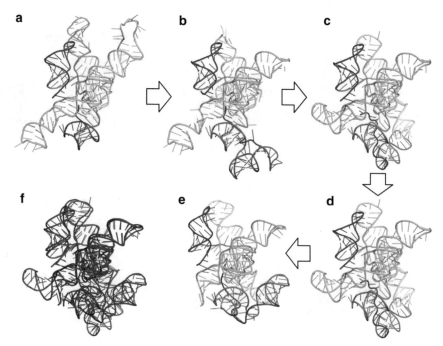

Fig. 2 Snaphots of the modeling process: (**a**) 3D structure of the Azoarcus group I intron (PDB ID: 1ZZN) used as the modeling template; (**b**) template-based model of phage Twort group I intron RNA built with ModeRNA; (**c**) template-based model of phage Twort group I intron RNA refolded with SimRNA; (**d**) SimRNA-generated model of phage Twort group I intron RNA optimized with QRNAS; (**e**) experimentally determined structure of phage Twort group I intron RNA (PDB ID: 1Y0Q). All RNA structures are shown in the simplified cartoon representation, with the backbone shown as a *ribbon* and base moieties as *sticks*; the residues are colored as a spectrum from 5′ (*blue*) to 3′ (*red*). (**f**) Superposition of the final model of phage Twort group I intron RNA shown in panel **d** (in *red*) with the experimentally determined structure shown in panel **e** (in *blue*)

template, to the initial homology model, to refolding and refinement, and finally to comparison of the final model with the experimentally determined structure.

The quality of the models geometry was evaluated using the MolProbity suite web-server (available at http://molprobity.biochem.duke.edu/) [17] using default parameters. After the initial parsing of the models, we used the "Add hydrogens" option of the server (required for the analysis of steric clashes), followed with the "Analyze all-atom contacts and geometry" tool . The template structure and all models were also superimposed onto the reference structure, and their similarity was calculated by means of the RMSD with an in-house program. Table 1 presents the results of evaluation.

Models presented here exhibit relatively large RMSD (>10 Å) from the reference structure. However, given the large size of the modeled RNA molecule (233 residues in the reference structure), such models should be considered as relatively accurate. The statistical significance of these models, according to [18], is high, with p-value of the prediction: <10^{-6} in all cases. Comparison of structures

Table 1
Assessment of structures considered in the modeling exercise presented in this work

Model quality indicators	Template structure (1ZZN)	Initial model generated with ModeRNA	Model refolded locally with SimRNA	Model optimized with QRNAS	Reference structure (1Y0Q)
Clashscore (MolProbity)	50.7	124.09	184.69	0.37	59.05
Bad bonds (MolProbity)	0.08%	1.90%	4.12%	0.00%	0.00%
Bad angles (MolProbity)	0.72%	1.63%	6.53%	0.88%	0.41%
RMSD from the reference structure (1y0q)	28.31 Å	15.70 Å	10.9 Å	11.0 Å	0.00 Å

Clashscore refers to the number of serious steric overlaps (>0.4 Å) per 1000 atoms. RMSD has been calculated for all pairs of homologous residues (without any distance threshold)

at different stages of the modeling reveals that the initial comparative model of the Twort group I intron RNA generated with ModeRNA is the farthest away in RMSD from the reference structure and that it exhibits problems with geometry and packing. The local refolding with SimRNA improves the accuracy of the model in terms of its similarity to the reference structure; however, it also introduces additional problems with geometry and packing. These problems can be almost completely alleviated (to the level of quality observed for experimentally determined structures) thanks to the geometry optimization with QRNAS, at negligible cost of accuracy.

The analysis of the models demonstrates that the procedure described in this chapter enables the generation of a useful 3D structural prediction, which has not only a correctly modeled conserved core, but also the peripheral elements have native-like orientation with respect to the core and to each other. Of course, peripheral elements exhibit a much larger deviations from the reference structure than regions in the core; however, it is also in the periphery were the local refolding with SimRNA brings about largest improvement of accuracy. Ultimately, refinement with QRNAS does not introduce significant changes of overall accuracy, but removes local errors introduced at earlier stages of modeling and ensures that the model is stereochemically correct.

The analysis of inaccuracies and shortcomings of the models suggests that computational predictions by themselves can only deliver an approximate estimation of the structure, particularly the details. While the methods presented herein are by no means perfect, they provide a useful toolbox for the generation of practically useful models of RNA 3D structure. The critical analysis of models and their comparison with experimentally determined structures is useful for the development of better modeling tools in the future.

Installation of ModeRNA

The standalone version of ModeRNA (currently version 1.7.1) requires Python 2.6 or higher and the BioPython library, and can be downloaded from http://genesilico.pl/moderna/download.

For inserting larger fragments (as shown in this tutorial) an additional package, called Larger Linker Libraries, is required. Download LIRdb_100 package from http://genesilico.pl/moderna/download/ and replace file data/LIR_fragments.lib with the downloaded file (rename the downloaded file LIRdb_100 as LIR_fragments.lib).

Using a standalone version of ModeRNA from Python is the most flexible and versatile way. Not only does it allow for advanced operations like editing secondary structure or exchanging single bases, but also makes it possible to automate repetitive tasks, e.g., when a user wants to remove modifications in hundreds of RNA structures. The Python interface is also the only way to use the ModeRNA v. 1.7.1 to build a model from more than one template.

The web server version of ModeRNA is available at http://genesilico.pl/modernaserver/. The online version provides tools that facilitate the process of homology modeling — from template selection and generating sequence alignment to the creation of the final model. All the options are available for a point-and-click user interface and do not require any programming knowledge. However, the most advanced options are available only with the standalone version.

Installation of SimRNA

Download the SimRNA package (available from http://genesilico.pl/software/stand-alone/simrna/) to a specified folder. Make sure the folder data/ is in the directory where the simulations are to be run. The folder data/ contains necessary energy functions for SimRNA optimization. SimRNA can be run by specifying the path on the command line or by setting the path variable, e.g., with the following command:

```
export PATH="${PATH}:/path/to/SimRNA/executable/directory"
```

The clustering program is distributed together with the SimRNA package. The clustering method can be run from the directory or from elsewhere if the path variable is set e.g., with the following command:

```
export    PATH="${PATH}:/path/to/clustering/
executable/directory"
```

Installation of QRNAS

Download the QRNAS package from http://genesilico.pl/qrnas/, unzip the archive, and compile it with the following command:

```
./qrnamake sequential
```

This should create an executable version of QRNAS.

Acknowledgements

We would like to thank Wayne Dawson for critical reading of the manuscript and valuable comments and suggestions. This work was supported mainly by the National Science Centre (NCN) [2012/04/A/NZ2/00455 to J.M.B.]. D.K. was supported by the Foundation for Polish Science (FNP) [grant MPD/2010/3 to Prof. Artur Jarmolowski, project cofinanced by the European Union Regional Development Fund]. M.M. was supported by the National Science Centre (NCN)[2014/12/T/NZ2/00501]. J.M.B. and J.M.K. were also supported by the European Research Council [ERC, StG grant RNA + P = 123D to J.M.B.] and J.M.B. was supported by the "Ideas for Poland" fellowship from the FNP.

References

1. Doudna JA (2000) Structural genomics of RNA. Nat Struct Biol 7(Suppl):954–956

2. Rother K et al (2011) RNA and protein 3D structure modeling: similarities and differences. J Mol Model 17(9):2325–2336

3. Magnus M et al (2014) Computational modeling of RNA 3D structures, with the aid of experimental restraints. RNA Biol 11(5):522–536

4. Rother M et al (2011) ModeRNA server: an online tool for modeling RNA 3D structures. Bioinformatics 27(17):2441–2442

5. Rother M et al (2011) ModeRNA: a tool for comparative modeling of RNA 3D structure. Nucleic Acids Res 39(10):4007–4022

6. Tozzini V (2009) Multiscale modeling of proteins. Acc Chem Res 43(2):220–230

7. Kolinski A (2004) Protein modeling and structure prediction with a reduced representation. Acta Biochim Pol 51(2):349–371

8. Boniecki M et al (2003) Protein fragment reconstruction using various modeling techniques. J Comput Aided Mol Des 17(11):725–738

9. Kolinski A, Bujnicki JM (2005) Generalized protein structure prediction based on combination of fold-recognition with de novo folding and evaluation of models. Proteins 61(Suppl 7):84–90

10. Magnus M, Boniecki MJ, Dawson W, Bujnicki JM (2016) SimRNAweb: a web server for RNA 3D structure modeling with optional restraints. Nucleic Acids Res 44(W1):W315–319. doi:10.1093/nar/gkw279

11. Altschul SF et al (1990) Basic local alignment search tool. J Mol Biol 215(3):403–410

12. Nawrocki EP et al (2015) Rfam 12.0: updates to the RNA families database. Nucleic Acids Res 43(Database issue):D130–D137

13. Nawrocki EP, Eddy SR (2013) Infernal 1.1: 100-fold faster RNA homology searches. Bioinformatics 29(22):2933–2935

14. Zhou Y et al (2008) GISSD: group I intron sequence and structure database. Nucleic Acids Res 36(Database issue):D31–D37

15. Wilm A, Higgins DG, Notredame C (2008) R-Coffee: a method for multiple alignment of non-coding RNA. Nucleic Acids Res 36(9):e52

16. Cruz JA et al (2012) RNA-Puzzles: A CASP-like evaluation of RNA three-dimensional structure prediction. RNA 14(4):610–625

17. Chen VB et al (2010) MolProbity: all-atom structure validation for macromolecular crystallography. Acta Crystallogr D Biol Crystallogr 66(Pt 1):12–21

18. Hajdin CE et al (2010) On the significance of an RNA tertiary structure prediction. RNA 16(7):1340–1349

Chapter 15

Exploring Alternative RNA Structure Sets Using MC-Flashfold and db2cm

Paul Dallaire and François Major

Abstract

We created an accelerated version of MC-Fold called MC-Flashfold that allows us to compute large numbers of competing secondary structures including noncanonical base pairs. We visualize the base pairs in these sets using high quality intuitive dot plots and arc plots. Our new tools allow us to explore RNA dynamics by visualizing the competing structures in free energy bands. Here we describe how to use these tools to generate dot plots that reveal the postulated anti-terminator stem in the *E. coli* trp operon leader sequence. These plots show the anti-terminator hairpin loop during transcription and as a minor population of the full-length leader sequence. This is a case of switching RNA structure that had been originally postulated based on short dyad inverted repeats. Other switching RNA sequences can be analyzed by using our method.

Key words MC-fold, RNA noncanonical pairs, RNA tertiary structure

1 Introduction

The set of base pairs in an RNA molecule is its secondary structure (often called 2D structure), and many computer programs are available to predict 2D structures starting from sequence alone. This is done generally by maximizing a probability function (equivalently by minimizing a free energy function) or by sampling from the Boltzmann distribution. The most likely 2D structure is called the minimum free energy structure or MFE. There also exists many structures whose probabilities are less than optimal and we call these "suboptimal" structures.

RNA base pairs include the canonical AU and GC but a very large variety of pairing types occur in nature [1] with varying frequencies of occurrence. The software MC-Fold uses the catalog of known occurrences of base pairs types along with their immediate environments to compute the MFE and a set of likely suboptimal 2D structures for given RNA sequence [2].

Many RNAs change their structures dynamically notably by breaking and reforming their base pairing patterns [3]. The energy

Douglas H. Turner and David H. Mathews (eds.), *RNA Structure Determination: Methods and Protocols*, Methods in Molecular Biology, vol. 1490, DOI 10.1007/978-1-4939-6433-8_15, © Springer Science+Business Media New York 2016

required for these changes to happen and the frequencies at which they occur are likely determinants of the affinity of RNAs to other macromolecules during induced fit [4]. Recent NMR studies [5] have shown that the likeliness of RNA base pairs predicted using MC-Fold coincide with the observed frequencies.

Dot plots can be used to represent the canonical ensemble of secondary structures where the probabilities of all possible base pairs are computed using the so-called partition function. The RNAfold program distributed with the Vienna package computes structures consisting of canonical base pairs and outputs both the MFE as well as this dot plot [6]. In this context, the term 'dot plot' refers to a specialized type of 'contact map' widely used in protein structure analysis where only residues that form a base pair are considered as being close together without regards to physical distance; see for example the interactive tools CMView [7] and RNAmap2D [8]. The canonical ensemble may not always be the best representation of a set of the more likely structures. As we see here, the case of the anti-terminator loop is revealing of this. For some sequences, dot plots computed on increasing numbers of suboptimal structures or depths (1, 10, 1000, 1,000,000) show that very frequent base pairs that become prominent at larger depths flood the MFE structure.

In this chapter we use a new and much faster version of MC-Fold called MC-Flashfold [9] along with a visualization tool called db2cm to inspect the potential formation of the elusive anti-terminator that is rich in noncanonical base pairs in the terminator/anti-terminator transcription attenuating system of the trp operon from *E. coli* [10]. For this particular case, we mimic transcription of the leader sequence by folding increasing lengths of the trp-leader sequence while visualizing the results using the graphical representations rendered by db2cm. At some sequence lengths the anti-terminator and the terminator hairpins coexist. The stability of the terminator loop is sufficient to dwarf the stem of the predicted anti-terminator.

Note that although exemplified using the *E. coli* trp operon leader sequence, this approach can be applied to other switching RNAs. The purpose we had in mind with the development of db2cm was to explore RNA secondary structure dynamics accounting for noncanonical base pairs.

1.1 Secondary Structure Representations

Prediction software such as MC-Flashfold represents structures as words in the dot-bracket format. These *words* are composed of the symbols dot '.', opening parenthesis '(',and closing parenthesis ')', where dots represent unpaired nucleotides and pairs of matching parenthesis represent base pairs. But dot-bracket structures tend to be difficult to read for the untrained eye. The representation of numerous suboptimal structures in the dot-bracket format, although exact, is not adequate for analysis. Drawings of 2D layouts are much more friendly but only a few structures can be neatly plotted on a surface at the same time for comparison. When we are willing to sacrifice knowledge concerning which base pairs correspond to which structures, dot plots and arc plots (where curved lines join nucleotides participating in base pairs) can be used to represent all the base pairs in large sets of suboptimal structures along with their relative importance in an intuitive way (Fig. 1).

Dot plots are really symmetric matrices giving the frequency of occurrence of each base pair in the set of considered structures for a sequence. Here rows and columns are nucleotides. For example the base pair formed between the ith and the jth nucleotides occurs at the frequency represented at the ith row and jth column of the dot plot (because the matrix is symmetric, we show only the upper diagonal). Squares on the diagonal are the frequencies of unpaired nucleotides. The frequencies are converted to color intensities of dots in the squares so that the dot plot graph is very readable. The frequencies can be Boltzmann weighted for the energies of the structures to which the base pair belongs to or not. If Boltzmann

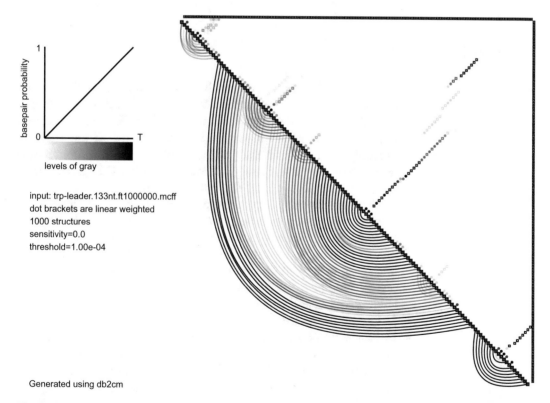

Fig. 1 db2cm output. The 133 nt long trp operon leader RNA sequence was folded using mcff. Shown is the image generated using db2cm on the resulting predictions. The *top left* graph is the sensitivity plot below which key call parameters are listed. The *right* area is composed of the dot plot above the main diagonal and the arc plot bellow. The exact command lines used are: 'mcff –n trp-leader –s $seq –ft 10000 > trp-leader.133 nt.ft1000000.mcff' and 'db2cm -f trp-leader.133 nt.ft1000000.mcff -size 0.1 -xdb 1000'

weighted, the frequency of a base pair corresponds to the sum of the probabilities of each structure which it is part of. If S' is the set of structures comprising the base pair considered and S is the set of all the structures considered, then the weighted frequency of the base pair is given by: $\dfrac{\sum\limits_{j \in S'} e^{-E_j}}{\sum\limits_{i \in S} e^{E_i}}$, otherwise, it is simply the ratio of the sizes of these sets: $\dfrac{|S'|}{|S|}$.

Because MC-Flashfold outputs canonical as well as non-canonical base pairs, it is interesting to generate dot plots that somehow distinguish these. The tool db2cm shows canonical base pairs as hollow squares and noncanonical ones as circles.

The frequencies can also be used to adjust the scale of gray used when drawing an arc plot. In an arc plot, nucleotides are disposed on a line and arced lines joining two bases represent base pairs. These plots are very easily understood. They become busier as the number of base pairs to represent grows excessively.

2   Materials

MC-Flashfold and db2cm must be installed on the user's personal computer to: (1) compute the MFE and suboptimal structures; and (2) generate the dot plots and arc plots. Some precompiled binaries are available for some operating systems. If the available precompiled binary files are not available for your computer system, installation is still straightforward. A recent C language compiler (such as GNU gcc) is the only requirement.

The graphs are generated as SVG files that can be viewed and printed using web browsers (we recommend the web browser Chrome from Google) and modified or converted using vector images manipulation software such as Illustrator from Adobe. The image file format SVG is an open standard for vector graphics. It was selected because, contrary to raster image formats, it allows for lossless scaling and rotation making for easier quality image preparation for any format and resolution.

These tools very portable and are expected to be easy to install on any Unix or Windows computer. They have been tested on Linux and Mac OS X. The code is simple to compile since it has no external dependency and is written in the language C.

3 Methods

3.1 Installing the Software

3.1.1 Obtaining the Software

Download the file MC-Flashfold.zip from http://www.major.iric. ca/ (select the MC-Tools tab to locate MC-Flashfold.zip) and save it on your Desktop. On Linux, decompress the archive using the utility zip. On Mac OS X right click on the file and choose 'Open with' ->'Unarchive App'. This will create a new folder called MC-Flashfold. You may now move the .zip file to trash. Navigate in this directory to the sub-directory called 'doc/' to a file called flashfold-fXX.pdf (where XX is the version number) comprising further installation instructions for the program mcff (short name for MC-Flashfold).

3.1.2 Understanding the Software Package

The package comprises the source code of three computer programs: mcff, flashScan, and db2cm.

MC-Flashfold

MC-Flashfold (or mcff) computes optimal and suboptimal RNA secondary structures. Its installation, compilation, and usage are fully described in flashfold-fXX.pdf.

FlashScan

FlashScan is a bash script that computes microRNA binding sites on mRNAs. mcff must be installed for flashscan to run. It requires no compilation. Once mcff is installed, typing 'flashScan –help' describes its usage.

db2cm

db2cm is a utility that produces dot plots and/or arc plots from the output of mcff. We describe its installation and use in the following steps.

3.1.3 Compiling db2cm

Note: precompiled binaries are distributed for some operating systems and if these work on your computer then you do not need to compile them from source, just copy them to their destination directory.

In a terminal window change to the 'source' directory under the just installed 'MC-Flashfold' (In Mac OS X, open the application 'Terminal.app') and type 'cd ~/MC-Flashfold/source' or 'cd /usr/local/bin/MC-Flashfold' according to the installation directory you chose during installation of mcff.

Compile the source with the following command: 'cc -lm -std=c99 -O3 db2cm.c -o db2cm'. Some compiler warnings may be generated at this step, pay no attention to them.

Now copy the new file called 'db2cm' from the current directory to its destination using either 'cp db2cm ~/bin' or 'cp db2cm /usr/local/bin' according to the choice you made while installing mcff.

3.2 Folding an RNA Sequence Using MC-Flashfold

In a terminal, create a *variable* to hold the first 133 nt of *E. coli* trp-operon leader sequence from start of transcription to the end of the terminator loop by typing the following:

'seq=AGUUCACGUAAAAAGGGUAUCGACAAUGAAAG
CAAUUUUCGUACUGAAAGGUUGGUGGCGCACUU
CCUGAAACGGGCAGUGUAUUCACCAUGCGUA
AAGCAAUCAGAUACCCAGCCCGCCUAAUGAGCGGGCU'
The following command will *fold* this sequence and output on screen the MFE accompanied by nine suboptimal structures:

'mcff –n trp-leader –s $seq –ft 10'

Here, the program mcff is asked to generate 10 suboptimal structures (parameter –ft 10) for the sequence whose data is contained in the variable seq and whose name is trp-leader.

We will require a much larger number of suboptimal structures to view alternative structures. We also need to store these in a format understood by db2cm in a file on the hard disk drive. This is done with the command:

'mcff –n trp-leader –s $seq –ft 1000 –v > trp-leader.ft1000. mcff'

Here the parameter –v tells mcff that we require a proper header to be included in the output and the output file name is located on the right side of the greater than sign. On a recent computer, this should take a few seconds. Now the file trp-leader. ft1000.mcff contains the secondary structure predictions as a text file. You can open this file using a text editor and look up the structures that it contains.

A summary of the parameters to mcff is obtained by typing: 'mcff –h'.

A complete explanation of the behavior of mcff is given in the document doc/flashfold-fXX.pdf in the MC-Flashfold/doc/ directory.

3.3 Creating Dot Plots and Arc Plots Using db2cm

In the simplest case we call the utility db2cm with default values for all parameters using as input the file of secondary structures generated in the previous section with mcff : 'db2cm –f trp-leader. ft1000.mcff'. This generates an image file in the SVG format called trp-leader.ft1000.mcff.svg in the current directory.

3.4 Viewing the Plots Using Chrome

SVG files are quite powerful and are defined in a W3C open standard. The software engines that are used to view SVG files are not all equal. As of this writing, we find that viewing db2cm generated SVG files is best done using the Internet browser chrome. This software is freely available for all common operating system in use today and can be downloaded from at http://www.google.com/ chrome/. To use chrome to view a SVG file that you have generated, in a terminal window, type 'pwd' to obtain the full path to your current directory and copy the resulting string in the textbox where you normally type a web address. This should list the contents of your directory in a clickable format.

3.5   Tailoring the Plots

db2cm images have the following elements:

(a) A left panel providing relevant information about the source of the data, the value of some key parameters used during the run and a graph showing the sensitivity curve and the threshold value used in the mapping of base pairs occurrences to intensities of gray used in the plots.

(b) A right panel showing the RNA sequence annotated by its dot plot on one side and by its arc plot on the other side. The dot plot is further annotated by the RNA sequence on its two edges.

A filled circle in the dot plot indicates a noncanonical base pair whereas a hollow square indicates a canonical base pair. The darkness of dots and arcs is more pronounced when the corresponding base pair occurs more frequently in the set of secondary structures. The frequency of base pairs is determined in one of two ways, selectable via the command line parameter –b. When –b is not set (or when it is set as '–b 0') the frequency of a base pair is the normalized sum of its occurrences in the secondary structures predictions. When '–b 1' is specified, each base pair occurrence is weighted by the exponential of the energy of the structure to which it participates. We interpret this value as the probability of the base pair. Often and especially for small numbers of structure predictions these two values yield very similar plots.

3.5.1   Adjusting the Contrast

Without correction, the frequency/probability of base pairs is translated linearly to levels of gray. This is not always adequate and the parameter '–sensitivity X' is used to adjust the contrast. The value of X determines the level of gray (g) of a base pair by adjusting its frequency (f) according to $g = f^{2^{-X}}$. When $X = 0$, $g = f$. We find that a reasonable range for X is $[-4 \ldots 4]$. The corresponding mapping curve is always printed as a five cm square image at the top left corner of the generated SVG image.

3.5.2   Choosing the Threshold

If a base pair occurs only very rarely, its corresponding darkness level is very low and hardly visible. db2cm avoids drawing points and arc for base pairs that occur less frequently than a fixed threshold and this results in much smaller files. By default this value is set to 1/10,000. The user can modify this value at will by setting a value for the parameter '–threshold X', where X is some value chosen in the interval $[0 \ldots 1[$. The graph plotted in the top-left corner of the file comprises a horizontal dashed line that shows the value for –threshold used in the computation of the file. A grayed box is also drawn showing the levels of gray that are prevented from being used in the dot plot and the arc plot.

3.5.3   Controlling Which Elements Get Plotted

The following parameters will prevent db2cm from drawing the corresponding elements in the SVG file:

'-arcs 0' tells db2cm to refrain from drawing the arc plot.

'-dotPlot 0' tells db2cm to refrain from drawing the dot plot.

'-seqd 0' tells db2cm to refrain from drawing the RNA sequence on the main diagonal.

'-seqs 0' tells db2cm to refrain from drawing the sequences on the axes of the dot plot.

'-legend 0' tells db2cm to refrain from drawing the left panel (no sensitivity graph and no additional data).

3.5.4 Customizing Image Size, Rotation and Zoom Level

The parameter '-size X' can be used to adjust image size. Setting '-size 1' makes each nucleotide in the plots 1 cm wide and 1 cm tall (unless rotation or zoom are changed also). db2cm defaults to '-size 0.2'. If the value for '-size' is unchanged between runs of db2cm on RNA sequences of varying lengths then comparing the images pixel for pixel is sound. The drawing of the left portion of the image is unaffected by this parameter.

Setting '-rotate X' rotates the plots X degrees clockwise. When this is done the size of each nucleotide may be reduced so that the main diagonal fits in the drawing area.

Setting '-zoom X' enlarges the plots by a factor X. The use of −zoom may be required if some arcs do not fit in the given plotting square window given the active rotation. The default for −zoom is 0.9.

3.5.5 Editing the Plots in Adobe Illustrator

Besides specifying command line parameters when you run db2cm you can edit the graph in a vector image editing software such as Illustrator. The geometric elements in the file are grouped according to their visual function so that selecting related groups of items is straightforward via Illustrator's *layers panel*.

Files generated from long RNA sequences and using low values of −threshold can comprise large numbers of graphical elements making its manipulation in Illustrator quite burdensome with today's computers. For example a dot plot produced for an RNA sequence of 1000 nt with the db2cm parameter −threshold set to 0.0 would generate well into the millions of graphical elements and editing such a file could prove difficult. By properly choosing the parameters when calling db2cm, much smaller files can be generated while conserving the data semantics.

3.6 Viewing the trp-operon Leader Anti-terminator and Terminator Stem-Loops

We use the already defined bash variable (that we called 'seq') to hold the sequence in order to simplify its manipulation. Earlier we computed 10^3 suboptimal structures. For this example we compute 10^6.

First, we obtain the secondary structure predictions (we say that we *fold* the sequence) using: (a) the full-length sequence of 133 nt; and, (b) a shorter version of 125 nt that is less likely to form the terminator loop.

3.6.1 Folding the Sequences

Fold the sequence using mcff (the computation takes a couple of minutes):

'mcff -n trp-leader -s $seq -v -ft 1000000 > trp-leader.133 nt.
ft1000000.mcff'

Here '-n' sets the sequence name, '-s' sets the sequence to the value of *seq*, '-v' tells mcff to output header information (so that db2cm can recognize it) and '- ft' tells mcff to compute roughly the first million structures. The greater than symbol tells the OS to direct the output to a file. trp-leader.133 nt.ft1000000.mcff is the output file name.

Fold the shorter version of the sequence (up only to nucleotide 125):

'mcff -n trp-leader-125 nt -s ${seq:0:125} -v -ft 1000000 > trp-leader.125 nt.ft1000000.mcff'

The expression ${seq:0:125} says that we want the first 125 nt of the sequence that we have placed in the variable *seq*.

3.6.2 Generating the Plots

Now we can call db2cm to generate the dot plots and arc plots. These commands will generate the files trp-leader.133 nt. ft1000000.mcff.svg and trp-leader.125 nt.ft1000000.mcff.svg

'db2cm -xdb 1 -f trp-leader.133 nt.ft1000000.mcff -arcs 0 -seqs 0'

'db2cm -xdb 1 -f trp-leader.125 nt.ft1000000.mcff -arcs 0 -seqs 0'

'-xdb 1' tells db2cm to consider only 1 secondary structure from the file. That 1 structure is an MFE in every case. '-f trp... mcff' is the input file name (there are other ways to specify the name of input file and we will see that soon).

Using a vector graphics package such as Illustrator, we can easily combine this data to a single image such as Fig. 2 (note: use reflect in Illustrator around a -45° plane on one file's relevant grouped elements).

Note that the file trp-leader.125 nt.ft1000000.mcff.svg clearly shows the anti-terminator loop that forms when the terminator loop sequence is absent (Fig. 2).

3.6.3 Drawing the Full Plots for Different Numbers of Structures

Here, the list of input files is given via 'stdin' by using the *vertical bar operator*. What happens is that the files in the current directory whose name end in *.mcff* are listed in a way that db2cm can read them. This way, a large number of files can be specified to db2cm in a very easy way.

This command creates the files trp-leader.125 nt.ft1000000. mcff.xdb10.svg and trp-leader.133 nt.ft1000000.mcff.xdb10.svg: 'ls *.mcff | db2cm -b 1 -xdb 10 -extra '.xdb10''

'-b 1' tells db2cm to use Botzmann normalization. '-xdb 10' tells db2cm to use the first 10 structures. '-extra '.xdb10'' tells db2cm to add the word '.xdb10' somewhere in the output file name. If you do not add -extra 'something' then previous files prepared with different parameters may be overwritten if you are not careful.

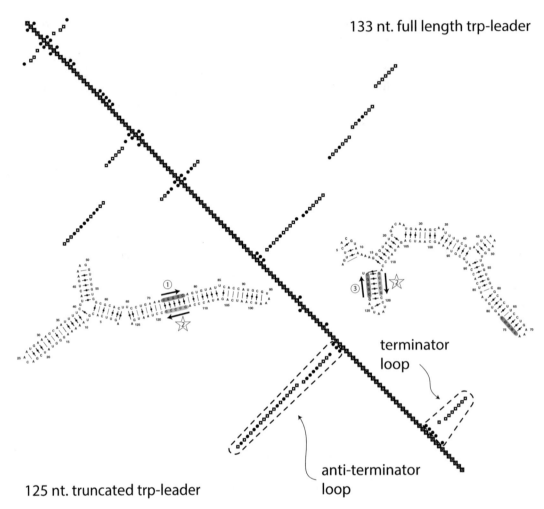

Fig. 2 Dot plots and secondary structures for truncated and full-length trp-leader MFEs. Dot plots for the full-length (133 nt) (*top-right*) and truncated (125 nt) (*bottom-left*) trp operon leader sequence from *E. coli*. The location of the anti-terminator and terminator loops are shown. Sub-sequences numbered 1, 2, and 3 shown in *circles* and *stars* indicate the positions of the dyad inverted repeats that led to the postulation of the terminator/anti-terminator hypothesis

Repeat with larger numbers of predictions

'ls *.mcff | db2cm -b 1 -xdb 100 -extra '.xdb100''
'ls *.mcff | db2cm -b 1 -xdb 1000000 -extra '.xdb1000000''

Figure 3 shows the changes in the plots when the depth is augmented. From the differences between the images produced with 10 and 10^6 structures that the best energy structures are misrepresented in a dot plot of larger ensembles of structures.

3.6.4 Revealing the Anti-terminator Loop in the Full-Length trp-leader

We can ask if the anti-terminator ever forms in the full-length sequence? Could it be that anti-terminator loops are simply infrequent in the full-length leader sequence?

Inspecting the figure trp-leader.133 nt.ft1000000.mcff. xdb1000.svg shows no sign of the anti-terminator loop, except for

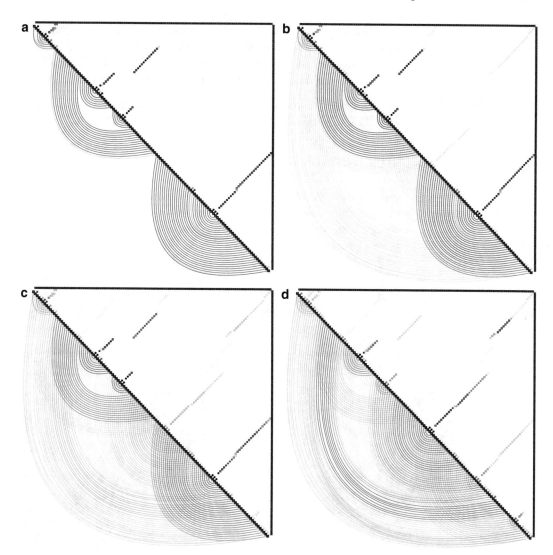

Fig. 3 Effect of depth on the visibility of the best energy structures. As per protocol 3.6.3, the *E. coli* trp operon leader RNA sequence was truncated to 125 nt, then folded using mcff to 10^6 suboptimal structures and four plots were computed using db2cm. The number of suboptimal structures used in the calculation of the plots (value of parameter –xdb) was varied: (**a**) 10 best structures, (**b**) 100, (**c**) 10^3 and (**d**) 10^6. These plots show the apparent loss of importance of the anti-terminator hairpin loop as the depth of analysis is increased

a very few base pairs at the tip (Fig. 1). We can modify db2cm parameters to reveal further details from the computed plots as follows. First, let us try just to set the threshold at 0.0 because we will now try to amplify low signals.

'db2cm -f trp-leader.133 nt.ft1000000.mcff -threshold 0 -b 1 -xdb 1000000 -extra '.xdb1000000.t0.b1''

However this image is not at all different than the one with a default threshold. We can augment the sensitivity:

'db2cm -f trp-leader.133 nt.ft1000000.mcff -threshold 0 -b 1 -sensitivity 1 -xdb 1000000 -extra '.xdb1000000.t0.b1.s1''

This does not show the anti-terminator much more. Finally, let us push the system somewhat more to see what happens. The following command should certainly show the anti-terminator loop in the dot plot of the full-length sequence if it exists at all.

'db2cm -f trp-leader.133 nt.ft1000000.mcff -b 1 -xdb 1000000 -sensitivity 4 -extra '.xdb1000000.s4.b1''

Now it is clear that there is some signal from the anti-terminator in the full-length sequence (Fig. 4).

3.6.5 Simulating Transcription Elongation

Simulating transcription elongation of the leader sequence further clarifies the relationship between the anti-terminator and the terminator. The script doc/examples/elongation/elongateTrpLeader. bash computes the dot plots for six RNA sequences of lengths 113 nt, 118 nt, 123 nt, 128 nt, and 133 nt and generates a single HTML file showing the images side by side. We can see from Fig. 5 that the anti-terminator hairpin loop has too little of its sequence synthesized to form in the shorter sequence and is not stable enough to compete with the terminator loop in the longest sequence.

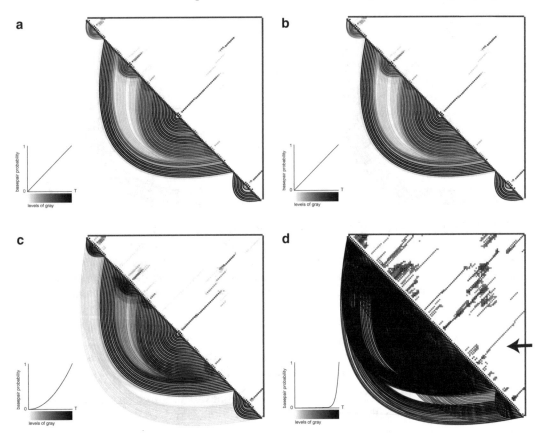

Fig. 4 Full-length sequence of the anti-terminator hairpin loop by increasing the threshold and sensitivity. The results of protocol 3.6.4 are shown. (**a**) default parameter values. (**b**) Threshold=0. (**c**) Threshold=0 and sensitivity=1. (**d**) Threshold=0 and sensitivity=4. The *black arrow* shows the location of the anti-terminator loop

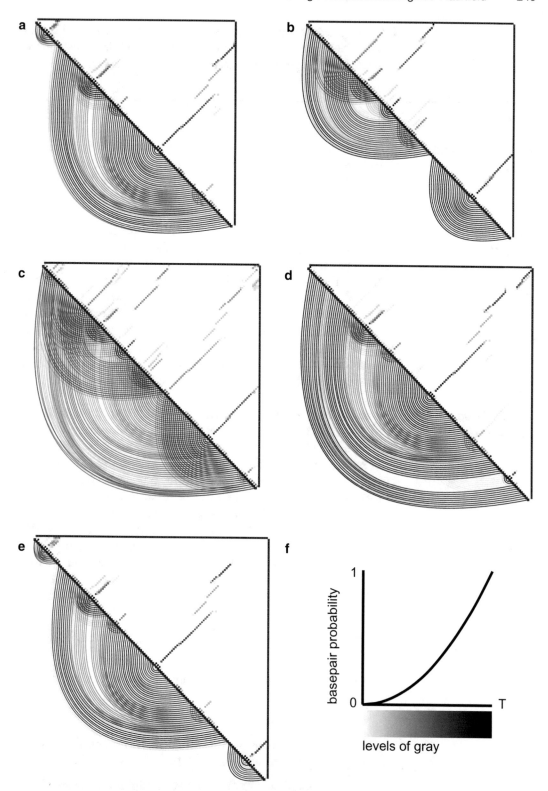

Fig. 5 Simulation of trp-leader transcription shows stable transient anti-terminator loop. The results of protocol 3.6.5 are shown. Trp-leader sequences of increasing lengths are folded using mcff to depth of 10^3 suboptimals. Sequence lengths are (**a**) 113 nt, (**b**) 118 nt, (**c**) 123 nt, (**d**) 128 nt, and (**e**) 133 nt. (**f**) All the plots were generated using –sensitivity of 1. The anti-terminator hairpin loop is clearly visible in panels **b** and **c**

However, the anti-terminator loop is clearly defined in the other panels. You can easily edit the provided script to replace the sequence or to change the parameters to perform other analysis.

---

4 Notes

4.1 Updating Your Software

It is good practice to verify that your software is up to date before engaging in investigations. In particular, mcff relies on databases that may be updated at any time. If this happens or if the software is improved, then its version number will reflect this change.

4.2 Fixing Copy and Paste of Commands

When executing the commands in your computer's terminal, you may need to retype all characters by hand instead of using copy and paste. That seems to be due to a reinterpretation of the dash ("-") character that is encoded in different ways according to its typographical properties. The MC-Flashfold software package comprises a text file called commandExamples.txt under the directory doc/examples/. In a separate terminal window set to the MC-Flashfold/doc/directory, list the contents of this file using the command 'cat commandExamples.txt'. Copy pasting those command lines should be a breeze.

4.3 Exploring Command Line Tools

The so-called *command line* tools are very powerful companions to mcff and db2cm. These tools are included in any Mac OS X or linux/unix distributions and are worth exploring. Of particular interest are bash (the terminal application), sed (a line oriented editor), and grep (a pattern recognition software). Here we give a few examples of one-liners that can be great time savers.

Converting HTML outputs generated using former versions of MC-Fold [2] to .db files. Suppose that you have a run of MC-Fold predictions that were performed over the Internet at http://www.major.iric.ca/MC-Fold/ and saved in the file run.mcfold.html and that you want to visualize its contents using db2cm. Type the following in a terminal and the resulting file will be recognizable by db2cm:

'cat run.mcfold.html | sed -n '1,/Explored/{d};/BP/{q};/^>/,${p}' | cut -f 1,2 -d ' ' > run.mcfold'

Creating a file that contains only the second best structure from a mcff run:

'cat input.mcff | sed -n '1,3p;5p' > output.mcff'

Extracting lines 1000–2000 from a mcff run and keeping the header lines so that db2cm can recognize the output file:

'cat input.mcff | sed -n '1,3p;1004,2003p' > output.mcff'

4.4 Using Folding Masks

mcff supports a considerable variety of *user masks*. These can be used to specify prior knowledge to the folding algorithm or to identify results that conform to base pairing constraints that you specify. For example if you are folding a tRNA sequence, you could specify that the anticodon nucleotides should not be paired in any way. If you fold a loop that is known to interact with a protein only when a certain noncanonical base pair forms you can set a mask for the bound state and another for the unbound state, or if you wish to simulate the presence of a binding protein on some segment, you could use a mask to prevent a segment of the RNA from participating to the folding. Details of how masks are used with mcff are found in the manual flashfold-fXX.pdf.

4.5 Forgetting the –v Parameter

If db2cm does not produce any result. Verify that you have used the parameter –v when running mcff. When you do not specify –v, the output from mcff does not include the necessary header in its output file.

References

1. Leontis NB, Stombaugh J, Westhof E (2002) The non-Watson-Crick base pairs and their associated isostericity matrices. Nucleic Acids Res 30(16):3497–3531

2. Parisien M, Major F (2008) The MC-Fold and MC-Sym pipeline infers RNA structure from sequence data. Nature 452(7183):51–55. doi:10.1038/nature06684

3. Al-Hashimi HM, Walter NG (2008) RNA dynamics: it is about time. Curr Opin Struct Biol 18:321–329

4. Williamson JR (2000) Induced fit in RNA-protein recognition. Nat Struct Biol 7(10):834–837. doi:10.1038/79575

5. Dethoff EA, Petzold K, Chugh J, Casiano-Negroni A, Al-Hashimi HM (2012) Visualizing transient low-populated structures of RNA. Nature 491(7426):724–728. doi:10.1038/nature11498

6. Lorenz R, Bernhart SH, Honer Zu Siederdissen C, Tafer H, Flamm C, Stadler PF, Hofacker IL (2011) ViennaRNA Package 2.0. Algorithms Mol Biol 6:26. doi:10.1186/1748-7188-6-26

7. Vehlow C, Stehr H, Winkelmann M, Duarte JM, Petzold L, Dinse J, Lappe M (2011) CMView: interactive contact map visualization and analysis. Bioinformatics 27(11):1573–1574. doi:10.1093/bioinformatics/btr163

8. Pietal MJ, Szostak N, Rother KM, Bujnicki JM (2012) RNAmap2D—calculation, visualization and analysis of contact and distance maps for RNA and protein-RNA complex structures. BMC Bioinformatics 13:333. doi:10.1186/1471-2105-13-333

9. Dallaire P (2015) Une signature du polymorphisme structural d'acides ribonucléiques non-codants permettant de comparer leurs niveaux d'activités biochimiques. Université de Montréal, Montréal

10. Kolter R, Yanofsky C (1982) Attenuation in amino acid biosynthetic operons. Annu Rev Genet 16:113–134. doi:10.1146/annurev.ge.16.120182.000553

Chapter 16

NMR Methods for Characterization of RNA Secondary Structure

Scott D. Kennedy

Abstract

Knowledge of RNA secondary structure is often sufficient to identify relationships between the structure of RNA and processing pathways, and the design of therapeutics. Nuclear magnetic resonance (NMR) can identify types of nucleotide base pairs and the sequence, thus limiting possible secondary structures. Because NMR experiments, like chemical mapping, are performed in solution, not in single crystals, experiments can be initiated as soon as the biomolecule is expressed and purified. This chapter summarizes NMR methods that permit rapid identification of RNA secondary structure, information that can be used as supplements to chemical mapping, and/or as preliminary steps required for 3D structure determination. The primary aim is to provide guidelines to enable a researcher with minimal knowledge of NMR to quickly extract secondary structure information from basic datasets. Instrumental and sample considerations that can maximize data quality are discussed along with some details for optimal data acquisition and processing parameters. Approaches for identifying base pair types in both unlabeled and isotopically labeled RNA are covered. Common problems, such as missing signals and overlaps, and approaches to address them are considered. Programs under development for merging NMR data with structure prediction algorithms are briefly discussed.

Key words Nuclear magnetic resonance, NMR, Secondary structure, Base pair identification, Nuclear Overhauser effect

1   Introduction

Knowledge of RNA secondary structure can provide a basis for insight into structure–function relationships and design of therapeutics [1–5]. Secondary structure determination is also a first step toward determination of 3D structure. X-ray crystallography provides definitive structures for RNA in crystals. Procedures for generating suitable crystals for X-ray analysis are not always successful, however. Chemical mapping provides insights into which nucleotides are not base paired, but interpretation can be ambiguous, especially for pseudoknots and multiple folding [6, 7]. Nuclear magnetic resonance (NMR) can identify nucleotides that are base paired and thus limit possible secondary structures. It can also

Douglas H. Turner and David H. Mathews (eds.), *RNA Structure Determination: Methods and Protocols*, Methods in Molecular Biology, vol. 1490, DOI 10.1007/978-1-4939-6433-8_16, © Springer Science+Business Media New York 2016

reveal multiple conformations [8, 9]. Like X-ray diffraction, NMR data can also provide full 3-dimensional structures of RNA, although it is limited to structures of about 100 nucleotides. Unlike X-ray diffraction, however, NMR analysis is carried out on biomolecules in solution, not in single crystals. Thus, NMR experiments can be initiated as soon as the biomolecule is expressed and purified. While this is a great advantage, a disadvantage is that acquisition and analysis of NMR data for a 3D structure requires greater time and effort than crystallography.

NMR structure determination is based primarily on detection of short-range magnetic interactions known as the *nuclear Overhauser enhancement*, or NOE, between hydrogen atoms. [10] As many NOEs as possible are detected, typically 8–15 per nucleotide, and used as restraints in constructing a molecular model. Other structural NMR measurements include scalar coupling constants that provide estimates for dihedral angles, and residual dipolar couplings (RDCs) that provide information about relative orientation of molecular bonds. Interesting approaches for using comparisons between chemical shift assignments and predicted 3D models are being developed [11]. For coverage of NMR methods for complete RNA chemical shift assignment and 3D structure determination, the reader is referred to the literature [12–16].

This chapter summarizes NMR methods that permit rapid identification of RNA secondary structure and other structural features—information that can be used as supplements to chemical mapping, and/or as preliminary steps required for 3D structure determination. The aim is to provide guidelines to enable a researcher with minimal knowledge of NMR to quickly extract secondary structure information and recognize some common internal loop structures in basic datasets. Some details of optimal acquisition and processing parameters for these datasets will be discussed, but not the details of spectrometer operation. It is presumed that the researcher has this ability or has access to either a local or national facility collaborator who can acquire such data.

2   Experimental Considerations

A number of factors should be considered to maximize the information that can be deduced from NMR data. The first consideration is the instrument itself. State-of-the-art instruments for biomolecular studies use magnetic field strengths typically between 11.7 and 21.1 Tesla (500–900 MHz for proton Larmor frequency). A higher magnetic field provides greater NMR signal intensity and spectral resolution. Another important factor is whether the instrument has a standard room-temperature probe, or a cryo-probe. A cryo-probe will typically yield two to three-fold greater signal than the same sample in a room-temperature probe. Thus, the time required to produce a given signal-to-noise ratio is reduced by 4- to 9-fold. The combination of highest field and a cryo-probe will give the best data. Most instruments are configured to accept NMR sample tubes with a 5 mm diameter and hold liquid sample volume of 0.25–0.5 mL with the smaller volume range only being possible if "susceptibility matched" tubes are used.

Sample amount is a critical factor. The RNA concentration required to achieve sufficient signal-to-noise ratio depends not only on the instrument, but also on the experiments to be performed. For instance, to monitor RNA interactions/changes during a titration, only 1D spectra of RNA imino protons (Fig. 1) are required and concentrations as low as 10 μM may be sufficient (~2.5 nmol) [17]. For 2D/3D NOESY experiments, required for secondary structure identification, a concentration of 0.5–1.0 mM is desirable, but 0.1–0.2 mM may be sufficient to answer many secondary structure questions if an 800–900 MHz spectrometer with cryo-probe is available.

Ionic strength of the buffer must also be considered because small, mobile ions reduce the sensitivity of signal detection. Cryo-probes are particularly sensitive to ionic strength, so buffers with very low or no added salts are often employed. Phosphate buffer is most commonly used as it has no protons to interfere with the ^{1}H NMR signal. Sample pH should be kept as low as possible without influencing the native conformation of the RNA. This is because

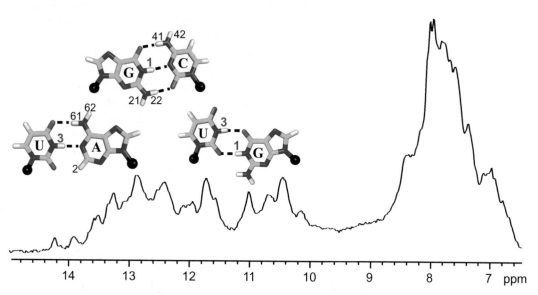

Fig. 1 The most common Watson–Crick base pairings found in helical stems of RNA shown with standard numbering of hydrogen atoms most relevant in identifying secondary structure by NMR. Imino protons, GH1 and UH3, have pink labels. The base pairs are shown above the imino proton region of the ^{1}H NMR spectrum of 5S ribosomal RNA from *Escherichia coli* (119 nucleotides). Each base pair is positioned above the portion of the ^{1}H NMR spectrum where the imino protons for that pair type most commonly resonate. Aromatic proton region of the ^{1}H NMR spectrum of the same RNA sample is also included, demonstrating spectral crowding in this region

exchange of imino hydrogens with solvent hydrogens results in line broadening and reduction of NOE cross-peak intensity. Hydrogen exchange is catalyzed by hydroxyl ions so pH less than 7.0 is desired; less than 6.5 will provide better detection of signals from loops that are not as stable as Watson–Crick stems. The experiments described here pertain to samples dissolved in H_2O as solvent; in D_2O solvent the imino protons exchange with deuterons and disappear from the proton spectrum.

3   Revealing Canonically Base Paired Stems

NMR can provide a rapid and early assessment of base pairing. The majority of this information comes from the region of a proton NMR spectrum where only imino protons of G and U residues are observed (Fig. 1). The imino protons of G and U resonate well down field (higher chemical shifts in parts per million, ppm) of all other protons in biological macromolecules with the exception of tryptophan and histidine sidechain protons. These resonances exhibit fairly characteristic chemical shift and NOE patterns depending on whether they are in GC, AU, or GU pairs, or unpaired. Generally, G imino protons in GC pairs are found 12.0–13.5 ppm and U iminos in AU pairs are found 13.0–14.5 ppm (Fig. 1). Thus when only one conformation is present, the 12.0–14.5 ppm region will have at most only one resonance for each GC or AU pair. In contrast, the aromatic region of H8/H6/H2 protons (6.5–8.5 ppm) is more crowded because GC and AU pairs have two or three resonances, respectively. More importantly, aromatic protons lack structurally characteristic chemical shift or NOE patterns. In addition, this region of the spectrum overlaps with the amide and aromatic protons of proteins. There are two imino protons in GU wobble pairs with the U imino primarily between 11 and 12.5 ppm and the G imino between 10 and 11.5 ppm (Fig. 1). G iminos that are not hydrogen bonded typically have chemical shifts lower than (upfield of) 11.5 ppm and often are broad and exchange readily with water protons rendering them invisible in NOESY spectra. Consequently, the 10–14.5 ppm region of the spectrum is relatively uncrowded even in fairly large RNAs or in the presence of protein. These aspects of the 1D imino ^1H spectrum make it useful for conveniently monitoring changes in structural properties or intermolecular interactions when buffer conditions are changed (addition of Mg^{2+}, for example), or proteins are added.

The fundamental measurement for structure determination by NMR is the nuclear Overhauser effect (NOE) which is usually detected in 2D spectra (2D NOESY). In a 2D NOESY spectrum, a "cross-peak" is observed at the intersection of frequencies of two protons that are within about 5 Å of each other. The cross-peak intensity varies as $1/r^6$, where r is the distance separating the two protons. NOESY cross-peaks between the imino protons of adjacent base pairs in an A-form helix are readily observed, so one cross-peak between two imino protons represents adjacent base pairs (Fig. 2), with the common exception of the strong cross-peak between two imino protons in a GU wobble pair. An imino resonance exhibiting cross-peaks to two different imino peaks identifies a "walk" representing three sequential base pairs. An additional cross-peak to the imino of one of the flanking base pairs indicates an even longer helical region. Thus, imino walks identify helixes important for secondary structure. Since the distance between imino protons of adjacent base pairs is typically 3.5–5.5 Å resulting in medium to weak NOE cross-peak intensities, a relatively long NOESY mixing time (100–300 ms) is generally recommended for these spectra. Recommended mixing time and other parameters are discussed in more detail later and in Table 1.

Identifying the type of base pair (GC, AU, GU) corresponding to each imino resonance further characterizes the secondary structure. AU, GC, and GU pairs can often be identified in unlabeled samples by a distinctive NOE pattern to their pairing partner. The imino protons in GC and AU pairs have strong NOEs to amino or aromatic proton peaks between 6.5 and 8.5 ppm (Fig. 2). These are best identified in short mixing time (25–75 ms) NOESY experiments.

GC pairs. The typical ^{1}H-^{1}H NOESY pattern in a short mixing time NOESY for a G imino (G-H1) in a GC pair includes two strong peaks to the amino protons of the paired C residue (C-H41 and C-H42). The peak to the downfield amino (C-H41) may be stronger than the peak to the upfield amino (C-H42) as the former is hydrogen bonded to G-O6 and, therefore, closer to G-H1. The peak from G-H1 to C-H42 is primarily due to spin-diffusion through C-H41 or flips of the amino group. Two strong cross-peaks between the G imino proton and the intrabase amino protons are also commonly observed, although these are usually broader than C amino signals. Spectra at elevated temperatures (20–30 °C) may distinguish C aminos from G aminos better than at low temperature (0–5 °C).

AU pairs. The typical NOE pattern in a short mixing time NOESY for a U imino (U-H3) in a AU pair includes one strong peak to the H2 proton of the paired A residue (A-H2). Peaks to the A amino protons may also be observed, but these signals are typically exchange broadened, so the cross-peaks are much less pronounced than the H2 cross-peak. Again, elevated temperatures exaggerate distinction of A-H2 and A amino protons. The C amino signals in GC pairs are also broader than A-H2 signals, but are typically narrower than A amino signals.

GU pairs. G and U imino protons in a GU wobble pair are identified by a very strong NOE between the two imino protons (Fig. 2), which are separated by only ~2.5 Å. In contrast to GC and AU pairs, neither of the iminos in a GU pair exhibit intense

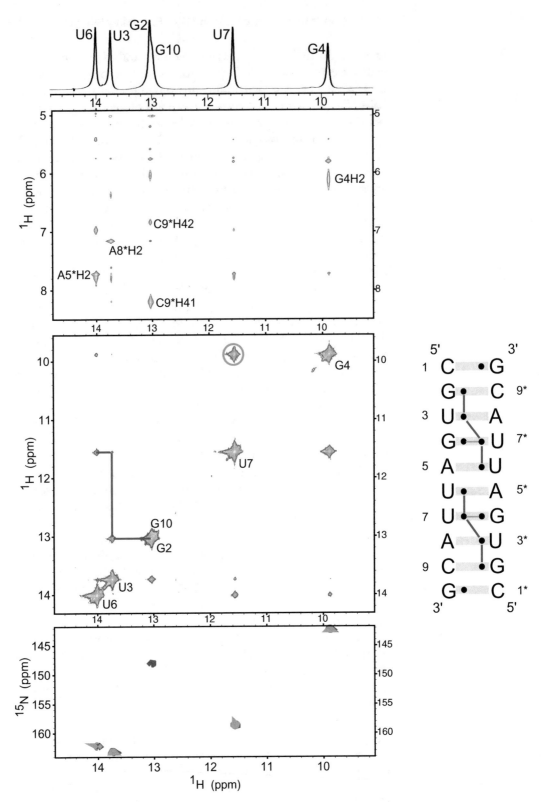

Fig. 2 NMR spectra of the self-complementary RNA duplex (CGUGAUUACG)$_2$ in 80 mM NaCl, 20 mM phosphate buffer at pH 6.5, and 95 % H$_2$O/5 % D$_2$O solvent. The *horizontal axis* of all spectra spans the imino proton region. The *top panel* is a 1D spectrum. The *second* and *third panels* are from a 2D NOESY spectrum acquired at 0 °C with a mixing time of 100 ms and a WATERGATE readout pulse [35]. The *bottom panel* is a ^{1}H-^{15}N HSQC

Table 1

NMR experiments most useful for identifying secondary structure in RNA

Experiment	Information
1D ^{1}H spectrum	Peak count; buffer conditions; solvent exchanging peaks
2D ^{1}H-^{1}H NOESY[a]	
Mix Time[b]	
25–75 ms	Base pair type from strong cross-peaks
100–300 ms	Find adjacent base pairs from imino–imino walk
2D ^{1}H-^{15}N HSQC	Assign imino protons as G or U (base pair type)
2D HNN-COSY	Identify imino hydrogen-bonding by correlation to two ^{15}N (base pair type)
2D/3D ^{13}C HMQC-NOESY[a]	Identify strong imino NOEs as H2, H6/H8, or NH$_2$ (base pair type)

[a]NOESY experiments should use water-suppression readout pulses optimized for excitation of the imino proton region (9–15 ppm)

[b]Within each range of mixing times, the shorter times are more appropriate for large RNAs (>~60 nts), while the longer times of the range are more appropriate for small RNAs (<~25 nts)

cross-peaks in the amino/aromatic region, although the G imino may show a broad cross-peak to its own amino protons below 6.5 ppm. The two amino protons show the same chemical shift because no hydrogen bonds restrict the NH$_2$ group from rotation about the C-N bond resulting in an identical averaging of the chemical shift environment experienced by these two protons. The G imino in a GU wobble pair is usually upfield of the U imino although the G imino chemical shift is particularly dependent on the orientation of the flanking base pairs and for some orientations the G and U iminos can be nearly overlapped [18]. The dependence of non-exchangeable proton chemical shifts on the orientation of the flanking base pairs has been closely examined [19].

Fig. 2 (continued) spectrum (natural abundance ^{15}N). The ^{15}N chemical shifts indicate which iminos are G and which are U. An "imino-walk" of NOESY cross-peaks is indicated with *blue lines* in the *third panel*. The *three step walk* indicates four sequential base pairs, represented in the diagram to the *right*. (Note that because the duplex is symmetric, nucleotide 1 is the same as 1*, etc.) In the diagram, *shaded boxes* represent base pairing and *black dots* represent imino protons. In the spectrum and diagram, respectively, the strong NOE between imino protons of the GU wobble pair is indicated with a *green circle* and *line*. The *second panel* (*vertical axis* region includes aromatic, amino, and H1′ protons) highlights strong cross-peaks that are characteristic of the different pair types. These include UH3-AH2 cross-peaks in Watson–Crick UA pairs and GH1-CH41 cross-peaks in Watson–Crick GC pairs. Also shown is the upfield shift and degeneracy of G amino protons that are not involved in hydrogen bonds, as for G4H2 in the G4-U7* wobble pair. Cross-peaks to G10H1 are weak as the terminal GC pair is exposed to solvent resulting in rapid exchange with solvent protons

As an alternative to identification of base pair type by NOESY pattern, imino protons can also be distinguished by identifying the chemical shift of the directly bonded imino nitrogen-15 (^{15}N). The imino nitrogen (N3) of U residues resonates between 155 and 165 ppm, while the imino nitrogen (N1) of G residues resonates between 140 and 150 ppm. These ^{15}N shifts are minimally influenced by hydrogen-bonds or neighboring residues (Fig. 2). Thus, U iminos and G iminos are unambiguously identified. ^{1}H-^{15}N correlation experiments, HSQC or HMQC (Heteronuclear Single/Multiple Quantum Correlation), are used for this purpose. In these 2D experiments, magnetization is transferred "through-bond" between the ^{1}H and ^{15}N nuclei. The natural abundance of ^{15}N nuclei is only 0.15%, so unless the sample is isotopically enriched, signal sensitivity is very low. It is possible to do the experiment at natural abundance if the sample concentration is greater than 1 mM and the molecule's size is less than ~25 nucleotides. Through-bond magnetization transfer is inefficient for large molecules or signals that are broad due to conformational or chemical exchange such as imino protons that exchange with solvent protons when base pair hydrogen bonding is weak or absent. Generally, it is preferable to isotopically enrich the sample for heteronuclear experiments. Isotopic enrichment with ^{15}N and/or ^{13}C opens the possibility of other experiments which can provide characterization of base pairs. A 2D HNN-COSY experiment can correlate an imino proton not only with the covalently attached imino-nitrogen detected in the HSQC, but also the imino nitrogen of the hydrogen-bonded base (e.g., C or A for GC or UA, respectively) [20–22]. In this experiment, magnetization is transferred between nitrogens "through-bond" via weak scalar coupling in the N–H$\cdots$N hydrogen bond. In other words, magnetization is transferred between nitrogen atoms that share electron density with one hydrogen atom. Because the transverse relaxation properties of ^{15}N are favorable compared to ^{13}C and because the transfers in this experiment involve only ^{15}N, this experiment can give surprisingly reasonable signals in large RNAs [23].

A 3D or 2D ^{13}C-edited HMQC-NOESY experiment can also aide in distinguishing base pair type in larger, labeled RNA. The HMQC-NOESY is a combination of through-bond correlation of ^{1}H and ^{13}C (HMQC) followed by ^{1}H-^{1}H NOESY. This experiment can identify whether an imino NOESY cross-peak in the aromatic/amino region (6.5–8.5 ppm) involves an adenine H2 proton or another aromatic (H8/H6) or amino proton. This is possible because the ^{13}C chemical shift of adenine C2 is distinct from C8 and C6 in any nucleobase [16]. Amino groups do not pass through the HMQC edit. So, for example, the 2D/3D ^{13}C-edited HMQC-NOESY can distinguish the UH3-AH2 cross-peak of a WC/WC UA pair from the UH3-AH8 cross-peak of a WC/Hoogsteen UA pair such as found in a UAU triple [24]. The 2D HNN-COSY distinguishes the same two base pairs via UH3 cross-peaks to the characteristic AN1 (WC/WC) or AN7 (WC/Hoogsteen) ^{15}N chemical shifts [25]. Another pair that can be similarly identified includes WC/WC GA pairs characterized by a strong GH1 to AH2 NOESY cross-peak (^{13}C-edited HMQC-NOESY with ^{15}N-^{1}H HSQC), or a GH1 to AN1 cross-peak (HNN-COSY) [26].

For small to medium-sized constructs (defined here as ~12 ~ 50 nucleotides) a simple one-dimensional spectrum and a two-dimensional NOE spectrum (typically 12–36 h of data collection) can often provide a full assessment of secondary structure without the need for isotopic labels. At the very least these simple initial spectra provide insight into the suitability of the construct and buffer conditions for a more complete study.

Despite the low density of peaks in the imino region, spectral overlaps will occur, especially in RNA larger than ~50–60 residues. Correlation with ^{15}N nuclei in an HSQC spectrum can identify many overlaps, or an HNN-COSY if the RNA is isotopically labeled. In unlabeled samples, overlapped imino peaks can sometimes be identified in the aromatic/amino region of a NOESY spectrum if more than the expected number of cross-peaks to one imino chemical shift are observed. For instance, three or four strong cross-peaks in the aromatic/amino region to an imino proton may indicate an overlap. Chemical shifts are temperature dependent, so spectra at more than one temperature can often resolve overlaps. In general, 2D NOESY spectra are acquired at room temperature or slightly higher, and at 0–10 °C. A short and a long mixing time NOESY is acquired at each temperature (Table 1).

Missing imino–imino cross-peaks in a WC stem walk are not uncommon. Some imino protons, even in WC stems, exchange readily with water protons due to unstable hydrogen-bonding. This occurs near helix ends, in short helices, and particularly often in AU pairs. NOESY cross-peaks are reduced by this exchange and the imino–imino NOE pathway along the helix may be broken. Hydrogen exchange can be slowed by low temperature and low pH. In some cases even subzero temperatures can recover rapidly exchanging imino protons. Buffer pH should generally not be above 6.5 unless necessary. In the case of an unstable UH3 in an AU pair, however, it is still usually possible to identify the strong UH3-AH2 cross-peak, and the NOE pathway along the stem can often be found through an NOE from the AH2 of the unstable AU pair to a stable imino of an adjacent base pair (GC or AU). Because this is not a strong NOE, 2D ^{13}C-HMQC-NOESY of an A-labeled sample will differentiate it from the strong amino cross-peaks, especially for larger RNAs. Some imino–imino cross-peaks are weaker than others simply because the distance is longer. Imino-to-imino distances in WC stems range approximately from 3.5 to 5.5 Å [18]. NOEs for the longer distances are aided by "spin-diffusion" through a third involved proton (e.g., NH$_2$ or adenine H2 proton) that is between the two imino protons. Spin-diffusion is often a problem in NMR as it causes NOE volumes that are not proportional to $1/r^6$, but sometimes, as in the case of enhancing the longer distances of the imino walk, it has a desirable influence.

4 Data Acquisition

Acquisition of 2D NOESY spectra of RNA is much the same as for proteins, but a few points are worth considering. RNA secondary structure characterization is primarily accomplished through observation of imino ^1H signals at 10–14 ppm (Fig. 1). Water suppression pulses and the spectral carrier frequency are usually centered on the water resonance near 5 ppm. Thus, a spectral width of 20 ppm (±10 ppm from center) is required to cover the range –5 to +15 ppm. However, since no RNA protons are found further upfield than approximately 3.5 ppm, there is "empty space" from 3.5 ppm to the upfield edge of the spectrum at –5 ppm. This empty space can be used to "wrap" NOESY spectra in the indirect dimension. If the indirect dimension spectral-width is reduced from 20 to 12 ppm (covering the range –1 to 11 ppm), then imino peaks that were previously at 11–15 ppm are "aliased" to the upfield portion of the indirect dimension (now at –1 to 3 ppm) without overlapping other peaks. Reduction of the spectral width means fewer t1 time-increments are required to obtain the same resolution as in a full-width spectrum, resulting in reduced total time for data acquisition. Alternatively, the same number of t1 increments yields higher resolution than in a full-width spectrum. t_1-wrapping is not useful in ^1H-^1H NOESY spectra of proteins because the ^1H shifts are distributed approximately equally on either side of the water signal.

The configuration of the water-suppression pulse used to read out the ^1H signal is also worth considering. Since imino ^1H signals are far from the water signal, very narrow-band water-suppression pulses that would allow direct detection of protons close to the water signal (e.g., H1′ protons at 5–6 ppm) are not required. Narrow-band excitation pulses typically require a few milliseconds, during which time signals decay via transverse relaxation processes. RNA imino proton signals often decay rapidly due to solvent exchange and would suffer losses during millisecond pulses. The large chemical shift difference between water and imino signals, along with no need to directly detect protons that are spectrally near water, means that broad-band shorter duration (<0.5 ms) water-suppression pulses can be used. NOESY cross-peaks from H1′ to imino protons can, nonetheless, still be observed along the indirectly detected dimension of the 2D spectrum. The pulses surrounding the indirect evolution time do not need to be water-suppression pulses.

5   Secondary Structure Prediction

The stretches of base pairs identified by NMR are complementary to information provided by chemical mapping. Further, the NMR findings can be entered into secondary structure prediction programs that have been modified to use the data to limit folding space or distinguish correct structures from a list of predicted structures. NAPSS (NMR-Assisted Prediction of Secondary Structure), discussed in the next chapter, and RNA-PAIRS (Probabilistic Assignment of Imino Resonance Shifts) are two examples currently being developed [7, 18, 27]. The combination of stretches of base pairs with algorithms for prediction of secondary structure allows assignment of resonances to individual nucleotides, a first step in determination of 3D structure.

6   3D Structure Determination

Global Structure. Identification of secondary structure elements as discussed here is important, but it is worth considering solution methods for rapidly characterizing the three-dimensional arrangements of these elements. Assignment of imino protons in elements of secondary structure as described above opens the possibility of using ^{1}H-^{15}N HSQC spectra of ^{15}N-labeled RNA to measure ^{1}H-^{15}N residual dipolar couplings (RDCs) if the RNA is suspended in an appropriate alignment medium [28]. ^{1}H-^{13}C RDCs can also be measured for easily assigned ^{1}H-^{13}C HMQC peaks, such as for the adenine H2/C2 in an AU pair. However, the RDC data alone cannot distinguish between several possible orientational arrangements of the helices. While the degeneracy can be resolved if multiple alignment media are used, Wang et al. have described a protocol using SAXS data to break the degeneracy [29, 30]. They demonstrate the combined NMR/SAXS method in RNA of 100 nucleotides.

Complete 3D Structure. Solution of a full 3D RNA structure by NMR involves measurement of hundreds to thousands of NOE cross-peaks, scalar-couplings, and RDCs. This requires assignment of not only imino protons but also all amino, aromatic, and sugar protons. Most of these experiments require that the solvent be changed from 95% H_2O/5% D_2O to 100% D_2O. Methods for making these unambiguous assignments and measurements are not discussed here, but the reader is referred to the books and reviews mentioned earlier [11–16]. In addition, novel isotopic labeling chemistry, including selective deuteration, is improving the assignment process and allowing studies of ever larger RNA molecules [31–34].

Acknowledgements

The efforts of Jim Hart in making the 5S rRNA sample of Fig. 1 are gratefully acknowledged.

References

1. Velagapudi SP, Gallo SM, Disney MD (2014) Nat Chem Biol 10:291–297

2. Kukol A, Hughes DJ (2014) Virology 454–455:40–47

3. DiGiusto DL, Krishnan A, Li L, Li H, Li S, Rao A, Mi S, Yam P, Stinson S, Kalos M, Alvarnas J, Lacey SF, Yee JK, Li M, Couture L, Hsu D, Forman SJ, Rossi JJ, Zaia JA (2010) Sci Transl Med 2:36ra43

4. Evdokimov AA, Mazurkova NA, Malygin EG, Zarytova VF, Levina AS, Repkova MN, Zagrebelnyi SN, Netesova NA (2013) Mol Biol (Mosk) 47:83–93

5. Blakeley BD, McNaughton BR (2014) ACS Chem Biol 9:1320–1329

6. Kierzek E, Kierzek R, Moss WN, Christensen SM, Eickbush TH, Turner DH (2008) Nucleic Acids Res 36:1770–1782

7. Hart JM, Kennedy SD, Mathews DH, Turner DH (2008) J Am Chem Soc 130:10233–10239

8. Hammond NB, Tolbert BS, Kierzek R, Turner DH, Kennedy SD (2010) Biochemistry 49:5817–5827

9. Salmon L, Yang S, Al-Hashimi HM (2014) Annu Rev Phys Chem 65:293–316

10. Wuthrich K (1986) NMR of proteins and nucleic acids. Wiley, New York

11. Sripakdeevong P, Cevec M, Chang AT, Erat MC, Ziegeler M, Zhao Q, Fox GE, Gao X, Kennedy SD, Kierzek R, Nikonowicz EP, Schwalbe H, Sigel RK, Turner DH, Das R (2014) Nat Methods 11:413–416

12. Wijmenga SS, van Buuren BNM (1998) Prog Nucl Magn Reson Spectrosc 32:287–387

13. Wu H, Finger LD, Feigon J (2005) Methods Enzymol 394:525–545

14. Lukavsky PJ, Puglisi JD (2005) Methods Enzymol 394:399–416

15. Dominguez C, Schubert M, Duss O, Ravindranathan S, Allain FH (2011) Prog Nucl Magn Reson Spectrosc 58:1–61

16. Furtig B, Richter C, Wohnert J, Schwalbe H (2003) Chembiochem 4:936–962

17. Martin-Tumasz S, Richie AC, Clos LJ II, Brow DA, Butcher SE (2011) Nucleic Acids Res 39:7837–7847

18. Chen JL, Bellaousov S, Tubbs JD, Kennedy SD, Lopez MJ, Mathews DH, Turner DH (2015) Biochemistry 54:6769–6782

19. Barton S, Heng X, Johnson BA, Summers MF (2013) J Biomol NMR 55:33–46

20. Dingley AJ, Grzesiek S (1998) J Am Chem Soc 120:8293–8297

21. Dingley AJ, Nisius L, Cordier F, Grzesiek S (2008) Nat Protoc 3:242–248

22. Dingley AJ, Masse JE, Feigon J, Grzesiek S (2000) J Biomol NMR 16:279–289

23. Zuo X, Wang J, Yu P, Eyler D, Xu H, Starich MR, Tiede DM, Simon AE, Kasprzak W, Schwieters CD, Shapiro BA, Wang YX (2010) Proc Natl Acad Sci U S A 107:1385–1390

24. Holland JA, Hoffman DW (1996) Nucleic Acids Res 24:2841–2848

25. Cash DD, Cohen-Zontag O, Kim NK, Shefer K, Brown Y, Ulyanov NB, Tzfati Y, Feigon J (2013) Proc Natl Acad Sci U S A 110:10970–10975

26. Wohnert J, Dingley AJ, Stoldt M, Gorlach M, Grzesiek S, Brown LR (1999) Nucleic Acids Res 27:3104–3110

27. Bahrami A, Clos LJ II, Markley JL, Butcher SE, Eghbalnia HR (2012) J Biomol NMR 52:289–302

28. Getz M, Sun X, Casiano-Negroni A, Zhang Q, Al-Hashimi HM (2007) Biopolymers 86:384–402

29. Wang YX, Zuo X, Wang J, Yu P, Butcher SE (2010) Methods 52:180–191

30. Burke JE, Sashital DG, Zuo X, Wang YX, Butcher SE (2012) RNA 18:673–683

31. D'Souza V, Dey A, Habib D, Summers MF (2004) J Mol Biol 337:427–442

32. Alvarado LJ, LeBlanc RM, Longhini AP, Keane SC, Jain N, Yildiz ZF, Tolbert BS, D'Souza VM, Summers MF, Kreutz C, Dayie TK (2014) Chembiochem 15:1573–1577

33. Davis JH, Tonelli M, Scott LG, Jaeger L, Williamson JR, Butcher SE (2005) J Mol Biol 351:371–382

34. Lu K, Miyazaki Y, Summers MF (2010) J Biomol NMR 46:113–125

35. Sklenar V, Piotto M, Leppik R, Saudek V (1993) J Magn Reson Ser A 102:5

Chapter 17

The Quick and the Dead: A Guide to Fast Phasing of Small Ribozyme and Riboswitch Crystal Structures

Jermaine L. Jenkins and Joseph E. Wedekind

Abstract

Ribozymes and riboswitches are examples of non-protein-coding (nc)RNA molecules that achieve biological activity by adopting complex three-dimensional folds. Visualization of such molecules at near-atomic resolution can enhance our understanding of how chemical groups are organized spatially, thereby providing novel insight into function. This approach has its challenges, which mainly entail sample crystallization followed by the application of empirical, structure-determination methods that often include experimental "phasing" of X-ray diffraction data. A paucity of high-quality crystals or a low symmetry space group are factors that demand rapid assessment of phasing potential during an ongoing experiment in order to assure a successful outcome. Here we describe the process of evaluating the anomalous signal-to-noise as a prelude to single wavelength or multiwavelength anomalous diffraction (SAD or MAD) phasing. Test cases include an autolytic 62-mer RNA enzyme known as the hairpin ribozyme, and a 33-mer riboswitch that binds the modified guanine metabolite $preQ_1$. The crystals were derivatized with iridium (III) hexaamine and osmium (III) pentaammine triflate, respectively. Each data set was then subjected to the XPREP and SHELX programs to assess the anomalous signal-to-noise and to locate the heavy-atom substructure. Subsequent noise filtering was conducted in SHELXE or RESOLVE. The methods described are applicable to the rapid phasing of RNA X-ray diffraction data, and contrast the efficacy of in-house X-rays with those attainable from synchrotron-radiation sources in terms of the potential to plan for and execute an experimental structure determination.

Key words RNA, Riboswitches, Ribozymes, X-ray crystallography, Single-wavelength anomalous diffraction, Iridium (III) hexaamine, Osmium (III) pentaammine, Autobuilding, Density modification, Substructure determination, Phasing

1 Introduction

In the old west, gunslingers fought with six-shooters blazing and only *the quick* prevailed. The stakes are not quite as high for structural biologists but the ability to make snap decisions to judge data quality on the fly can be essential. Here the battle is won with wit rather than hot lead. In the area heavy-atom phasing for RNA structure determination, significant inroads have been made to

Douglas H. Turner and David H. Mathews (eds.), *RNA Structure Determination: Methods and Protocols*, Methods in Molecular Biology, vol. 1490, DOI 10.1007/978-1-4939-6433-8_17, © Springer Science+Business Media New York 2016

surmount this major methodological bottleneck. First, new mimics of hydrated Mg^{2+} provide more options for heavy atom derivatization. Second, the identification of preferred binding sites for such metal provides a rational recourse to traditional "soak-and-pray" tactics [1]. Third, and perhaps most significant, fast computational approaches allow rapid analysis of diffraction data during an ongoing experiment. In this chapter, we provide a brief overview of first-choice heavy atom derivatives for RNA phasing and a step-by-step guide to assess data quality in terms of the anomalous diffraction signal. This is a preface to single wavelength or multiwavelength phasing, and is intended for graduate students or postdoctoral fellows. The more seasoned user may find it helpful as a practical companion for phasing.

1.1 Rationale for the Choice of Iridium and Osmium Amines for RNA Phasing

Mg^{2+} is a prevalent ion in plasma as well as in cells where it has been measured at concentrations of 0.8 mM and 2.5 mM, respectively [2]. Mg^{2+} is of central importance in RNA folding where it is frequently observed in coordination with the negatively charged phosphate backbone or in the major groove at the base edge of tandem guanines [3]. Mg^{2+} prefers octahedral geometry and may adopt a fully hydrated coordination sphere, $Mg(H_2O)_6^{2+}$ (Fig. 1a), or a partially hydrated shell in which inner-sphere contacts are provided by the RNA [3]. From the vantage point of the crystallographer, $Mg(H_2O)_6^{2+}$ offers little in the way of solving the phase problem. However, a handful of non-physiological ions have been exploited for phasing due to their similarity to the $Mg(H_2O)_6^{2+}$ making them useful for RNA binding. Key ions used to date include hexammine salts of Co(III), Os(III) and Ir(III) (Fig. 1a). Each of these magnesium mimics adopts strict octahedral geometry, and exhibits nearly the same coordination distance between the ion and the amine, as Mg^{2+} and water. However, the NH_3 group is incapable of accepting a hydrogen bond unlike H_2O, which causes the amine coordination shell to gravitate to negatively charged environments. Another important difference is that the amine groups within the coordination sphere of $Co(NH_3)_6(III)$ resist exchange relative to the rapid exchange observed for water in the coordination sphere of $Mg(H_2O)_6^{2+}$ [4]. This implies that hexammine complexes of Co(III)—and possibly Os(III) and Ir(III)—bind almost exclusively to the RNA via outer sphere contacts.

Among the hydrated $Mg(H_2O)_6^{2+}$ mimics, osmium (III) hexammine has had a distinguished history in the experimental phase determinations of leviathan RNA and RNA-protein complexes such as the P4-P6 domain of the group I intron, the 30S ribosome, and RNase P [5–7]. The complexities of $Os(NH_3)_6(III)$ synthesis, as well as its lack of commercial availability, led some researchers to seek out related compounds such as osmium (III) pentaammine triflate, which is commercially available and was used by the authors in the preQ$_1$ riboswitch structure determination [8]. Iridium (III) hexammine is even more promising because it is relatively easy to produce compared to its osmium counterpart and has demonstrated efficacy in RNA phasing [9]. A major breakthrough in the heavy-atom derivatization of RNA was the identification of sequences with the propensity to bind hexammine metals based on a systematic screening analysis of singlet and tandem GU wobble pairs [9]. These observations imply that hexammine metal binding sites can be engineered into any RNA helix for phasing purposes; representative successful sequences include: 5′-GUUC-3′ 3′-CGGG-5′, or 5′-GGC-3′ 3′-CUC-5′. Although the introduction of such sites seems ideal, this might not be necessary as a first-choice phasing technique. Our experience has shown that iridium (III) hexammine can bind at non-wobble positions, such as the Hoogsteen edge of guanine with additional coordination by the negatively charged phosphodiester backbone (Fig. 1b). Similarly, osmium (III) pentaammine targeted a location comprising multiple oxygen atoms contributed from the sugar edges of adjacent uridines (Fig. 1c). Unfortunately, such binding sites cannot be predicted a priori but might be identifiable through heavy atom co-crystallization or by soaking of compounds into RNA crystals as described [1]. If these methods fail, the use of engineered sites is highly recommended.

1.2 Observed Metal Binding Sites in Case Studies

In the case of the hairpin ribozyme, we succeeded in growing crystals by substituting $Ir(NH_3)_6(III)$ for $Co(NH_3)_6(III)$ in the crystallization medium. Our prior analysis revealed that $Co(NH_3)_6(III)$ coordinates at a major site that utilizes the Hoogsteen edge of G21, and a minor site at the tandem guanine bases G12 and G13 [10]. The Ir(III)-containing crystals were isomorphous with those prepared from Co(III), and binding of $Ir(NH_3)_6(III)$ was observed at the major site (Fig. 1b) as well as the minor site (data not shown). The major site produced a 16σ anomalous signal for Ir(III) based on a 30-fold redundant data set collected in-house (f'' 6.6 e−) using an X8 Prospector system with an IμS microfocus X-ray source and an Apex II CCD detector (Bruker AXS Inc, Madison, WI). However, the signal-to-noise for the anomalous difference was limited to ~6.0 Å resolution, which was insufficient for a de novo SAD phasing structure determination. Nonetheless, the iridium substructure could be located using the program SHELX [11], and a molecular envelope was generated for the correct image of the known 62-mer RNA [12]. The results suggested that a high-resolution SAD phasing solution should be attainable with optimized anomalous using synchrotron radiation. Such methods were also applied to the 33-mer, preQ₁ metabolite-sensing riboswitch. The results revealed that SAD phasing from $Os(NH_3)_5(III)$ using optimized anomalous at the L_{III} edge [8] was sufficient to produce a noise-suppressed electron-density map of comparable quality to that obtained from multiwavelength anomalous diffraction (MAD) phasing (Fig. 1d versus e) [8]. This map was Partially suitable for auto building of the RNA, which produced a Partially complete model.

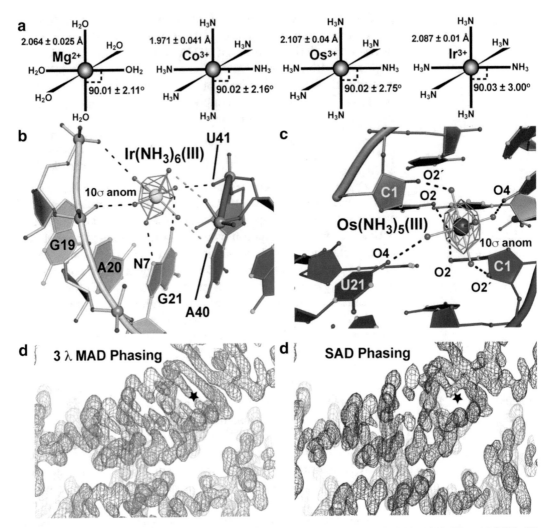

Fig. 1 Chemical and structural properties of $Mg(H_2O)_6(II)$ and its mimics $Co(NH_3)_6(III)$, $Ir(NH_3)_6(III)$ and $Ir(NH_3)_n(III)$ (where $n = 5$ or 6) that bind RNA. (**a**) Octahedral coordination geometry and coordination distances for various ions (adapted from [3]). (**b**) The major $Ir(NH_3)_6(III)$ binding site in the hairpin ribozyme, which is isomorphous to $Co(NH_3)_6(III)$. An anomalous difference electron-density map is shown as *orange* mesh. (**c**) Unrefined model for $Os(NH_3)_5(III)$ binding between two molecules of the preQ$_1$ riboswitch; the rotational averaging of the pentaammine gives the appearance of a hexammine. An anomalous difference electron-density map is shown as *orange* mesh. (**d**) MAD electron density map derived from PHENIX and density modified in RESOLVE (adapted from [8]). (**e**) SAD phasing electron-density map of the correct preQ$_1$ riboswitch image based on the peak wavelength for $Os(NH_3)_5(III)$ in panel (**d**). The substructure was located using SHELXD with subsequent density modification with SHELXE and RESOLVE. The density modified electron density map is contoured at the 1.0σ level. A *star* represents notable differences in quality between the map in **d** versus **e** that could confound model building by SAD phasing

Herein we describe the methods we utilized for rapidly assessing SAD- or MAD-phasing potential of site-bound Ir(III) and Os(III). The initial procedures are designed to be rapid in order to inform the user whether or not a heavy atom has the potential for phasing, or whether the conditions must be optimized for subsequent experiments. Metrics to assess phasing potential, including substructure determination, and electron-density map visualization are discussed with respect to the SHELX programs. Finally, alternative methods for density modification are provided, as well as a brief discussion of automated RNA building.

2 Materials

1. A demo version of XPREP is available upon request from Bruker AXS Inc (Madison, WI) at demolicense@rt.bruker-axs.nl. XPREP can be run on Windows or Linux-based operating systems. The program suite SHELXL can be downloaded from http://shelx.uni-ac.gwdg.de/SHELX/, and the programs SHELX can be used via the CCP4i graphical interface [13] on Windows, Linux or Mac OS X operating systems. Representative computer systems in the authors' labs include: a Windows® XP Pro desktop system with a 2.1 GHz Intel Core 2 Duo processor, 2 GB DDR2 RAM, and a 0.5 Tb HD connected to a 19 in. LCD monitor; HP Windows® 7 laptop with a 2.2 GHz AMD Dual-Core processor, 8 GB DDR2 RAM, 0.5 Tb HD, and a 15.6 in. LED monitor with a second Zalman Trimon ZM-M220W stereo monitor.

2. PHENIX (**P**ython based **H**ierarchical **EN**vironment for Integrated **X**tallography) suite of programs is a multiplatform (Linux and Mac) software suite available to academic users (www.phenix-online.org). The suite evolves rather quickly so the current version available for download will not be the version, 1.6-289, used by the authors herein. We chose to give command line arguments, as these are not as likely to change as rapidly as the GUI-based interface. PHENIX comes bundled with versions of SOLVE [14] and RESOLVE [15].

3. The Collaborative Computational Project No. 4 (CCP4) crystallography software suite [16] can be downloaded from http://www.ccp4.ac.uk and will run on Linux, Mac OS X, and Windows operating systems. This will include the CCP4i graphic interface and the molecular model-building program COOT [17].

4. The heavy atom derivative pentaammine(trifluoromethanesulfonato)osmium(III) triflate is available from Sigma-Aldrich (St Louis, MO).

5. Iridium (III) hexammine can be synthesized as described in Keel et al. 2007 starting from the iridium chloride salt (Sigma-Aldrich) [9].

3 Methods

3.1 Finding Anomalous Signal-to-Noise Ratios as a Function of Resolution

XPREP (*see* **Note 1**) is a program developed by George M. Sheldrick (Universität Göttingen) for analysis of X-ray diffraction data. Analyses include: space group assessment, generation of Patterson maps, and evaluation of anomalous signal-to-noise ratios, as well as features to prepare the diffraction data and command files for heavy-atom substructure determination in the context of a macromolecule. A major advantage of Sheldrick's approach compared to others is the simplicity of the XPREP interface—which is non-graphical—and the rapidity of calculations. What follows here is an outline of the fundamental steps required to assess whether an X-ray data set exhibits a discernable anomalous diffraction signal-to-noise ratio as a function of resolution. With a sufficient signal, the data can be subjected to SAD phasing techniques, whereas the lack of signal can inform the user to revise experimental conditions to encourage a more successful outcome. In this chapter, we worked with XPREP version 2008 (Bruker AXS). The reader is cautioned that other versions of XPREP may exhibit slightly different menu or name options, but the fundamental outcome should be the same.

1. XPREP reads various reflection file formats including *.hkl* files from programs such as PROTEUM2 (Bruker AXS), XDS [18], and *.sca* from HKL2000 [19]. To take full advantage of XPREP's capabilities an unmerged data set should be used.

   A. In the SCALEPACK module of HKL2000 select the "*Anomalous*" radio button to have recorded intensities (I (+) and I (−)) (*see* **Note 2**) for Bijvoet pairs treated equally during scaling but output separately to the *.sca* file. SCALEPACK also gives the option to separate Bijvoets I (+) and I (−) in both scaling as well as output by specifying the "*Scale Anomalous*" radio button; note; this feature should be used with caution when Bijvoet pairs are not recorded with appreciable redundancy.

   B. In PROTEUM2 within the "*Scaling: Setup tab*" choose "*Output file type = Unmerged.hkl file*". You will also have the option later in the "*Space Groups and Statistics*" module to output a *.sca* file that will also have your unmerged data.

2. To execute the program open a terminal in the your working directory and type:

   % xprep

3. A new window should appear. At the prompt type in the name of the reflection file (a *.hkl* file will be used here as an example):

   my_data

4. Next it is necessary to confirm the file type. XPREP—whose text is depicted below in bold italics—will give a best guess in square

brackets but the information must be confirmed by the user by hitting the return key as necessary:

Option [4]

i. The number of reflections and the mean intensity of all data divided by its error (*Mean (I/sigma)*) is calculated.

Enter the unit cell dimensions (the format is *a b c α β γ*)

ii. Next the "*Lattice exceptions*" will be displayed based on the cell dimensions input. The primitive (P) lattice will always be a choice but the correct lattice should be chosen based on prior knowledge.

5. The main menu should display the following: current data set name, cell dimensions, and wavelength. XPREP will automatically change the setting for unconventional unit cells (e.g., monoclinic *c* unique), so the user should check that the desired cell is displayed. To continue working within XPREP the user must "*Determine or input the Space Group*".

Select option [S]

i. If the correct space group had been indentified previously, one could simply choose option [I] on the next screen and type in the information. However, it is reassuring to use option [S] to see if XPREP independently confirms the previously assigned space group.

Select option [S] Determine the Space Group

ii. The user is then asked to reconfirm the *Crystal Lattice* and *Lattice type*.

iii. The calculated "*Mean (E*E− 1)*" value for the data will be displayed along with the expected theoretical values.

iv. "*Systematic absence exceptions*" will be displayed along with possible space group(s). Choose the space group carefully because there are often no statistical differences between space groups such as enantiomorphs.

   1. The "*space group No.*" is displayed from the International Tables for Crystallography.

   2. The frequency is given for the occurrence of the space group in the Cambridge Structural Database, "*CSD*".

   3. "*R(sym)*" not always helpful but the correct space group is expected to have the lowest value.

   4. "*CFOM*" (combined figure-of-merit) sums up all the criteria considered; the lower the value the higher the space group probability.

6. The user is then returned to the main menu were the Crystal system and Space group information are now visible. All the functions of XPREP—including detection of the anomalous signal-to-noise ratio as a function of resolution for SAD phasing—are available now.

A. Select option [A] "*Absorption, powder, SIR, SAD, MAD etc.*"

B. A new menu window will open with the current data set displayed at the top of the screen.

    i. Select option [A] MAD, SAD, SIR OR SIRAS

C. Several options will be displayed but for our purposes choose:

    i. Select option [A] SAD (Single-wavelength Anomalous Scattering)

    ii. Next the "*Target number of reflections in the local scaling sphere*" will be set.

        1. Choose the default value by hitting the return key.

D. The "*Anomalous signal-to-noise ratios*" will displayed in a table:

    i. Row 1 lists the resolution in shells

    ii. Row 2 has the ratios based on the input sigmas

    iii. Row 3, which is only displayed if the data input were unmerged, has the signal-to-noise ratios based on the differences between the Friedel-related amplitudes (F(+) and F(−)).

    iv. The user will be prompted to enter an effective B-value for normalization of the delta-F or F_A values. Choose the default value of no renormalization

E. Type in a file name and hit return.

F. For example, use *mydata001*—This *.hkl* file will contain the indices (H, K, L), Bijvoet differences (ΔF or F_A), $\sigma \Delta F$ or σF_A, and the initial estimates of the phase angle alpha (α). (*See* **Note 1**.)

G. To write an instruction file for SHELXD: Select Yes

    i. Hit the return key to choose a file name that matches the prefix name already assigned to the *.hkl* file in F (above).

        1. For example, this will have the form *mydata001. ins.*

    ii. Type in "Element type for Heavy atom" (e.g., Ir or Os).

    iii. Type in the expected "Number of unique heavy atoms" (e.g., 1 or 2).

1. Only a reasonable guess is required since SHELXD will search for up to 1.5 times this number.

    iv. Confirm or type in the "*Wavelength*" at which the data were recorded.

    v. Type in the "*Resolution cutoff in Ångstroms*".

        1. Choose the resolution cutoff such that the signal-to-noise is 1.3 or greater in the highest resolution shell based on the outcome in D (above).

H. The *mydata001.ins* file will be displayed in the window and contains the information in Fig. 2.

    i. The number of trials (NTRY) defaults to 1000 but a reasonable starting value would be 100.

    ii. A *.prp* file will be written automatically that includes the results of the space group determination and the anomalous signal-to-noise ratios.

3.2 Locating Heavy Atom Sites with the SHELxD Program (Called XM by Bruker)

1. To use the SHELxD program [11], set the terminal directory to where your *.ins* and *.hkl* files are located.

2. To execute the program type:

% XM mydata001 - file extension is not necessary if the *.ins* and *.hkl* (ΔF or F_A) files have the same unique prefix name.

```
TITL mydata001 in P6(3)22
CELL 1.13960 110.5000 110.5000 59.3000 90.000 90.000 120.000 !(λ in Å and cell dimensions)
ZERR 24.00 0.0156 0.0156 0.0119 0.000 0.000 0.000 !(# asymmetric units, errors in the unit cell dimensions)
LATT -1 !(type of crystal lattice, 1 for primitive cells, negative for non-centrosymmetric)
SYMM -Y, X-Y, Z !(symmetry operators the operator X,Y,Z is always assumed)
SYMM -X+Y, -X, Z
SYMM -X, -Y, 0.5+Z
SYMM Y, -X+Y, 0.5+Z
SYMM X-Y, X, 0.5+Z
SYMM Y, X, -Z
SYMM X-Y, -Y, -Z
SYMM -X, -X+Y, -Z
SYMM -Y, -X, 0.5-Z
SYMM -X+Y, Y, 0.5-Z
SYMM X, X-Y, 0.5-Z
SFAC Os !(or any other single element even if there are several heavy atom types)
UNIT   48 !(approximate number of heavy atoms per cell multiplied by 4)
SHEL 999 4.30 !(the resolution at which to truncate the data)
PATS !(Patterson seeding)
FIND   2 !(number of sites to search for, should be within 20% for best results)
MIND -1.5 -0.1 !(min allowed dist in Å between sites with crossword table caluated; the 2nd parameter allows use of atoms on special positions)
NTRY 100 !(Number of trys)
HKLF 3 !(3 indicates format in which F will be read rather than F * F)
END
```

Fig. 2 Representative instruction file for osmium substructure determination for the preQ$_1$ riboswitch. Comments are shown in *parentheses*

3. The SHELXD program outputs three files:

    A. The *mydata001.res* file contains the space group, unit cell information, symmetry operators, and the location of anomalous scatters. The highest scoring solution is written on the first line of the file along with the CC (correlation coefficient, *see* **Note 3**), which should be a large value but typically a $CC \geq 30\%$ and CC(weak) $\geq 15\%$ indicate a possible solution.

    B. The *mydata001.lst* file is described in Subheading 3.3, step **2.A.i**.

    C. The *mydata001.pdb* file has the *xyz* coordinates of the anomalous scatters.

3.3 Phase Calculations and Noise Suppression Using the SHELXE Program

The SHELXE program [20] will calculate phases quickly based on the heavy atom substructure search, and then conduct density modification to suppress the image of the incorrect structure, which is necessary for the SAD method [21]. The output files contain the noise-filtered SAD phases. These can be read into an interactive graphics program such as COOT for inspection of the electron density map for an interpretable RNA structure suitable for model building (Fig. 1d).

1. To execute the program type:
   % *XE my_data mydata001 -s0.50 -m100 -h -r3.2 -b* (Note; no prefix is necessary if the file has a unique name). The command-line arguments for the program are:

   i. The native data set (*my_data.hkl*) must be input first followed by the native Bijvoet differences file (*mydata001.hkl*) written by XPREP. The program will then search the working directory for the *mydata001.res* file, which contains the heavy atom sites that must be read in as well (described above in Subheading 3.2, **step 3.A**).

   ii. *-s*—Estimate of the solvent fraction. Generally crystals with higher solvent content result in better density modification outcomes.

   iii. *-m*—Defines the number of trials to be run but the program can be stopped at any point, by pressing *control-c*.

   iv. *-h*—Tells SHELXE that the anomalously scattering atoms are present in the data file (*my_data.hkl* or *.sca*) that was input into XPREP in Subheading 3.1, **step 1**.

   v. *-r*—Allows you to set the high-resolution cutoff for map calculation.

   vi. *-b*—Stipulates that an anomalous difference map (*.pha*) will be output and a peaksearch of that map will be carried out. The input heavy atom sites and any additional sites will be written to a *.hat* file.

2. SHELXE should be run a second time with the "-*i*" command added to invert the hand of the substructure and the space group in the case of the 22 enantiomorphic space groups.

A. The SHELXE program outputs:

i. A *mydata001.lst* file that contains a copy of the commands input along with definitions of the commands. SHELXE calculates several statistics during each density modification cycle that are helpful to determine the quality of the phases for structure determination. Significant factors to consider are: *Connectivity*—the fraction of adjacent pixels that are either both located in the solvent or the RNA; *Contrast*—the variance of the electron density averaged over all pixels [20]. *Pseudo-CC*—a pseudo correlation coefficient is calculated every five cycles of noise suppression (the default) based on 10% of the data that were randomly omitted from the map calculations. For all three statistics, larger numeric values indicate a better result. These factors can be used to judge when the density modification process has converged.

ii. The output file *mydata001.phs* has indices *hkl*, F^2, σF^2, figure-of-merit (FOM), and phase (PHI) that can be used to generate an electron density map. Note; the file *mydata001.pha* is an anomalous difference map that should reveal only the locations of anomalously scattering atoms.

1. These files can be read into COOT but first the symmetry and unit cell information must be added by loading the .*res* (*mydata001.res*) file output by SHELXD (Subheading 3.2, **step 3.A**). Then the .*phs* or .*pha* file can be opened using the "*Open MTZ, mmcif, fcf, or phs…*" option. This opens the "*Choose a symmetry and Cell for the Phases*" file window where the available symmetry information is selected by clicking *OK*.

iii. The output file *mydata001.hat* contains the refined anomalous scattering sites and may also contain weak anomalous sites that were not initially found by SHELXD.

iv. The second run using the "-*i*" option produces the same file types but with "_*i*" before the file extension such as *mydata001_i.phs*.

B. The anomalous scattering sites in the .*hat* file can alternatively be read back into SHELXE with the goal of improving the occupancies of weak sites, as well as the overall *contrast* and *connectivity*. This can be accomplished by moving the .*hat* file to a new directory and renaming it to .*res*. Then copy the required .*hkl* files to the new directory and rerun SHELXE using the same commands in Subheading 3.3,

step 1. If correct sites are known then running one more time should be sufficient.

C. To determine which SHELXE solution is correct the first step entails inspection of the *.lst* and *_i.lst* files. Typically there is a pronounced difference between the *contrast, connectivity*, and *pseudo-CC* values between the two solutions, with the better solution having the larger quality indicator values. The higher the *pseudo-CC*, the easier it is to interpret the electron-density map. Examination of either the *.phs* or *_i.phs* electron-density maps should reveal density that resembles a folded RNA with clear solvent channels (Fig. 1d or e). Visual inspection of the two anomalous difference maps (output as *.pha* and *_i.pha*) should also help to discern the correct solution, since one should have substantially better coverage of the anomalous scatters (*mydata001.res or .pdb*) as illustrated in Fig. 1b, c.

3.4 Options for Converting Files SHELX (.hkl) or SCALEPACK (.sca) Format to .mtz Format

1. To convert a *.hkl* (SHELX) file to a *.mtz* (CCP4) formatted file one can use the program reflection_file_converter from the *P*henix software suite [22]. Although the GUI can be used the command line interface is convenient:

   % phenix.reflection_file_converter my_data_1m.hkl = intensities --symmetry = P6122 --unit_cell = 92.7,92.7,130.1,90,90,120 --label = Iobs, SigIobs --write-mtz-amplitudes --mtz-root-label = FOBS --mtz = FILE

   i. The argument =*intensities* signifies that the file is a SHELX file.

   ii. The commands *--symmetry* and *--unit_cell* must be specified since there is no symmetry or unit cell info in the *.hkl* file.

   iii. The command *--label* defines the input column types (Iobs, SigIobs).

   iv. The intensities are converted into amplitudes with the command *--write-mtz-amplitudes*.

   v. The command *--mtz-root-label = FOBS* defines a new label for the amplitudes. If an unmerged file was input, it will have (+) and (−) FOBS but some programs will not recognize these labels.

   vi. The command *--mtz = FILE* is used to name the new output file where the argument FILE can be any name the user chooses.

   vii. The resulting *FILE.mtz* dataset can be used as output or a test set can be added using the PHENIX *Reflection tools* editor located in the main GUI.

2. To convert a SCALEPACK (*.sca*) to an *.mtz* file convert the intensities to amplitudes by use of the following command line arguments in PHENIX:

     i. **% phenix.reflection_file_converter my_data_1m.sca --write-mtz-amplitudes --mtz-root-label = FOBS --generate-r-free-flags --mtz = my_data_1m**

    ii. The default percentage of R_{free} flags generated is 10% but it can be altered using variations of the command: *--r-free-flags-fraction = 0.05*.

3. *As an alternative to* PHENIX, the program, *F2MTZ* from CCP4 (*Convert to/modify/extend .mtz files*) can be used in the context of the CCP4i GUI interface [13], which allows the use of the program CTRUNCATE [23] to convert intensities to amplitudes (negative intensities will be converted to positive amplitudes) as well as the generation of helpful statistics that describe the quality of the diffraction data (Wilson plots, twinning tests, etc.). The output *.mtz* file will contain both the amplitudes and the original intensities.

     i. The space group and unit cell information are absent from the *.hkl* file and will require manual input.

    ii. For Wilson scaling the number of nucleotides in the asymmetric unit must be input.

   iii. Check that the *Data labels* make sense (i.e., H index for H, K, L, intensity for I, and standard deviation for SIGI).

3.5 Using RESOLVE for Further Density Modification and PHENIX/RESOLVE for Optional RNA Autobuilding

RESOLVE [15] is robust maximum-likelihood based density modification program that can be used to improve initial maps calculated by programs such as SHELXE. RESOLVE when used with PHENIX AutoBuild [24] represents a powerful iterative model building and refinement option.

1. To run the standalone version of RESOLVE to improve the electron density map from SHELXE, but without autobuilding, one can use a simple script csh or tcsh shell script:

```
# !/bin/csh
setenv CCP4_OPEN UNKOWN
setenv     SYMOP=/usr/local/phenix-1.6-289/solve_
resolve/ext_ref_files/symop.lib
setenv     SYMINFO=/usr/local/phenix-1.6-289/solve_
resolve/ext_ref_files/syminfo.lib
phenix.resolve < <EOD> > resolve.log
hklin mydata001.mtz
LABIN     FP = FP     PHIB = PHIB     FOM = FOM
SIGFP = SIGFP
Solvent_content 0.71
no_build
EOD
```

i. To find the location of the SYMOP and SYMINFO libraries in your PHENIX environment in a terminal window type **phenix.resolve** and copy the information from the window to the above script. This implies that the file phenix_env has been located and "sourced" in the csh or tcsh during login or it can be sourced from the command line:

1. **%   source   /Applications/PHENIX-1.6-289/ Contents/phenix-1.7.1-743/phenix_env**

2. Be sure to make the csh script executable by resetting the permission:

a. **% chmod a + x resolve.csh**

ii. The SHELXE *mydata001.phs* file was converted to *.mtz* format using CCP4i (Subheading 3.4 *my_data_1m.mtz*) to serve as input for RESOLVE. By default the full resolution of the data will be used for calculations. RESOLVE will output the files *resolve.log* and *resolve.mtz*. The latter file contains *hkl*, FP, SIGFP, FOMM (figure-of-merit of the phase), PHIM (modified phase), FreeR_flag, FC (calculated amplitude), and Hendrickson–Lattman coefficients (HLAM, HLBM, HLCM, HLDM). To view the new density modified electron density map the resolve.mtz file can be opened in COOT using the "Open MTZ ..." menu; check the "Use Weights?" button in the "Column Label Assignment" window.

2. PHENIX Autobuild can use the RESOLVE density-modified map as input to iteratively build and refine an RNA model; this may require several hours.

% phenix.autobuild data = my_data_1m.mtz map_file = resolve. mtz seq_file = my_seq.dat chain_type = RNA resolution = 2.8 solvent_fraction = 0.71 &

i. The specified data file is based on the experimentally derived *my_data_1m.hkl* that was converted to *MTZ* format wherein the intensities were converted to amplitudes (Subheading 3.4). If the data file does not include a test set (FreeR_flags), then AutoBuild will choose one (default is ~10 % of the total reflections). AutoBuild will then start from the RESOLVE density modified map but will use the experimental data for refinement.

ii. The sequence file must be in one letter format and have individual chains separated by the greater than sign (>) or a blank line.

iii. Solvent fraction (0–1) of the crystal should be input to ensure proper bulk solvent calculation but PHENIX will automatically calculate this if it is not input.

iv. Even if Autobuild fails to build a complete model it still often outputs useful partial models with corresponding maps that can be loaded into COOT.

    a. The *overall_best.pdb* file is the best-refined model built by PHENIX.

    b. There will be two MTZ files with map coefficients: a density modified map *overall_best_denmod_map_coeffs.mtz* and an *overall_best_refine_map_coeffs.mtz* from *phenix.refine* that can be used generate a *2mFo-DFc* and *Fo-Fc* map in COOT.

    c. The AutoBuild_run_1_1.log file has a record of all the model-building and refinement results.

v. If AutoBuild runs to completion (may take several hours) an AutoBuild.summary.dat file will be written that includes a summary of the output files for the best solution and information about the model-building results of each cycle. A file with a list of all the parameters used during the run will be output as AutoBuild_Facts.dat. The best solution is listed first.

4   Notes

1. In the case of SAD phasing the phase angle alpha (α) is initially assigned a value of $270°$ if $F(+) < F(-)$, and $90°$ if $F(+) > F(-)$.

2. The recorded intensity (I) or its associated structure factor amplitude (F) is used throughout this chapter. These terms are often used without distinction due to the ability of most programs to accept either. Instances where one is required over the other are specified.

3. In SHELXD the correlation coefficient (CC) [25] is the difference between normalized structure factors E_{obs} and E_{calc} for all data and CC_{weak} is this difference for 30% of the unused reflections [11].

Acknowledgments

We thank Prof. Clara L. Kielkopf and Dr. Matthew M. Benning for helpful discussions on crystallographic phasing. We thank Prof. Robert T. Batey for the gift of $Ir(NH_3)_6Cl_3$. We thank the staff of SSRL for assistance with X-ray data collection. This work was supported in part by NIH grants GM063162 and RR026501 to J.E.W. SSRL is operated by Stanford on behalf of the US DOE. The SSRL Structural Molecular Biology Program is supported by the DOE, and by NIH/NCRR and NIGMS.

References

1. Wedekind JE, McKay DB (2000) Purification, crystallization, and X-ray diffraction analysis of small ribozymes. Methods Enzymol 317:149–168

2. Laires MJ et al (2004) Role of cellular magnesium in health and human disease. Front Biosci 9:262–276

3. Wedekind JE (2011) Metal ion binding and function in natural and artificial small RNA enzymes from a structural perspective. Met Ions Life Sci 9:299–345

4. Jou RW, Cowan JA (1991) Ribonuclease-H activation by inert transition-metal complexes—mechanistic probes for metallocofactors—insights on the metallobiochemistry of divalent magnesium-ion. J Am Chem Soc 113:6685–6686

5. Cate JH et al (1996) Crystal structure of a group I ribozyme domain: principles of RNA packing. Science 273:1678–1685

6. Clemons WM Jr et al (2001) Crystal structure of the 30 S ribosomal subunit from Thermus thermophilus: purification, crystallization and structure determination. J Mol Biol 310:827–843

7. Kazantsev AV et al (2005) Crystal structure of a bacterial ribonuclease P RNA. Proc Natl Acad Sci U S A 102:13392–13397

8. Spitale RC et al (2009) The structural basis for recognition of the PreQ0 metabolite by an unusually small riboswitch aptamer domain. J Biol Chem 284:11012–11016

9. Keel AY et al (2007) A general strategy to solve the phase problem in RNA crystallography. Structure 15:761–772

10. Alam S et al (2005) Conformational heterogeneity at position U37 of an all-RNA hairpin ribozyme with implications for metal binding and the catalytic structure of the S-turn. Biochemistry 44:14396–14408

11. Sheldrick GM (2008) A short history of SHELX. Acta Crystallogr A 64:112–122

12. MacElrevey C et al (2007) A posteriori design of crystal contacts to improve the X-ray diffraction properties of a small RNA enzyme. Acta Crystallogr D Biol Crystallogr 63:812–825

13. Potterton E et al (2003) A graphical user interface to the CCP4 program suite. Acta Crystallogr D Biol Crystallogr 59:1131–1137

14. Terwilliger TC, Berendzen J (1999) Automated MAD and MIR structure solution. Acta Crystallogr D Biol Crystallogr 55:849–861

15. Terwilliger TC (2000) Maximum-likelihood density modification. Acta Crystallogr D Biol Crystallogr 56:965–972

16. Collaborative Computational Project, Number 4 (1994) The CCP4 suite: programs for protein crystallography. Acta Crystallogr D Biol Crystallogr 50:760–763

17. Emsley P, Cowtan K (2004) Coot: model-building tools for molecular graphics. Acta Crystallogr D Biol Crystallogr 60:2126–2132

18. Kabsch W (2010) Xds. Acta Crystallogr D Biol Crystallogr 66:125–132

19. Otwinowski Z, Minor W (1997) Processing of X-ray diffraction data collected in oscillation mode. Methods Enzymol 276:307–326

20. Sheldrick GM (2010) Experimental phasing with SHELXC/D/E: combining chain tracing with density modification. Acta Crystallogr D Biol Crystallogr 66:479–485

21. Wang BC (1985) Resolution of phase ambiguity in macromolecular crystallography. Methods Enzymol 115:90–112

22. Adams PD et al (2010) PHENIX: a comprehensive Python-based system for macromolecular structure solution. Acta Crystallogr D Biol Crystallogr 66:213–221

23. Evans PR (2011) An introduction to data reduction: space-group determination, scaling and intensity statistics. Acta Crystallogr D Biol Crystallogr 67:282–292

24. Terwilliger TC et al (2008) Iterative model building, structure refinement and density modification with the PHENIX AutoBuild wizard. Acta Crystallogr D Biol Crystallogr 64:61–69

25. Fujinaga M et al (1987) Crystal and molecular structures of the complex of alpha-chymotrypsin with its inhibitor turkey ovomucoid third domain at 1.8 A resolution. J Mol Biol 195:397–418

INDEX

Douglas H. Turner and David H. Mathews (eds.), *RNA Structure Determination: Methods and Protocols*, Methods in Molecular Biology,
vol. 1490, DOI 10.1007/978-1-4939-6433-8, © Springer Science+Business Media New York 2016

Printed in the United States
By Bookmasters